OXFORD MEDICAL PUBLICATIONS

Methods for the Economic Evaluation of Health Care Programmes

Second Edition

Methods for the Economic Evaluation of Health Care Programmes

Second Edition

Michael F. Drummond
Professor and Director, Centre for Health Economics
University of York, England

Bernie J. O'Brien
Associate Professor, Centre for Evaluation of Medicines
Department of Clinical Epidemiology and Biostatistics
McMaster University, Ontario, Canada

Greg L. Stoddart
Professor, Centre for Health Economics and Policy Analysis
Department of Clinical Epidemiology and Biostatistics
McMaster University, Ontario, Canada
and Fellow, Canadian Institute for Advanced Research

George W. Torrance
Professor, Centre for Health Economics and Policy Analysis
Centre for Evaluation of Medicines
Department of Clinical Epidemiology and Biostatistics
McMaster University, Ontario, Canada

OXFORD NEW YORK TORONTO

OXFORD UNIVERSITY PRESS

1997

Oxford University Press, Great Clarendon Street, Oxford OX2 6DP

Oxford New York
Athens Auckland Bangkok Bogota Bombay Buenos Aires
Calcutta Cape Town Dar es Salaam Delhi Florence Hong Kong
Istanbul Karachi Kuala Lumpur Madras Madrid Melbourne
Mexico City Nairobi Paris Singapore Taipei Tokyo Toronto Warsaw

and associated companies in
Berlin Ibadan

Oxford is a trade mark of Oxford University Press

Published in the United States
by Oxford University Press Inc., New York

First edition published 1987
Reprinted 1988 (twice), 1989, 1990, 1992, 1993, 1994 (twice), 1995, 1996
Second edition published 1997
Reprinted 1997

A catalogue record for this book is available from the British Library

Library of Congress Cataloging in Publication Data

Methods for the economic evaluation of health care programmes /
Michael F. Drummond . . . [et al]. – 2nd ed.
(Oxford Medical publications)
Includes bibliographical references and index.
1. Medical care—Cost effectiveness. 2. Medical care, Cost of—Evaluation.
I. Drummond, M. F. II. Series
RA410.5.D77 1997   338.4'33621–dc21   97-10273

ISBN 0 19 262774 0 (hbk)
ISBN 0 19 262773 2 (pbk)

Printed in Great Britain by
Biddles Ltd, Guildford & King's Lynn

Preface to the first edition

We regard this book as a truly joint effort arising from our common concern to improve the quality of economic evaluation in the health care field.

For a number of years we have been independently engaged in teaching, research, and consultancy in this area. In particular we have offered advice to colleagues from other disciplines and on many occasions have been part of multidisciplinary teams undertaking evaluations of programmes or treatments. These experiences have convinced us of the need for a book which discusses the methodological principles of economic evaluation in health care in a way that would benefit those who plan to undertake such studies.

The book has two particular roots. First, the MS737 course (Economic Analysis for the Evaluation of Health Services) in the Faculty of Health Sciences at McMaster University, which we all have instructed at some stage, attempts to provide a basic gounding in economic evaluation methodology. During the course, the students undertake an evaluation of a programme or health care treatment of their choice. The course assessment is based on the completion of the project.

Second, the Seminex Workshop Series, coordinated by the Faculty of Business at McMaster, has provided the impetus for us to polish our course materials and to make them more free-standing.

What you see here is the result of these roots. The material has been tried and tested both in graduate and continuing education settings. We hope that it meets the needs of the wide readership that is envisaged.

Birmingham, UK   M.F.D
and Hamilton, Canada   G.L.S
June 1986   G.W.T.

Acknowledgements

A number of colleagues in the health economics field have commented on an earlier draft of this book. Some have read the whole manuscript; others have commented on particular sections. In all instances their comments have been constructive, but we have not been able to take on board all suggestions, as not everyone agrees on all points. Therefore, whilst acknowledging their help, we want to make it clear that the following individuals are in no way responsible for what follows!

With this caveat we are grateful to Gordon Blackhouse, John Brazier, Martin Buxton, Paul Dolan, Cam Donaldson, Amiram Gafni, Ron Gueree, Magnus Johannesson, Bengt Jönsson, Göran Karlsson, Alistair McGuire, Frans Rutten, Kevin Schulman, Mark Sculpher, and Milt Weinstein for the comments received.

Finally we would like to thank our secretaries, Nancy Bishop, Christine Henderson, and Vanessa Windass, for their help with the preparation of the manuscript and for generally humouring us on bad days. All three were indispensable, but Vanessa in particular has made a major input to the production of the book.

Preface to the second edition

Much has happened in economic evaluation in health care since the publication of the first edition of this book in 1987. There are now many more empirical studies and there is a greater acknowledgement of the usefulness of economic evaluation in health care decision-making. In addition, there have been a number of methodological developments, particularly in cost–utility and cost–benefit analysis.

In producing this second edition our general aim has been to meet the need that the first edition was intended to meet 10 years ago; namely to serve as an introductory text for those contemplating undertaking, commissioning, or using an economic evaluation. As the field has moved on so, we hope, has the book. It is greatly enlarged and, in some places, more technical than the first edition.

We have been appreciative of the positive feedback to the first edition and have retained the critical appraisal framework, since this underpins many of the official guidelines to economic evaluation methodology that have been published in recent years. Also, we have added many new examples, whilst retaining some of the original ones that served us well.

Reactions to the writing style in the first edition have generally been favourable. However, we have tried to improve further the layout of the book, including boxes containing illustrations or points of particular interest. The prime mover in these changes was Bernie O'Brien, our new co-author, who had used our first edition with his own students. Bernie joined the faculty at McMaster a few years ago and has taught both on the graduate course in economic evaluation and on the two-day workshop for health care professionals, our informal 'prerequisite' for being a co-author.

The content of the book has changed in a number of ways, to reflect the advances in economic evaluation methodology. In Chapter 2 we have clarified the terminology and pointed out that there are many components, of building blocks for an economic evaluation that can be assembled in a number of different ways. There have also been substantial changes to the chapters on cost-effectiveness, cost–utility, and cost–benefit analysis. In particular, the chapters on cost–utility and cost–benefit analysis reflect the rapid expansion in the literature and the new approaches being proposed for the evaluation of health outcomes.

We have also added completely new chapters. Chapter 8, on the collection and analysis of data, discusses the pros and cons of basing economic evaluation on trials versus models. It also discusses the application of statistical analysis in economic evaluation. Chapter 9, on the presentation and use of data, discusses issues in the comparison of economic evaluation results, in cost-effectiveness rankings or 'league tables', and in the transferability or portability of economic data.

Another feature of the methodological debate over the past 10 years is that of whether or not economic evaluation should be solely based on the principles of welfare economics, or more particularly those of Paretian welfare economics. We have decided to adopt a broadly-based approach, including discussion of methods that some would not wish to call 'economic evaluation'. This perspective is evident in our debate amongst three analysts in Chapters 2 and 9. Our general approach has been to outline the advantages and disadvantages of particular methodologies, rather than to prescribe one 'correct' methodology.

Finally, we were conscious from feedback received that many readers refer to the first edition as 'the little blue book'. Therefore we asked the publishers to retain the same colour scheme for the new edition. Perhaps this will be referred to as 'the big blue book' in the future! We hope you enjoy reading the new edition.

York, UK   M.F.D.
and Hamilton, Canada   B.J.O.
May 1997   G.L.S.
                                                  G.W.T.

Contents

1

How to use this book

There is a growing literature on economic evaluation in health care. Studies have been conducted by economists, medical researchers, clinicians, and multidisciplinary teams containing one or more of these parties. The studies go under a confusing range of labels, such as *cost-effectiveness analysis, cost–benefit analysis, and cost–utility analysis*. They also vary greatly in quality, as methodological critiques have shown (Warner and Hutton 1980; Drummond 1981; Drummond *et al.* 1986; Adams *et al.* 1992; Gerard, 1992; Udvarhelyi *et al.* 1992; Donaldson and Shackley 1997).

Several good introductions to economic evaluation in health care already exist (Drummond 1980; Weinstein 1981; Warner and Luce 1982; Luce and Elixhauser, 1990; Kamlet, 1992; Gold *et al.* 1996). All of these give the reader a basic appreciation of the nature of economic evaluation and its relevance to health care decision-making at all levels. This book is intended as a supplement to, and not a replacement for, such texts. It aims to take the reader past the stage of general appreciation of the methodological steps involved, and towards preparing him or her for some *hands-on* experience in undertaking an evaluation, perhaps as part of a multidisciplinary team including economists, epidemiologists, and clinicians. We do not claim that we provide a comprehensive methodological 'cookbook', nor that after reading this book the uninitiated could work without support. Rather, we seek to provide a well-equipped 'tool-kit' which, based on our own experience of undertaking economic evaluations, we believe will result in the reader being better prepared to meet most situations.

The next two chapters are concerned with equipping the reader to appraise the quality of the existing literature, an important precursor to one's own study. In Chapter 2, we establish a baseline by discussing the kinds of questions economic evaluations seek to answer, and the basic forms of evaluation. Then in Chapter 3, we present a check-list of questions to ask about any economic evaluation published in the literature. As well as providing a method of systematically appraising the quality of existing evidence, this chapter sets out, in an organized manner, the main methodological issues that would need to be resolved by anyone undertaking an economic evaluation in the health care field.

In Chapters 3, 5, and 6, this critical appraisal exercise is applied to published papers. It should be emphasized that it is not our intent to present the critical appraisals as our own expert assessment of the authors of published studies, nor to counsel perfection. Rather, these studies have been chosen because they demonstrate the complexity of economic evaluation and are generally extremely well-done pieces. (In including critical appraisals of some of our own work we have also demonstrated a willingness to swallow some of our own medicine!) There are a number of potential ways of using the critical appraisal exercises, including self-study while reading this book, or as the basis for critical appraisal workshops for health care professionals (Chambers *et al.* 1983). The original articles are not reproduced here for copyright reasons. They should be easily accessible to the reader, however.

The remainder of the book gives exercises or examples dealing with the main methodological issues raised by the various forms of economic evaluation. In all forms the general approach is to compare the consequences of health care programmes with their costs. For purposes of exposition it is considered that there are four main forms of economic evaluation, each dealing with costs but differing in the way that the consequences of health care programmes are measured and valued (see Table 1.1).

Table 1.1. Measurement of costs and consequences in economic evaluation

Type of study	Measurement/ valuation of costs in both alternatives	Identification of consequences	Measurement/ valuation of consequences
Cost-minimization analysis	Dollars	Identical in all relevant respects	None
Cost-effectiveness analysis	Dollars	Single effect of interest, common to both alternatives, but achieved to different degrees	Natural units (e.g. life-years gained, disability-days saved, points of blood pressure reduction, etc.)
Cost–utility analysis	Dollars	Single or multiple effects, not necessarily common to both alternatives	Healthy years or (more often) quality-adjusted life-years
Cost–benefit analysis	Dollars	Single or multiple effects, not necessarily common to both alternatives	Dollars

The first form considered, *cost analysis*, is discussed in Chapter 4 and deals only with costs. Therefore this represents a partial form of economic appraisal, unless it can be shown that the consequences of the programmes or treatments being considered are equivalent. (Where the consequences of two or more alternatives are examined alongside costs in the same study, and are shown to be equivalent, the study is sometimes called a *cost-minimization analysis*. However, we consider this to be a special form of cost-effectiveness analysis (see below).

Chapter 5 examines *cost-effectiveness analysis* (CEA). In this form of economic evaluation the consequences of programmes are measured in the most appropriate natural effects or physical units, such as 'years of life gained' or 'cases correctly diagnosed'. No attempt is made to *value* the consequences, so implicitly it is assumed that the output concerned is in some sense 'worth having'. (It should be pointed out, however, that in estimating the costs of obtaining different amounts of the output in question, many cost-effectiveness studies do begin to raise this broader question.)

In its classical form, CEA considers a single measure of output, such as life-years gained. However, some CEAs may present an array of output measures alongside cost and leave it to the decision-maker to form his own view of the relative importance of these. Some analysts have used the term *cost–consequences analysis* for this variant of CEA (CCOHTA 1994). The presentation of an array of output measures is a useful approach, even if the analyst then goes on to *value* the outcomes relative to one another (as discussed below).

Cost–utility analysis (CUA) is discussed in Chapter 6. In this form of economic evaluation the consequences of programmes are adjusted by health state preference scores or *utility* weights. That is, states of health associated with the outcomes are valued relative to one another. In general terms this means that one can assess the quality of (for example) life-years gained, not just the crude number of years. This approach is particularly useful for those health treatments or programmes that extend life only at the expense of side effects (e.g. antihypertensive drug therapy or chemotherapy for certain types of cancer) or produce reductions in morbidity rather than mortality.

Cost–utility analysis is therefore a broader form of analysis than cost-effectiveness analysis, but is a variant of that general approach. Some authors (Gold *et al.* 1996) prefer not to make a distinction between CEA and CUA, since they are so similar. We retain the two labels here for pedagogic reasons, since CUA involves additional analytic procedures which we discuss in Chapter 6. In particular, it incorporates *valuation* of the outcomes obtained.

Chapter 7 deals with *cost–benefit analysis*. In this form of economic evaluation attempts are made to value the consequences of programmes in money terms, so as to make them commensurate with the costs. Therefore, potentially this is the broadest form of analysis, where one can ascertain whether the beneficial consequences of a programme justify the costs. However, as will be seen, measurement problems often mean that the range of benefits valued in money terms is fairly limited. Thus, whilst in theory it is a broad form of evaluation, in practice many of the cost–benefit analyses published to date are more restricted than cost–utility or cost-effectiveness analyses and are limited to a comparison of those costs and consequences that can easily be expressed in money terms. This problem is being addressed by the developments in valuing the benefits of health care programmes in terms of individuals' willingness-to-pay, as discussed in Chapter 7.

It should be stressed that these clear distinctions among forms of analyses are made purely for pedagogic reasons. In real life the distinctions are often blurred, as evidenced by many of the examples we shall discuss. Certainly it is not always possible for analysts at the beginning of a study, to be clear on the most appropriate form of analysis to use. Sometimes they may decide to use more than one form. However, the main advantage of subdividing the material in this way is that in each chapter further methodological issues can be introduced in a logical, cumulative manner. Of course most, if not all, of the issues dealt with under cost analysis are also relevant to the other forms of economic evaluation discussed. The same applies to many of the issues first raised under cost-effectiveness analysis. Therefore *Chapters 4 through 7 are not free-standing* and should not be read on that basis.

Chapters 8 and 9 discuss practical aspects of undertaking and using economic evaluations. Chapter 8 discusses data collection and analysis, including the pros and cons of trial-based and modelling studies. Chapter 9 discusses the presentation and use of economic evaluation results, including the interpretation of cost-effectiveness league tables.

Chapter 10 concludes this book with some thoughts on how to take matters further. It contains some hints on issues to clarify before undertaking an economic evaluation (our 'survival guide') and some further sources on the more thorny methodological issues.

REFERENCES

Adams, M. E., McCall, N. T., Gray, D. T., *et al.* (1992). Economic analysis in randomized control trials. *Medical Care*, **30**, 231–43.

Canadian Coordinating Centre for Health Technology Assessment (1994). *Guidelines for economic evaluation of pharmaceuticals: Canada* (1st ed) CCOHTA, Ottawa.

Chambers, L. W., Stoddart, G. L., and Sullivan, B. (1983). Continuing education for health professionals and administrators: workshops on becoming a critical user of health care research. *Can. J. Public Health*, 74(1), 29–34.

Department of Clinical Epidemiology and Biostatistics (1984*a*). How to read clinical journals: VII. To understand an economic evaluation (part A). *Can. Med. Assoc. J.*, **130**, 1428–33.

— (1984*b*). How to read clinical journals: VII. To understand an economic evaluation (part B). *Can. Med. Assoc. J.*, **130**, 1542–9.

Donaldson, C., Shackley, P. (1997). Economic evaluation. In: R. Detels, W. W. Holand, J. McEwen, and G. S. Omenn (eds.). *Oxford textbook of public health (third edition)* Volume 2: the methods of public health. Oxford University Press, Oxford (pp 949–71).

Drummond, M. F. (1980). *Principles of economic appraisal in health care.* Oxford University Press, Oxford

— (1981). *Studies in economic appraisal in health care.* Oxford University Press, Oxford.

—, Ludbrook, A., Lowson, K. V., and Steele, A. (1986). *Studies in economic appraisal in health care (Volume 2).* Oxford University Press, Oxford.

Gerard, K. (1992). Cost–utility in practice: a policy makers guide to the state of the art. *Health Policy,* 21, 249–79.

Gold, M. R., Siegel, J. E., Russell, L. B., and Weinstein, M. C. (ed.) (1996). *Cost-effectiveness in health and medicine.* Oxford University Press, New York.

Kamlet, M. S. (1992). *The comparative benefits modeling project: a framework for cost-utility analysis of government health care programs.* US Department of Health and Human Services, Public Health Service, Washington DC.

Luce, B., and Elixhauser, A. (1990). *Standards for socioeconomic evaluation of health care products and services.* Springer-Verlag, Berlin Heidelberg.

Udvarhelyi, I. S., Colditz, G. A., Rai, A., and Epstein, A. M. (1992). Cost-effectiveness and cost–benefit analyses in the medical literature. Are methods being used correctly? *Annals of Internal Medicine,* 116, 238–44.

Warner, K. E. and Hutton, R.C. (1980). Cost–benefit and cost-effectiveness analysis in health care: growth and composition of the literature. *Medical Care,* 18(11), 1069–84.

— and Luce, B. R. (1982). *Cost–benefit and cost-effectiveness in health care: principles, practice and potential.* Health Administration Press, Ann Arbor, Michigan.

Weinstein, M. C. (1981). Economic assessment of medical practices and technologies. *Medical Decision-Making,* 1(4), 309–30.

2

Basic types of economic evaluation

Those who plan, provide, receive, or pay for health services face an incessant barrage of questions such as:

- Should clinicians check the blood pressure of each adult who walks into their offices?
- Should planners launch a scoliosis screening programme in secondary schools?
- Should individuals be encouraged to request annual check-ups?
- Should local health departments free scarce nursing personnel from well-baby clinics so that they can carry out home visits on lapsed hypertensives?
- Should hospital administrators purchase each and every piece of new diagnostic equipment?
- Should a new, expensive drug be listed on the formulary?

These are examples of general, recurring questions about:

- who should do what to whom,
- with what health care resources, and
- with what relation to other health services?

The answers to these questions are most strongly influenced by our estimates of the relative merit or value of the alternative courses of action they pose. This book is concerned with the strategies and tactics whereby these estimates of relative value can be ascertained and interpreted, that is, with the evaluation of health services.

More specifically, the book focuses on one type of evaluation, sometimes referred to as *economic evaluation or efficiency evaluation* (the two terms are synonymous for our purposes). In this type of evaluation we are asking the questions:

1. Is this health procedure, service, or programme worth doing compared with other things we could do with these same resources?
2. Are we satisfied that the health care resources (required to make the

procedure, service, or programme available to those who could benefit from it) should be spent in this way rather than some other way?

It is imperative to note that although economic evaluation provides important information to decision-makers, it addresses only one dimension of health care programme decisions. Economic evaluation is most useful and appropriate when preceded by three other types of evaluation, each of which addresses a different question:

1. Can it work? Does the health procedure, service, or programme do more good than harm to people who fully comply with the associated recommendations or treatments? This type of evaluation is concerned with *efficacy*.
2. Does it work? Does the procedure, service, or programme do more good than harm to those people to whom it is offered? This form of health care evaluation, which considers both the efficacy of a service and its acceptance by those to whom it is offered, is the evaluation of *effectiveness* or usefulness.
3. Is it reaching those who need it? Is the procedure, service, or programme accessible to all people who could benefit from it? Evaluation of this type is concerned with *availability*.

Methodological criteria for assessing efficacy, effectiveness, and availability evaluations have been described elsewhere by Sackett (1980), from which the above questions have been drawn. These criteria will not be reviewed here.

2.1. WHY IS ECONOMIC EVALUATION IMPORTANT?

To put it simply, resources – people, time, facilities, equipment, and knowledge – are scarce. Choices must and will be made concerning their deployment, and methods such as 'what we did last time', 'gut feelings', and even 'educated guesses' are not always better than organized consideration of the factors involved in a decision to commit resources to one use instead of another. This is true for at least three reasons:

1. *Without systematic analysis, it is difficult to identify clearly the relevant alternatives.* For example, in deciding to introduce a new programme (rehabilitation in a special centre for chronic lung disease), all too often little or no effort is made to describe existing activities (episodic care by family physicians in their offices) as an alternative 'programme' to which the new proposal must be compared. Furthermore, if the objective is, indeed, to reduce morbidity due to chronic lung disease then preventive programmes (e.g. abatement of cigarette smoking) may represent a more efficient avenue and should be added to the set of programmes competing in the evaluation.

2. *The viewpoint assumed in an analysis is important.* A programme which looks unattractive from one viewpoint may look significantly better when other viewpoints are considered. Analytic viewpoints may include any or all of: the individual patient, the specific institution, the target group for specific services, the Ministry of Health budget, the government's overall budget position (Health plus other Ministries), and the community or societal viewpoint.

3. *Without some attempt at measurement, the uncertainty surrounding orders of magnitude can be critical.* For example, when the American Cancer Society endorsed a protocol of six sequential stool tests for cancer of the large bowel, most analysts would have predicted that the cost per case detected would increase markedly with each test. But would they have guessed that it would reach $47 million for the sixth test as Neuhauser and Lewicki (1975) have demonstrated? Admittedly, while this is an extreme example, it illustrates that without measurement and comparison of outputs and inputs we have little upon which to base any judgement about value for money. In fact, the real cost of any programme is not the number of dollars appearing on the programme budget, but rather the health outcomes achievable in some other programme which have been forgone by committing the resources in question to the first programme. It is this 'opportunity cost' which economic evaluation seeks to estimate and to compare with programme benefits.

2.2. WHAT DOES ECONOMIC EVALUATION MEAN?

Two features characterize economic analysis, regardless of the activities (including health services) to which it is applied.

First, it deals with both the inputs and outputs, sometimes called *costs* and *consequences*, of activities. Few of us would be prepared to pay a specific price for a package whose contents were unknown. Conversely, few of us would accept a package, even if its contents were known and desired, until we knew the specific price being asked. In both cases, it is the linkage of costs and consequences which allows us to reach our decision.

Second, economic analysis concerns itself with choices. Resource scarcity, and our consequent inability to produce all desired outputs (even efficacious therapies!), necessitates that choices must, and will, be made in all areas of human activity. These choices are made on the basis of many criteria, sometimes explicit but often implicit. Economic analysis seeks to identify and to make explicit one set of criteria which may be useful in deciding among different uses for scarce resources.

These two characteristics of economic analysis lead us to define economic evaluation as *the comparative analysis of alternative courses of action in terms of both their costs and consequences*. Therefore, the basic tasks of any economic evaluation are to identify, measure, value, and compare the costs and consequences of the alternatives being considered. These tasks characterize all economic evaluations, including those concerned with health services (see Box 2.1).

Box 2.1: Economic evaluation always involves a comparative analysis of alternative courses of action

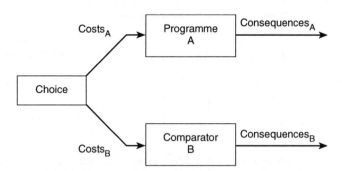

The diagram illustrates that an economic evaluation is usually formulated in terms of a choice between competing alternatives. Here we consider a choice between two alternatives, A and B. The comparator to Programme A, the programme of interest, does not have to be an active treatment. It could be doing nothing. Even when two active treatments are being compared, it may still be important to consider the baseline of doing nothing, or a low cost option. This is because the comparator (Programme B) may itself be inefficient.

   The precise nature of the costs and consequences to be considered, and how they might be measured and valued, will be discussed in Section 2.4 below. However, the general rule when assessing programmes A and B is that the *difference* in costs is compared with the *difference* in consequences, in an incremental analysis.

In fact, these two characteristics of economic analysis may be employed to distinguish and label several evaluation situations commonly encountered in the health care evaluation literature. In Table 2.1, the answers to two questions – (1) is there comparison of two or more alternatives and (2) are both costs (inputs) and consequences (outputs) of the alternatives examined – define a six-cell matrix for evaluation situations.

In cells 1A, 1B, and 2 there is no comparison of alternatives (i.e. a single service or programme is being evaluated). To put it more accurately, the service or programme is being *described*, since evaluation requires comparison. In cell 1A, only the consequences of the service or programme are examined, and thus the evaluation is labelled an *outcome description*. In cell 1B, because only costs are examined it is called a *cost description*. The large literature on *cost of illness*, or *burden of illness* falls into this category. These studies describe the cost of disease to society, but are not full economic evaluations because alternatives are not compared (Drummond 1992).

Basic types of economic evaluation

In cell 2, both outcomes and costs of a single service or programme are described and thus the evaluation is termed a *cost-outcome description*.

Table 2.1. Distinguishing characteristics of health care evaluation

Are both costs (inputs) and consequences (outputs) of the alternatives examined?

		NO		YES
		Examines only consequences	Examines only costs	
Is there comparison of two or more alternatives?	NO	1A PARTIAL EVALUATION 1B Outcome description	Cost description	2 PARTIAL EVALUATION Cost-outcome description
	YES	3A PARTIAL EVALUATION 3B Efficacy or effectiveness evaluation	Cost analysis	4 FULL ECONOMIC EVALUATION Cost-minimization analysis Cost-effectiveness analysis Cost-utility analysis Cost-benefit analysis

An example of this type of study is that by Reynell and Reynell (1972) on coronary care units. They presented data on the costs of one such unit and gave an estimate of the likely number of lives saved. However, there was no explicit attempt to compare the costs and consequences of the coronary care unit with an alternative, or the *status quo*. Reynell and Reynell describe their study as 'cost–benefit analysis'. As regular users of economic evaluation results may have recognized, and readers of this book will likely discover, the titles of published economic evaluations are not always accurate indicators of the type of evaluation actually performed!

Cells 3A and 3B contain evaluation situations in which two or more alternatives are compared, but in which the costs and consequences of each alternative are not examined simultaneously. In cell 3A, only the consequences of the alternatives are compared and thus we term these *efficacy* or *effectiveness evaluations*. This, of course, is the cell into which the large and important literature containing most randomized clinical trials falls. In cell 3B, only the costs of the alternatives are examined. In such situations the studies performed may be called *cost analyses*. An example of such a study is that by Lowson *et al.* (1981) on the comparative costs of three methods of providing long-term oxygen therapy in the home: oxygen cylinders, liquid oxygen, and the oxygen concentrator (a machine that extracts oxygen from air). The authors argued that a cost analysis was sufficient as the relative effectiveness of the three methods was not a contentious issue.

Note that none of the above-mentioned cells entirely fulfils both of the conditions for economic evaluation. For this reason they have all been designated *partial evaluations*. This does not imply that studies with these characteristics are unimportant, for they may represent important intermediate stages in our understanding of the costs and consequences of health services or programmes. However, the label *partial evaluation* does indicate that they will not allow us to answer efficiency questions. For this we need studies, employing the techniques listed in cell 4 under *full economic evaluation*. We now turn to a consideration of these four techniques.

2.3. DO ALL ECONOMIC EVALUATIONS USE THE SAME TECHNIQUES?

The identification of various types of costs and their subsequent measurement in dollars is similar across most economic evaluations; however, the nature of the consequences stemming from the alternatives being examined may differ considerably. Let us consider four examples to illustrate how the nature of consequences affects their measurement, valuation, and comparison to costs.

2.3.1. Example 1: cost-minimization analysis

Suppose we are comparing two programmes involving minor surgery for adults. Both accomplish the outcome of interest, and from an examination of effectiveness data differ in no other significant respects except that one requires hospital admission for at least one night while the other (a day surgery programme) does not. If we identified the common outcome of interest – operations successfully completed – we would find that it could be achieved to the same degree (i.e. identical number of surgeries) in either programme, though presumably at different costs. The economic evaluation is then essentially a search for the least cost alternative. Analyses such as this are often called *cost-minimization analyses*. We might also be interested in the distribution of costs (e.g. in this case to what extent does the day-surgery programme shift costs to the patient), but our principal efficiency comparison will be made on the basis of cost per surgical procedure.

Two examples of studies dealing with choices in minor surgery are those by Russell *et al.* (1977) on day-case surgery for hernias and haemorrhoids, and by Waller *et al.* (1978) on 48-hour postoperative stay following treatment for inguinal hernia or varicose veins. In both cases the short-stay alternative was compared with traditional in-patient treatment. An example of a cost-minimization study dealing with a different health care issue is that by Fenton *et al.*(1982) on home versus hospital treatment for psychiatric patients.

It was mentioned in Chapter 1 above that cost-minimization analysis (CMA) is really a special form of cost-effectiveness analysis, where the consequences of the alternative treatments being compared turn out to be equivalent. It can be seen from Fig 2.1 that there are nine possible outcomes when one therapy is being compared with another. In three of the nine cases the analysis reduces to a CMA. In fact, very few studies are designed, from the outset, to be cost-minimization analyses. Either they are designed as cost-effectiveness analysis and end up being simplified because the consequences turn out to be equivalent, or they are designed as cost analyses *in the knowledge that* previous clinical research has demonstrated equivalence in consequences.

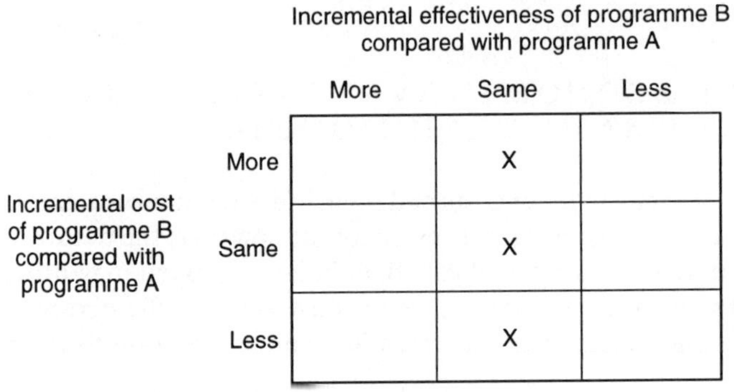

Incremental effectiveness of programme B
compared with programme A

	More	Same	Less
More		X	
Same		X	
Less		X	

(Row label to the left: Incremental cost of programme B compared with programme A)

X = here the study reduces from a cost-effectiveness analysis to a cost-minimization analysis.

Figure 2.1.   Nine possible outcomes in the comparison of incremental cost and incremental effectiveness of two programmes.

Therefore, in practice, whether or not a cost analysis constitutes a partial or full economic evaluation depends on what is already known about the relative clinical effectiveness of the alternatives. In the example cited above, the cost analysis by Lowson *et al.* (1981) could be considered a full evaluation (i.e. a cost-minimization analysis) since it was already known that the different methods of providing domiciliary oxygen were clinically equivalent.

2.3.2. Example 2: cost-effectiveness analysis

Suppose that our interest is now the prolongation of life after renal failure and that we are comparing the costs and consequences of hospital dialysis versus kidney transplantation. In this case the outcome of interest – life-years gained – is common to both programmes; however, the programmes may have differential success in achieving this outcome, as well as differential costs. Consequently we would not automatically lean toward the least cost programme unless, of course, it also resulted in a greater prolongation of life. In comparing these alternatives we would normally calculate this prolongation and compare cost per unit of effect (i.e. cost per life-year gained). Such analyses, in which costs are related to a single, common effect which may differ in magnitude between the alternative programmes, are usually referred to as *cost-effectiveness analyses*. Note that the results of such comparisons may be stated either in terms of cost per unit of effect, as in this example, or in terms of effects per unit of cost (life-years gained per dollar spent). The latter is a particularly useful approach when working within a given budget constraint, as long as the alternatives under consideration are not of radically different scale (Donaldson and Shackley 1997*a*).

Furthermore, although the alternatives used in this example are similar in that both could be considered variants of an overall renal programme, it should be noted that cost-effectiveness analysis can be performed on any alternatives which have a common effect. Thus kidney transplantation could be compared to heart surgery (or even mandatory bicycle helmet legislation!) if the common effect of interest was life-years saved. Similarly, an influenza immunization programme could be compared to a home care programme (or even a community safety education programme!) if a common effect of interest, perhaps disability days avoided, could be identified.

There are many examples of cost-effectiveness analysis in the literature. Ludbrook (1981) provided an estimate of the cost-effectiveness of treatment options for chronic renal failure. In addition, a number of studies compare the cost-effectiveness of actions which do not produce health effects directly, but which achieve other clinical objectives that can be clearly linked to improvements in patient outcome. For example, Hull *et al.* (1981) compared diagnostic strategies for deep vein thrombosis in terms of the cost per case detected. Similarly, Logan *et al.* (1981) compared work-site and regular (physician office) care for hypertensives in terms of the cost per mm Hg drop in diastolic blood pressure obtained.

2.3.3 Example 3: cost–benefit analysis

Often we cannot be assured that the consequences of alternative programmes are identical. In addition, it is frequently not possible to reduce the outcomes of interest to a single effect common to both alternatives. We may be interested in effects which, though common to both alternatives, are multiple. Or we may identify single or multiple effects which are not common to the alternatives. The first case is easy to see if we make two extensions to Example 2: (1) to include home dialysis in addition to hospital dialysis and kidney transplantation, and (2) to include quality of life (perhaps measured by the occurrence of marital disruption) and incidence of medical complications as consequences of interest in addition to life-years gained. In order to pursue cost-effectiveness analysis we would now have to compute cost-effectiveness ratios for three effects. In the event that one alternative was not clearly superior on all three counts, we would be faced with the task of either designating (implicitly or explicitly) a primary effect on which to base the comparison, or finding a method whereby the multiple common effects could be combined into one common denominator.

The need for a common denominator in order to measure the consequences of alternatives is even more apparent in the following example. Suppose we are attempting to compare a hypertension screening programme, aimed at preventing premature death, with an influenza immunization programme, aimed at preventing disability days. Here the outcome of interest differs between alternatives. Consequently, a meaningful cost-effectiveness comparison is impossible.

In situations like these, when we require a common denominator to facilitate comparison of outcomes, analysts frequently attempt to go beyond consideration of the specific effects themselves and to attach a measure of value to the set of effects resulting from a particular service or programme. One measure of value is dollars, and the consequences of a service or programme will often be expressed in terms of their dollar benefits in order to facilitate comparison to programme costs. This, of course, requires us to translate effects such as disability days avoided, life-years gained, medical complications avoided (and even marital disruptions avoided) into their dollar benefit. This is not always an easy task, but depending on the type of effect, it is sometimes both appropriate and feasible to attempt it. Analyses which measure both the costs and consequences of alternatives in dollars are called *cost–benefit analyses*. The results of such analyses might be stated either in the form of a ratio of dollar costs to dollar benefits, or as a simple sum (possibly negative) representing the net benefit (loss) of one programme over another.

It is perhaps worth noting that (at least in theory) cost–benefit analysis (CBA) provides information on the *absolute* benefit of programmes, in addition to information on their relative performance. That is, cost–benefit analysis provides an estimate of the value of resources used up by each programme compared to the value of resources the programme might save or create. This view of cost–benefit analysis implicitly assumes that each programme is being compared to a *do-nothing* alternative which entails no costs and no benefits. However, in practice cost–benefit analyses often amount to a comparison of those costs and benefits that can be easily expressed in money terms, so very few published analyses can aspire to this wider role. Also, there are very few instances where absolutely nothing is done to tackle a given health problem, so in most cost–benefit analyses the implicit do-nothing alternative has some costs and benefits attached to it. Notice the different treatment of the do-nothing alternative which is often implicit in cost-effectiveness analysis. Cost-effectiveness analysis implicitly assumes at the outset that a tenable do-nothing alternative does not exist and that one of the programme alternatives will therefore be undertaken regardless of its net benefit. While this may be quite a realistic position for health care decision-makers to adopt, it should be noted that cost-effectiveness analysis may lead to a decision to undertake a programme which does not pay for itself (i.e. a programme that entails a net resource cost instead of resource saving).

Implicitly, the assumption is that the output, in terms of health effects, is worth having and the only question is to determine the most cost-effective way to achieve it.

An example of a study which did attempt to quantify and value a wide range of costs and benefits is that by Weisbrod *et al.* (1980) on conventional hospital-oriented versus community-based programmes for mental illness. They found that although the community-based programme was more costly, this was more than offset by its extra value in terms of patients being able to take up or maintain employment. (Earnings were used as a dollar measure of these benefits.)

The recent literature contains a number of studies that assess individuals' *willingness-to-pay* for health benefits. For example, Johanneson and Jönsson (1991) give estimates for willingness-to-pay for antihypertensive therapy, Neumann and Johanneson (1994) give them for in vitro fertilization, and O'Brien *et al.* (1995) give them for a new antidepressant. A comprehensive cost–benefit analysis of health care interventions would use this approach to value the health benefits. Paradoxically, although there has been considerable progress in willingness-to-pay methodology in recent years, very few cost–benefit analyses incorporating these estimates have so far been published.

2.3.4. Example 4: cost–utility analysis

A second measure of value, preferred by those analysts who have reservations about valuing benefits in dollar terms, is *utility*. Here we use the term utility in a general sense to refer to the preferences individuals or society may have for any particular set of health outcomes (e.g. for a given health state, or a profile of states through time). Later, in Chapter 6, we shall be more specific about terminology, since utility has specific connotations in economics and the various methods to measure health state preferences may or may not estimate true utilities.

The notion that the utility of an outcome, effect, or level of health status is different from the outcome, effect, or level of health status itself can be illustrated by the following example. Suppose that twins, identical in all respects except occupation (one being a sign painter and the other a translator), both broke their right arm. While they would be equally disabled (or conversely, equally healthy), if we asked them to rank 'having a broken arm' on a scale of 0 (dead) to 1 (perfect health) their rankings might differ considerably because of the significance each one attaches to arm movement, in this case due to occupation. Consequently, we would expect that their assessments of the utility of treatment (i.e. the degree to which treatment of the fractures improved the quality of their lives) would also differ.

Utility analysis is viewed as a particularly useful technique because it allows for *quality of life* adjustments to a given set of treatment outcomes, while simultaneously providing a generic outcome measure for comparison of costs and outcomes in different programmes. The generic outcome, usually expressed as *quality-adjusted life-years (QALYs)*, is arrived at in each case by adjusting the length of time affected through the health outcome by the utility value (on a scale of 0 to 1) of the resulting level of health status (see Box 2.2). Other generic outcomes measures, such as the *healthy years equivalent* (HYE), have been proposed as alternatives to the QALY (Mehrez and Gafni 1989). These are discussed further in Chapter 6.

Box 2.2. QALYs Gained from an intervention

In the conventional approach to QALYs the quality-adjustment weight for each health state is multiplied by the time in the state (which may be discounted, as discussed in Chapter 5) and then summed to calculate the number of quality-adjusted life-years. The advantage of the QALY as a measure of health output is that it can simultaneously capture gains from reduced morbidity (quality gains) and reduced mortality (quantity gains), and integrate these into a single measure. A simple example is displayed in the figure below, in which outcomes are assumed to occur with certainty. Without the health intervention an individual's health-related quality of life would deteriorate according to the lower curve and the individual would die at time Death 1. With the health intervention the individual would deteriorate more slowly, live longer, and die at time Death 2. The area between the two curves is the number of QALYs gained by the intervention. For instruction purposes the area can be divided into two parts, A and B, as shown. Then part A is the amount of QALY gained due to quality improvements (i.e. the quality gain during time that the person would have otherwise been alive anyhow), and part B is the amount of QALY gained due to quantity improvements (i.e. the amount of life extension, but adjusted by the quality of that life extension).

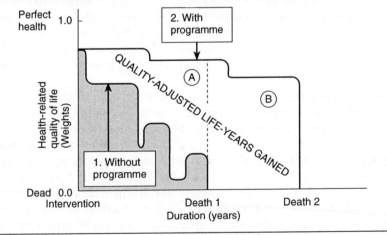

Analyses that employ utilities as a measure of the value of programme effects are termed *cost–utility analyses*. The results of cost–utility analyses are typically expressed in terms of the cost per healthy year or cost per quality-adjusted life-year gained by undertaking one programme instead of another.

Examples of cost–utility analyses include the study by Boyle *et al.* (1983) on neonatal intensive care for very-low-birth-weight infants and that by Oldridge *et al.* (1993) on a formal post-myocardial infarction rehabilitation programme.

In commenting on the different characteristics of the four main types of economic evaluation, two further points warrant emphasis. First, the main purpose of classifying study types is to illustrate the different analytic characteristics of completed studies, not to prescribe a particular study type in advance. Often at the beginning of a study the analyst may not be able to predict what form the final analysis might take, as this may depend on the results of an associated clinical evaluation. For example, it may not be known in advance that a clinical evaluation will show two treatments to be medically equivalent, thereby reducing a cost-effectiveness analysis to a cost-minimization analysis. Furthermore, the different approaches are sometimes used together to tackle a particularly thorny problem – Boyle *et al.* (1983) used all three of cost-effectiveness, cost–utility and cost–benefit analyses in their evaluation of neonatal intensive care, since each explores a different dimension of value.

2.4 WHAT ARE THE RELEVANT COSTS AND CONSEQUENCES IN THE ECONOMIC EVALUATION OF HEALTH CARE PROGRAMMES?

It was shown above that the different forms of economic evaluation measure and value the various costs and consequences to different extents. Which is the most appropriate form of analysis? The answer to this question depends not only on the problem being tackled, but also the institutional framework, the practical measurement challenges and the perspective the analyst takes on the role of economic evaluation.

Box 2.3 contains a hypothetical debate among three analysts. This illustrates that there is more than one perspective on the role of economic evaluation in health care, each having its underlying rationale. For example, Analyst A has a strong theoretical perspective. Welfare economics, the branch of economics underpinning economic evaluation, places considerable emphasis on the values individuals place on outcomes, since individuals are considered to be the best judges of their own welfare. (We discuss this in more detail in Chapter 7.) Analyst B adopts a health sector budget perspective, which may be close to that adopted by many health care decision-makers.

Analyst C is clearly a pragmatist, but his or her pragmatism may be at the expense of having a clear underlying theory for this approach to economic evaluation. Indeed, some economists feel that the term, economic evaluation, ought to be reserved only for evaluations whose methods are consistent with the underlying principles of welfare economics (Birch and Gafni 1996).

However, most economists use the term more broadly, to encompass all studies undertaking a systematic assessment of costs and consequences. (We return to this issue in Chapters 7 and 9.)

Box 2.3. The role of economic evaluation in health care: a conversation among three analysis

Analyst A
I think the best way to undertake an economic evaluation is to ascertain the total amount that individuals would be willing to pay for the programme. This amount can then be directly compared with the costs in order to assess whether the programme is worthwhile. My approach is consistent with economic theory and economic evaluation gives us the result we would have obtained from the market, had one been operating.

Analyst B
In my mind the purpose of economic evaluation is to help us allocate the health care budget. Therefore we should consider health care resources only and compare the resources consumed with the health improvement obtained. We might measure health improvements in natural units, or health effects, but health state preference scores would be better because this would allow us to make broader comparisons among programmes. I do not like willingness-to-pay valuations since these may be conditioned by individuals' ability to pay and may also reflect the non-health attributes of programmes, which I do not believe should be funded as part of the health care budget.

Analyst C
I think we should take a broad societal perspective, but some of the costs and consequences are easier to express in monetary terms than others. Also, like Analyst B, I am worried that willingness-to-pay valuations may reflect the prevailing income distribution, and in many countries ability to pay has been explicitly rejected as a method of allocating health care resources. Therefore I think we should measure and value a wide range of costs and consequences and present them in a way that helps health care decision makers form a better judgement.

Because of these perspectives on economic evaluation, it is useful to view the various costs and consequences of health care programmes as building blocks, which can be assembled in the evaluation in different ways. Figure 2.2 is an expansion of the diagram given in Box 2.1. Again we consider the costs and consequences of a health care programme (which is always evaluated in comparison with another programme, or the *status quo*). However, here we give a more detailed breakdown of the costs and consequences and show, through the use of formulae, the possible alternative approaches to economic evaluation.

In Figure 2.2 the resources consumed by the programme are considered to be in three sectors. In each case their quantities (q) would be measured and the total cost calculated by multiplying the quantities by the relevant prices (p). The resource consumption in the health care sector is relatively straightfor-

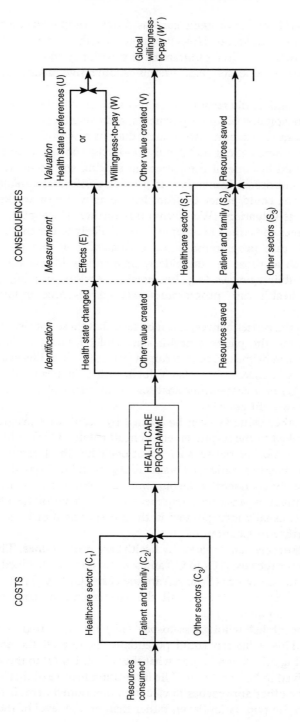

Figure 2.2. Components of economic evaluation in health care

ward and would consist of items such as drugs, equipment, hospitalization, physician visits, and so on. However, note that these include not only the costs of providing the initial programme (e.g. a kidney transplant) but also all the continuing care costs (e.g. immunosuppressive drugs, treatment of infections, etc.).

The patient and family resources could consist of out-of-pocket expenses in travelling to hospital, various co-payments, and expenditure in the home (e.g. adapting a room to accommodate a home dialysis machine). However, one of the most important patient and family resources consumed in treatment is *time*. This could be time of the patient in seeking and receiving care, or it could be the time of family members in providing informal nursing support at home. The time could either be from leisure activities or worktime, which would affect its valuation. (We discuss this further in Chapter 3.)

The resources consumed in other sectors are likely to depend on the nature of the health care programme being evaluated. For example, some programmes, such as those for the elderly or mentally ill, consume resources from other public agencies (e.g. homemaker services, nursing home care). Also, many health care programmes rely on resource inputs from the voluntary sector.

Turning to the consequences, it can be seen that these consist of three main categories. First, the patients health state will be changed (hopefully improved). This can be measured in terms of effects (E) (e.g. life-years gained or disability days reduced), but also valued, either in terms of health state preferences (U) in a cost–utility analysis, or in terms of willingness-to-pay (W) in a cost–benefit analysis.

Secondly, other value (V) can be created by health care programmes, not necessarily linked to the improvement in health state. This could include the value of information or reassurance about one's health. There is currently a debate about whether patients obtain utility or value from the process of receiving care, independent of the outcome (Donaldson and Shackley 1997*b*). Whilst potentially a separate component of the value of health care programmes, V is usually incorporated in the measurement of U or W. (This is discussed further in Chapter 7.)

Thirdly, resources can be saved by health care programmes. These savings (S_1 to S_3) mirror the costs (C_1 to C_3) and are measured and valued in a similar way. In fact, these savings (S_1 to S_3) are the costs (C_1 to C_3) not spent on the alternative programme. Indeed, all the assessments of consequences are comparative to an alternative.

Finally, the global willingness-to-pay (*W'*) for the programme may be ascertained. This valuation could potentially include all the consequences identified in Fig 2.2, depending on what the respondent(s) to the willingness-to-pay perceived to be important. The interesting feature of this approach, as opposed to the other approaches to valuation mentioned here, is that it could be applied on the population level, rather than on the level of the individual patient. For example, a representative sample of the population could be asked what additional amount they would be willing to pay in higher taxes for a new programme to be added to those already existing in a given country. (We discuss this approach further in Chapter 7 and distinguish among three approaches to willingness-to-pay assessment.)

Thus there are a number of possible formulations of economic evaluation depending on the perspective adopted by analysts and the estimation methods they employ (see Table 2.2).

Table 2.2. Possible formulations of economic evaluation

Cost-minimization analysis
$(C_1 - S_1)$
$(C_1 + C_2 + C_3) - (S_1 + S_2 + S_3)$

Cost-effectiveness analysis
$(C_1 - S_1) / E$
$[(C_1 + C_2 + C_3) - (S_1 + S_2 + S_3)] / E$

Cost-utility analysis
$(C_1 - S_1) / U$
$[(C_1 + C_2 + C_3) - (S_1 + S_2 + S_3)] / U$

Cost-benefit analysis
$(W') - (C_1 + C_2 + C_3)$
$[(W + V + S_1 + S_2 + S_3) - (C_1 + C_2 + C_3)]$

CBA results can also be expressed as ratios, although this is not recommended (see Box 2.4).

---

*Please note that E and U represent *changes* in effectiveness or health status, compared to an alternative.

Considering again the three hypothetical analysts in Box 2.3, Analyst A is arguing for a cost–benefit analysis to be undertaken, with the formulation $(W') - (C_1 + C_2 + C_3)$. If this approach were followed it would be important to make sure that W did indeed capture the total value of all the consequences. However, in a country with a publicly-financed health care system, individuals asked about their willingness-to-pay may not take account of the health care resource savings (S_1), or resource savings in other sectors (S_3). Therefore, the appropriate formulation for the evaluation might be $(W' + S_1 + S_3) - (C_1 + C_2 + C_3)$, and the estimation procedure for W' would be designed so as to explicitly exclude S_1 and S_3, in order to avoid double-counting.

Analyst B is clearly arguing for either a cost-effectiveness analysis, with the formulation $(C_1 - S_1) / E$, or a cost–utility analysis, with the formulation $(C_1 - S_1) / U$. However, these are not the only possible formulations of CEA or

CUA. Alternative formulations, assuming a societal viewpoint, would also consider C_2, C_3, S_2 and S_3 (see Table 2.2).

Analyst C, our pragmatist, does not appear to be set on a precise formulation for the analysis and might be satisfied by a display of all the costs and consequences, measured in the most appropriate units. (We called this a *cost–consequences analysis* in Chapter 1.) Alternatively, he or she may be happy with a CEA or CUA including a broad range of resource changes, e.g. $(C_1 + C_2 + C_3) - (S_1 + S_2 + S_3) / U$. One potential problem here would be double counting. That is, the health state preference scores (U) might incorporate individuals' valuations of time savings to themselves or their family (e.g. the ability to return to work and earn income). This was the view taken by the US Public Health Service Panel on Cost-Effectiveness in Health and Medicine (Gold *et al.* 1996). Therefore, if such a formulation were to be used, it would be important to ensure that the estimation of (U) was made so as to exclude the value of savings in patient and family time included in (S_2). The same double-counting problem could arise if willingness-to-pay was used to estimate the value of the change in health state (W) in money terms. Thus, the estimate would either have to be purged of the value of S_2, or S_2 should be excluded from the formulation of the evaluation.

The three different analytical perspectives typified by Analysts A–C also imply differing views on the inclusion of the other value created (V) This could be, for example, the value to pregnant mothers of seeing an ultrasound image of their unborn baby (Berwick and Weinstein 1985), or the pleasure of being cared for even if one's health state was not changed. Whether or not these items are viewed as legitimate, or whether or not they are classified as health-related, is for debate. However, it is clear that Analyst A would include them in an estimation of the global willingness-to-pay (*W'*), whereas Analyst B would definitely exclude them.

The purpose of this discussion is to illustrate that it is very difficult to outline one standard form of economic evaluation. First, there are different perspectives on the role of economic evaluation, as illustrated by Analysts A–C. Secondly, measurement difficulties may compromise any analytic approach. Finally, the institutional context may influence how the various 'building blocks' are assembled. For example, an analyst adopting the position of Analyst A may not attempt to capture all the benefits of the health care programme in the estimation of *W'* if he or she is operating in a setting where health care is provided free at the point of use. In such a case the element of value of the programme relating to savings in health care resources may best be handled separately. Therefore, the way in which each individual building block or component is measured may influence the measurement of others and also the way in which the various components are assembled in the analysis.

Two other points should be made about the alternative formulations for economic evaluation given in Fig 2.2. First, since some of the formulations are presented as ratios, it is worth noting that the size of the ratio depends on what goes into the numerator and denominator respectively (see Box 2.4). Whereas this is not a problem within a particular study, providing the analysts are clear on what they have done, it can be a major problem if the ratios from two or more studies are subsequently compared. (Birch and Donaldson 1987). (We return to this in Chapter 9.) This has led some to argue for a standard formulation of the cost-effectiveness ratio (Gold *et al.* 1996), but, as we discuss above, this is difficult.

Box 2.4. Be wary of ratios

Suppose a health care programme had costs and consequences as follows:

COSTS	CONSEQUENCES
C_1 Health care costs $1 000 000	Health state improvement
C_2 Patient/family resources $5 000	U (in preference scores) 10 QALYs
C_3 Costs in other sectors $50 000	W (in willingness-to-pay) $2 000 000
	S_1 Health care savings $25 000
	S_2 Savings in other sectors $20 000
	S_3 Savings in patient/family resources $12 000
	V (Other value created) $0

The following ratios could be calculated:
(i) *Cost-utility ratio (health care resources only)*
$$(C_1 + S_1) / U = \$75\,000 \text{ per QALY}$$

(ii) *Cost-utility ratio (all resource use)*
$$(C_1 + C_2 + C_3 - S_1 - S_2 - S_3) / U = \$77\,300 \text{ per QALY}$$

(iii) *Benefit–cost ratio (including all consequences in the numerator as benefits)*
$$[(W + S_1 + S_2 + S_3) / (C_1 + C_2 + C_3)] = 2.163$$

(iv) *Benefit–cost ratio (treating resource savings as cost-offsets, deducted from the denominator)*
$$[W / (C_1 + C_2 + C_3 - S_1 - S_2 - S_3)] = 2.004$$

Secondly, in describing the various formulations of economic evaluation here, we have avoided using the terms *direct, indirect,* and *intangible* costs and benefits. Box 2.5 illustrates how these terms, which are common in the existing literature, relate to the terminology used here.

From the user's point of view the most important consideration is whether the complexity of the analysis matches the breadth of the question posed. Cost-benefit and cost-utility analyses, since they address the issue of outcome valuation, enable us to assess broader choices. Cost-benefit analysis can also shed light on whether the treatments concerned are 'worthwhile' when compared to other programmes within and outside the health care sector. Cost-minimization and cost-effectiveness analyses tacitly assume that the treatment objective concerned is worth meeting, and generally address more restrictive questions. We would argue that to assess whether or not a particular evaluation has been appropriate to the question originally posed, the user needs to be aware of these analytic distinctions.

Second, the power of these analytic techniques should not be overstated. None of the approaches is intended to be a magic formula for removal of judgement, responsibility, or risk from decision-making activities, though each is capable of improving the quality and consistency of decision-making.

Box 2.5. New terms for old

The existing literature in economic evaluation in health care, including the first edition of this book, classifies costs and benefits as *direct, indirect,* or *intangible.* For the reasons outlined below, we do not use the terms here.

Direct costs and benefits
These terms have been used in the past to denote the resources consumed (costs) or saved (benefits) by the programme, when compared to an alternative (which could be no programme). In the main these would be resources in the health care sector, but sometimes would include patients' out-of-pocket expenses, resources from other statutory agencies and voluntary bodies. However, use of the terms is not consistent across studies, which sometimes causes confusion.

Indirect costs and benefits
These terms have been used in the past to denote the time of patients (or their families) consumed or freed by the programme. In the main the focus has been on worktime and indirect costs and benefits have been synonymous with productivity gains and losses. The term has often caused confusion as it is used by the accountancy profession to denote overhead costs.

Intangible costs and benefits
These terms have been used in the past to denote those consequences that are difficult to measure and value, such as the value of improved health *per se*, or the pain and suffering associated with treatment. However, the latter are not costs (i.e. resources denied other uses) and in any case these items are not strictly intangible as they are often measured and valued, through the utility or willingness-to-pay approach.

At root, they are methods of critical thinking, of approaching choices, and often of placing difficult choices out in the open for discussion. While they generate quantitative statements about the value of programme costs and consequences, qualitatively they are simply frameworks for comprehensive identification and display of (economic) factors involved in decision-making. Whether factors covered by the economic analyses are, in fact, the dominant concerns in a specific decision, and whether the limitations of economic evaluation (discussed in Chapter 3) significantly restrict its usefulness in a specific situation, are judgements which quite properly remain the responsibility of the final decision-maker.

In this sense, cost-minimization, cost-effectiveness, cost-benefit, and cost-utility analyses may represent only a partial analysis of any specific choice.

In this chapter, we have attempted to provide the reader with an introduction to the nature of economic evaluation itself, and the distinguishing characteristics of the principal types of economic evaluation which may be encountered. Of course, identifying an evaluation is one thing; deciding whether it has been soundly executed (and then whether it is potentially useful for a particular decision) is quite another! Therefore, in Chapter 3 we outline the elements common to sound economic evaluations.

REFERENCES

Berwick, D. M. and Weinstein, M. C. (1985). What do patients value? Willingness-to-pay for ultrasound in normal pregnancy. *Medical Care*, **23**, 881–93.

Birch, S., Donaldson, C. (1987). Applications of cost benefit analysis to health care: departures from welfare economic theory. *J. Health Economics*, **6**, 211–25.

Birch, S. and Gafni, A. (1996). Cost-effectiveness and cost utility analysis: methods for the non-economic evaluation of health care programmes and how we can do better. In *Managing technology in health care* (ed. E. Geilser and O. Heller), Chapter 4, pp. 51–68. Klewer Academic Publishers, Norwell, M. A.

Boyle, M. H., Torrance, G. W., Sinclair, J. C., and Horwood, S. P. (1983), Economic evaluation of neonatal intensive care of very-low-birth-weight infants. *N. Engl. J. Med.* **308**, 1330–7.

Donaldson, C., Shackley, P. (1997a). Economic evaluation. In: R. Detels, W. W. Holland, J. McEwen, G. S. Omenn (eds.) *Oxford textbook of public health (third edition)* Volume 2: the methods of public health (pp 949–71) Oxford University Press, Oxford.

Donaldson, C., Shackley, P. (1997b). Does 'process utility' exist? A case study of willingness to pay for laparoscopic cholecystectomy. *Social Science and Medicine*, **44**, 699–707.

Drummond, M.F. (1992). Cost of illness studies: a major headache? *PharmacoEconomics*, **2**(1), 1–4.

Fenton, F. R., Tessier, L., Contandriopoulos, A.-P., Nguyer, H., and Struening, E. L. (1982). A comparative trial of home and hospital psychiatric treatment: financial costs. *Can. J. Psychiatry* **27**, (3), 177–87.

Gold, M. R., Siegel, J. E., Russell, L. B., and Weinstein, M. C. (ed.) (1996). Cost-effectiveness in helath and medicine. Oxford University Press, New York.

Hagard, S., Carter, F., and Milne, R. G. (1976). Screening for spina bifida cystica: a cost-benefit analysis. *B. J. Soc Prevent Med.*,**30**, (1), 40–53.

Hull, R., Hirsh, J., Sackett, D. L., and Stoddart, G. L. (1981). Cost-effectiveness of clinical diagnosis, venography and non-invasive testing in patients with symptomatic deep-vein thrombosis. *N. Engl. J. Med.* **304**, 1561–7.

Johannesson, M. and Jönsson, B. (1991). Economic evaluation in health care: is there a role for cost-benefit analysis? *Health Policy*, 17, 1–23.

Logan, A. G., Milne, B. J., Achber, C., Campbell, W. P., and Haynes, R. B. (1981). Cost-effectiveness of a work-site hypertension treatment programme. *Hypertension*, **3**, (2), 211–18.

Lowson, K. V., Drummond, M. F., and Bishop, J. M. (1981). Costing new services: long-term domiciliary oxygen therapy. *Lancet*, **ii**, 1146–9.

Ludbrook, A. (1981). A cost-effectiveness analysis of the treatment of chronic renal failure. *Appl. Economics*, **13**, 337–50.

Mehrez, A., Gafni, A. (1989). Quality-adjusted life-years, utility theory and health years equivalents. *Medical Decision Making*, **9**, 142–9.

Neuhauser, D. and Lewicki, A. M. (1975). What do we gain from the sixth stool guaiac? *N. Engl. J. Med.*, **293**, (5), 226–8.

Neumann, P. and Johannesson, M. (1994). The willingness to pay for in vitro fertilization: a pilot study using contingent valuation. *Medical Care*, **32**, 686–699.

O'Brien, B. J., Novosel, S., Torrance, G. and Streiner, D. (1995). Assessing the economic value of a new antidepressant: a willingness-to-pay approach. *PharmacoEconomics*, **8**(1), 34–5.

Oldridge, N., Furlong, W., Feeny, D., Torrance, G., Guyatt, G., Crowe, J. *et al.* (1993). Economic evaluation of cardiac rehabilitation soon after acute myocardial infarction. *Amer. J. Cardiol.*, **72**, 154–61.

Reynell, P. C. and Reynell, M. C. (1972). The cost-benefit analysis of a coronary care unit. *Br. Heart J.*, **34**, 897–900.

Russell, I. T., Devlin, H. B., Fell, M., Glass, N. J., and Newell, D. J. (1977). Day-case surgery for hernias and haemorrhoids: a clinical, social and economic evaluation. *Lancet*, **i**, 844–7.

Sackett, D. L. (1980). Evaluation of health services In *Health and preventive medicine* (ed. J. M. Last), pp. 1800–23. Appleton-Century Crofts, New York.

Stason, W. B. and Weinstein, M. C. (1977). Allocation of resources to manage hypertension. *N. Engl. J. Med.*, **296**, 732–7.

Waller, J., Adler, M., Creese, A., and Thorne, S. (1977). Early discharge from hospital for patients with hernia or varicose veins. *Department of Health and Social Security (UK)*, HMSO, London.

Weisbrod, B. A., Test, M. A., and Stein, L. I. (1980). Alternatives to mental hospital treatment: economic cost-benefit analysis. *Arch. General Psychiatry*, **37**, 400–5.

3

Critical assessment
of economic evaluation

Those who receive or read an economic evaluation are often faced with the difficult task of assessing study results. The question that readers of evaluations are most likely to ask themselves is: *'Are these results useful to me in my setting?'* The answer to this question is determined by the answers to the following specific questions.

1. Is the methodology employed in the study appropriate and are the results valid?
2. If the results are valid, would they apply to my setting?

This chapter concentrates on question (1), and is designed to assist users of economic evaluation in assessing the validity of the results they encounter.

When assessing the validity of evidence, whether pertaining to efficacy, effectiveness, availability, or efficiency, we normally proceed by examining closely the methods employed to produce the evidence. Often it is helpful to separate the various elements of a methodology so that each can be scrutinized more closely. In this chapter we identify the key elements of any economic evaluation and discuss methodological characteristics which users may expect to find in well-executed studies. A brief summary of relevant questions to ask about an economic evaluation is provided in Box 3.1, and this critical appraisal check-list is then applied to a published article.

Of course, it is unrealistic to expect every study to satisfy all of the points; however, the systematic application of these points will allow readers to identify and assess the strengths and weaknesses of individual studies.

Box 3.1. A check-list for assessing economic evaluations

1. Was a well-defined question posed in answerable form?
1.1 Did the study examine both costs and effects of the service(s) or programme(s)?
1.2 Did the study involve a comparison of alternatives?
1.3 Was a viewpoint for the analysis stated and was the study placed in any particular decision-making context?

2. Was a comprehensive description of the competing alternatives given (i.e. can you tell who did what to whom, where, and how often)?
2.1 Were any important alternatives omitted?
2.2 Was (Should) a *do-nothing* alternative (be) considered?

3. Was the effectiveness of the programmes or services established?
3.1 Was this done through a randomized, controlled clinical trial? If so, did the trial protocol reflect what would happen in regular practice?
3.2 Was effectiveness established through an overview of clinical studies?
3.3 Were observational data or assumptions used to established effectiveness? If so, what are the potential biases in results?

4. Were all the important and relevant costs and consequences for each alternative identified?
4.1 Was the range wide enough for the research question at hand?
4.2 Did it cover all relevant viewpoints? (Possible viewpoints include the community or social viewpoint, and those of patients and third-party payers. Other viewpoints may also be relevant depending upon the particular analysis.)
4.3 Were capital costs, as well as operating costs, included?

5. Were costs and consequences measured accurately in appropriate physical units (e.g. hours of nursing time, number of physician visits, lost work-days, gained life-years)
5.1 Were any of the identified items omitted from measurement? If so, does this mean that they carried no weight in the subsequent analysis?
5.2 Were there any special circumstances (e.g. joint use of resources) that made measurement difficult? Were these circumstances handled appropriately?

6. Were costs and consequences valued credibly?
6.1 Were the sources of all values clearly identified? (Possible sources include market values, patient or client preferences and views, policy-makers' views and health professionals' judgements.)
6.2 Were market values employed for changes involving resources gained or depleted?
6.3 Where market values were absent (e.g. volunteer labour), or market values did not reflect actual values (such as clinic space donated at a reduced rate), were adjustments made to approximate market values?

6.4 Was the valuation of consequences appropriate for the question posed (i.e. has the appropriate type or types of analysis – cost-effectiveness, cost-benefit, cost-utility – been selected)?

7. Were costs and consequences adjusted for differential timing?
7.1 Were costs and consequences which occur in the future 'discounted' to their present values?
7.2 Was any justification given for the discount rate used?

8. Was an incremental analysis of costs and consequences of alternatives performed?
8.1 Were the additional (incremental) costs generated by one alternative over another compared to the additional effects, benefits, or utilities generated?

9. Was allowance made for uncertainty in the estimates of costs and consequences?
9.1 If data on costs or consequences were stochastic, were appropriate statistical analyses performed?
9.2 If a sensitivity analysis was employed, was justification provided for the ranges of values (for key study parameters)?
9.3 Were study results sensitive to changes in the values (within the assumed range for sensitivity analysis, or within the confidence interval around the ratio of costs to consequences)?

10. Did the presentation and discussion of study results include all issues of concern to users?
10.1 Were the conclusions of the analysis based on some overall index or ratio of costs to consequences (e.g. cost-effectiveness ratio)? If so, was the index interpreted intelligently or in a mechanistic fashion?
10.2 Were the results compared with those of others who have investigated the same question? If so, were allowances made for potential differences in study methodology?
10.3 Did the study discuss the generalizability of the results to other settings and patient/client groups?
10.4 Did the study allude to, or take account of, other important factors in the choice or decision under consideration (e.g. distribution of costs and consequences, or relevant ethical issues)?
10.5 Did the study discuss issues of implementation, such as the feasibility of adopting the 'preferred' programme given existing financial or other constraints, and whether any freed resources could be redeployed to other worthwhile programmes?

3.1. ELEMENTS OF A SOUND ECONOMIC EVALUATION

1. Was a well-defined question posed in answerable form?

Such a question will clearly identify the alternatives being compared and the viewpoint(s) from which the comparison is to be made. Questions such as, '*Is a chronic home care programme worth it?'* and, *'Will a community hypertension screening programme do any good?'* solicit the issues of *to whom and compared to what*. Similarly, questions such as, *'How much does it cost to run our intensive care unit?'*, and *'What are the costs and outcomes of adolescent counselling by social workers?'* are not efficiency questions because they fail to specify the alternatives for comparison. (See Chapter 2 for a review of the basic types of economic evaluation.) This is not to say that the questions do not provide important accounting or management information; they may do so, but the answers to them do not by themselves qualify as efficiency statements.

A well-specified question, for example, might look as follows: *'From the viewpoint of (a) both the Ministry of Health and the Ministry of Community and Social Services budgets, and (b) patients incurring out-of-pocket costs, is a chronic home care programme preferable to the existing programme of institutionalized, extended care in designated wards of general hospitals?'*. Note that the viewpoint for an analysis may be that of a specific provider or providing institution, the patient or groups of patients, a third-party payer (public or private), or society (i.e. all costs and consequences to whomsoever they accrue). Obviously it is difficult for the analyst to consider every single cost and consequence of a health care programme to all members of society. Indeed, the 'ripple effects' of some programmes may be far-reaching and consideration of some items may have to be excluded for practical reasons. However, it is important to recognize that in considering the use of the community's scarce resources, the viewpoint of the providing institution may often be too restrictive and a broader viewpoint should also be considered. For example, it may be that a programme is preferable from the societal viewpoint, but not from the viewpoint of the providing institution. In such a case the Ministry of Health may wish to consider giving an incentive to the providing institution to ensure that the socially preferred programme goes ahead. The existence of different viewpoints was highlighted by Weisbrod *et al.* (1980) in their study of community-oriented and hospital-based treatments for mental illness.

2. Was a comprehensive description of the competing alternatives given?

A clear and specific statement of the primary objective of each alternative programme, treatment, or service is critical in selecting among cost-effectiveness, cost–utility, and cost–benefit analysis as the type of evaluation to be undertaken. A full description of the competing alternatives is essential for three further reasons:

1. Readers must be able to judge the applicability of the programmes to their own settings.
2. Readers should be able to assess for themselves whether any costs or consequences may have been omitted in the analysis.

3. Readers may wish to replicate the programme procedures being described.

Therefore, readers should be provided with information allowing an identification of costs:

- who does what to whom,
- where, and
- how often,

and consequences:

- what are the results?

3. Was there evidence that the programmes' effectiveness had been established?

We are not interested in the efficient provision of ineffective services, i.e. those services which have been shown to do no more good than harm (by themselves, or compared with no treatment). In fact, we are not interested in the provision of such services under any conditions, efficient or otherwise. *If something is not worth doing, it is not worth doing well!* Therefore, if the economic evaluation assumes effectiveness, some indication of the prior validation of effectiveness should be given. It is also possible that the efficiency evaluation may have been conducted simultaneously with the evaluation of efficacy or effectiveness. This is the case in many randomized trials of therapies which also include a comparison of the costs of the experimental programme and a control, which may be a placebo or the currently existing programme. Note, however, that efficiency evaluations, by themselves, are incapable of establishing effectiveness. Precedent or simultaneous evidence of effectiveness is required. After all, there are efficient methods of worsening the quality of life as well as improving it! [Those wishing to know more about the methods of establishing whether a therapy does more good than harm should consult Sackett *et al.* (1991).]

4. Were all the important and relevant costs and consequences for each alternative identified?

Even though it may not be possible or necessary to measure and value all of the costs and consequences of the alternatives under comparison, a full identification of the important and relevant ones should be provided. The combination of information contained in the viewpoint statement and programme description should allow judgement of what specific costs and consequences or outcomes it is appropriate to include in the analysis.

An overview of the categories of costs and consequences that are relevant to an economic evaluation of health services and programmes was given in Fig 2.2. (This is presented again here as Fig 3.1.)

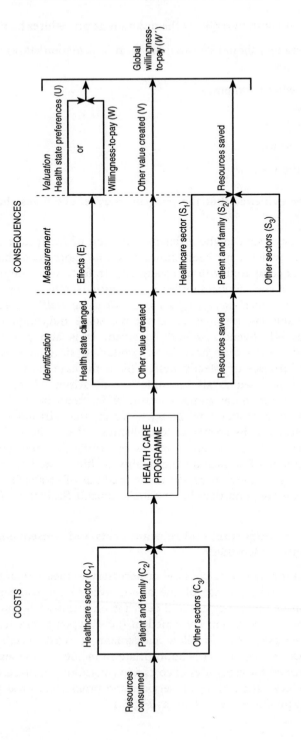

Figure 3.1. Components of economic evaluation in health care

Three categories of cost are identified. The health care resources consumed consist of the costs of organizing and operating the programme, including dealing with the adverse events caused by the programme. The identification of these costs often amounts to listing the *ingredients* of the programme – both variable costs (such as the time of health professionals or supplies) and fixed or overhead costs (such as light, heat, rent or capital costs). The ways of measuring and valuing these items are discussed in more detail in Chapter 4.

The patient and family resources consumed include any out-of-pocket expenses incurred by patients and/or family members as well as the value of any resources that they contribute to the treatment process. This would include the value of their time and sometimes patients and/or family members may lose time from work while seeking treatment or participating in a health care programme.

While the above two categories of costs cover most of the cost items relevant to economic evaluations of health services, a third category, resources consumed in other sectors, also warrants mention. As mentioned in Chapter 2, some programmes, such as those for care of the elderly, consume resources from other public agencies or the voluntary sector. Occasionally it may also be the case that the operation of a health service or programme changes the resource use in the broader economy. Examples of situations where these factors may be important are:

(1) an occupational health and safety programme (perhaps legislated by government) that changes the production process in an automobile manufacturing plant, thereby using up more resources, perhaps in a more labour-intensive way. These costs are passed on in the increased price of cars and are borne by the purchasers of cars, who are likely not the workers for whom the programme was initiated;

(2) a 55-mile-per-hour speed limit policy which reduces morbidity and mortality due to accidents, but increases the price of, for example, fruit which now takes longer to arrive (i.e. a higher wage bill for the truck driver).

In principle, these factors should be considered in the economic evaluation, though for many health care programmes they may be insignificant. (Few economic analyses of alternative health care programmes take them into account.)

Three categories of consequences of health services or programmes are also shown in Fig 3.1. The changes in health state relate to changes in the physical, social or emotional functioning of individuals. In principle, such changes can be measured objectively, and refer only to an individuals ability to function and not to the significance, preference or value attached to this ability by the individual, or by others. However, as indicated in Fig 3.1 and discussed later, values can be attached either by health state preference scores or willingness-to-pay.

In addition, other value may be created by the programme (e.g. reduction in anxiety) and resources may be freed. For example, a vaccination programme may free resources if fewer individuals contract the disease and thus require treatment. This was discussed in Chapter 2.

Given the wide range of costs and consequences indicated above, it may be unrealistic to expect all relevant items to be measured and valued in the analysis, due to their small size or influence relative to the effort required to measure or value them accurately; however, it is helpful to users to identify as many relevant items as possible. It is particularly important that the outcomes of interest be identified clearly enough for a reader to judge the appropriateness of the type (or types) of economic evaluation chosen. That is, it should be apparent:

- whether a single outcome is of primary interest as opposed to a set of outcomes;
- whether the outcomes are common to both alternatives under comparison, and;
- to what degree each programme is successful in achieving each outcome of interest.

Similarly, it is important to know whether the consequences of primary interest are the therapeutic effects themselves (thus implying cost effectiveness analysis if possible), the change in quality of life of patients and their families (cost–utility analysis), or the overall value created (cost–benefit analysis).

5. Were costs and consequences measured accurately in appropriate physical units?

While identification, measurement, and valuation often occur simultaneously in analyses, it is a good practice for users of evaluation results to view each as a separate phase of analysis. Once the important and relevant costs and consequences have been identified, they must be measured in appropriate physical and natural units. For example, measurement of the operating costs of a particular screening programme may yield a partial list of *ingredients* such as 500 physical examinations performed by physicians, 10 weeks of salaried nursing time, 10 weeks of a 1000 square foot clinic, 20 hours of medical research librarian time from an adjoining hospital, etc. Similarly, costs borne by patients may be measured, for instance, by the amount of medication purchased, or the number of times travel was required for treatment, or the time lost from work while being treated.

Notice that situations in which resources are jointly used by one or more programmes present a particular challenge to accurate measurement. How much resource use should be allocated to each programme? And on what basis? A common example of this is found in every hospital, where numerous clinical services and programmes share common overhead services (e.g. electric power, cleaning, and administration), provided centrally. In general, there is no non-arbitrary solution to the measurement problem; however, users of results should satisfy themselves that *reasonable* criteria (number of square feet, number of employees, number of cases, etc.) have been used to distribute the common costs. Users should definitely ascertain that such shared costs have been allocated, in fact, to participating services or programmes, as this is a common omission in evaluations! Clinical service directors often argue that small changes in the size of their programmes (up or down) do not affect the consumption of central services. Sometimes it is even argued that overhead costs are unaffected by the service itself. However, though this argument may be intuitively appealing from the viewpoint of a particular programme or service director, the extension of this method to each service in the hospital would imply that the totality of services could be operated without light, heat, power, and secretaries! (The allocation of overhead costs is discussed further in Chapter 4.)

With respect to the measurement of consequences, if the identification of outcomes of interest has been clearly performed, then selection of appropriate units of measurement for programme effects should be relatively straightforward. For example, effects might relate to mortality and be measured in life-years gained or deaths averted; they might relate to morbidity and be measured, for example, in reductions in disability days or improvements on some index of health status measuring physical, social, or emotional functioning; they may be even more specific, depending upon the alternatives under consideration. Thus, percentage increase in weight-bearing ability may be an appropriate natural measurement unit for an evaluation of a physiotherapy programme, while the number of correctly diagnosed cases may be appropriate for a comparison of venography with leg scanning in the diagnosis of deep-vein thrombosis.

Changes in resource use resulting from the effects will be measured in physical units similar to those employed for costs. Thus the changes in utilization resulting from any particular programme will likely be recorded in numbers of procedures, or amounts of time, space, or equipment. Changes in the resource use by patients will continue to be measured in amounts of medication purchased, trips taken for treatment, and so forth.

While the nature of changes in the quality of life may be described, this is one case where measurement in objective, physical, or natural units is difficult, although the consequence of some surgical interventions may be quantified in number of complications. However, the adjustment of effects for quality of life is usually a matter of valuation, although we also discuss the use of quality of life scales in cost-effectiveness analysis in Chapter 5.

6. Were costs and consequences valued credibly?

The sources and methods of valuation of costs, benefits, and utilities should be clearly stated in an economic evaluation. Costs are normally valued in units of local currency, based on prevailing *prices* of, for example, personnel, commodities, and services, and can often be taken directly from programme budgets. All current and future programme costs are normally valued in constant dollars of some base year (usually the present), in order to remove the effects of inflation from the analysis.

It should be remembered that the objective in valuing costs is to obtain an estimate of the worth of resources depleted by the programme. This may necessitate adjustments to some apparent programme costs (e.g. the case of subsidized services or volunteer labour received by one programme instead of another). In addition, valuation of the cost of a day of institutional care for a specific condition is particularly troublesome in that the use of an average cost per day (the widely quoted *per diem*), calculated on the basis of the institution's entire annual case-load, is almost certainly an overestimate or underestimate of the actual cost for any specific condition, sometimes by quite a large amount.

In principle and (with great effort) in practice, it is possible to identify, measure and value each depleted resource (e.g. drugs, nursing time, light, food, etc.) in treating a specific patient or group of patients. While this yields a relatively accurate cost estimate, the detailed monitoring and data collection are usually prohibitively expensive. The other broad alternative costing strategy is to start with the institution's total costs for a particular period and then to improve upon the method of simply dividing by the total patient-days to produce an average cost-per-day. Quite sophisticated methods of cost allocation to individual hospital departments or wards have been developed, as illustrated by Boyle *et al.* (1982) with respect to neonatal intensive care. An intermediate method involves acceptance of the components of the general *per diem* relating to *hotel* costs (since these are relatively invariant across patients) combined with more precise calculation of the medical treatment costs associated with the specific patients in question. For an example of this intermediate approach see Hull *et al.* (1982). Of course, the effort devoted to accurate *per diem* estimates depends upon their overall importance in the study; however, unthinking use of *per diems* or average costs should be guarded against. (This is discussed further in Chapter 4.)

In valuation of preferences or utilities, we are basically attempting to ascertain how much better the quality of life is in one health situation or 'state' compared with another (e.g. dialysis at home with help from a spouse or friend versus dialysis in hospital). Several techniques are available for making the comparison; the important thing to note is that each will produce an adjustment factor with which to increase or decrease the value of time spent in health situations or 'states', resulting from the alternative in question relative to some baseline. The results of these analyses are usually expressed in *healthy years* or *quality-adjusted life-years* gained, as a result of the programmes being evaluated.

Two broad approaches to estimating health state preferences can be found in the literature. The first approach, outlined by Torrance (1986), emphasizes the development of measurement methods and empirical testing on different populations. The other approach, outlined by Weinstein (1981), places emphasis on the estimation of preference scores by a quick (and inexpensive) consensus-forming exercise, and then undertaking extensive sensitivity analysis on the chosen scores to see whether study results change if the chosen estimates are varied. We see a role for both approaches. The latter approach is useful in getting decision-makers to think about resource allocation problems and is, in fact, relatively quick and inexpensive. The measurement approach is useful in highlighting the fact that different actors (doctors, policy-makers, patients, and the general public as taxpayers) may have different preferences, and is clearly crucial in situations where the study result is sensitive to the preference scores assigned. (An example of such a case arose in the study by Stason and Weinstein (1977) on the economics of hypertension therapy. The study result was sensitive to whether it was assumed that the side effects of antihypertensive drugs constituted a one or two per cent reduction in health status.)

Since the measurement of preferences in health is still a relatively new field, there are many unresolved issues which readers of cost–utility analyses should note. Users of such analyses will probably want to know, at minimum, *whose* preferences were used to construct the adjustment factor – the patient's, the provider's, the taxpayer's or the bureaucrat's? If patients' preferences have not been employed, we may want to assure ourselves further that the persons whose preferences did count clearly understood the characteristics of the health state, either through personal experience or through a description of the state presented to them. These issues are taken up in Chapter 6.

Many of the same issues arise when estimating willingness-to-pay, either for a change in health state or for the overall impact of the programme in question. These issues are taken up in Chapter 7.

One of the important consequences of health care programmes is the creation of healthy time. The valuation of this item poses difficulties. Indeed, its categorization, under changes in health state or patient and family resources freed is uncertain. The reasons for this are as follows.

The value of healthy time can manifest itself in a number of ways. First, living in a better health state has a value to the individual in its own right (e.g. less pain, better quality of life). Secondly, healthy time can be used in leisure. Thirdly, healthy time can be used for work, which generates income for the individual and productive output for society.

In a CEA, the measurement of the effects (E) does not capture the value of healthy time. Therefore, if it is to be included it would have to be estimated separately, as an element of the patient and family resources freed. In a CUA or CBA, where we are attempting to *value* the consequences of the programme, we might expect that the value of living in a better health state is captured in the preference score (U), or the willingness-to-pay (W). The value of healthy time in leisure is probably also captured in (U) or (W), as it is closely linked with improved quality of life.

Whether or not the value of using healthy time for work is also included in (U) or (W) probably depends on how the scenario (used for valuation) is written. It may be possible, for example, to ask individuals to imagine that their income would not be affected by their health state, since this is covered by unemployment insurance. In such a case, an analyst undertaking an evaluation from a societal viewpoint may wish to include a separate estimate of productivity gains to society if a persons health state is improved. If so, it would be important to ensure that the person did *not* include this in their own valuation, so as to avoid double counting.

Of course, healthy time can also be consumed by a programme if it requires the individual to spend time seeking or undergoing treatment, perhaps in hospital. In a CEA, the value of healthy time lost would have to be estimated separately.

In a CUA or CBA, the way forward would again depend on how the health state scenario is described. If the description contained elements of the process of undergoing care (e.g. you will be admitted to hospital for seven days for treatment), this may be reflected in the preference score (U) or willingness-to-pay (W). Otherwise, the value of healthy time lost in therapy may have to be estimated separately.

Therefore, we have another example of where the assembly of components (building blocks) in the analysis is partly dependent on how they are measured and valued. In conducting an economic evaluation from a societal perspective, it is important to avoid both zero-counting and double-counting. Of course, the estimation of global willingness-to-pay (W') avoids the problem of categorizing the value of healthy time, either as a component of the change in health state or as a component of patient and family resources freed. Rather, the challenge of this approach is to ensure that individuals appreciate *all* the elements of value created and resources consumed by a health care programme, so that this is reflected in their valuation (W').

7. Were costs and consequences adjusted for differential timing?

Since comparison of programmes or services must be made at one point in time (usually the present), the timing of programme costs and consequences which do not occur entirely in the present must be taken into account. Different programmes may have different time profiles of costs and consequences. For example, the primary benefits of an influenza immunization programme are immediate while those of hypertension screening occur well into the future. The time profile of costs and consequences may also differ within a single programme; the costs of the hypertension screening programme would be incurred in the present. Therefore, future dollar cost and benefit streams are reduced or 'discounted' to reflect the fact that dollars spent or saved in the future should not weigh as heavily in programme decisions as dollars spent or saved today. This is primarily due to the existence of *time preference*. That is, individually and as a society we prefer to have dollars or resources now as opposed to later because we can benefit from them in the interim. This is evidenced by the existence of interest rates (as well as the popular wisdom about 'a bird in the hand'). Moreover since *time preference* is not exclusively a financial concept, discounting of outcomes should also be undertaken in cost-effectiveness and cost–utility studies (Weinstein and Stason 1977). The mechanics of discounting and the choice of discount rate are discussed in Chapter 4.

8. Was an incremental analysis of costs and consequences of alternatives performed?

For meaningful comparison, it is necessary to examine the additional costs that one service or programme imposes over another, compared with the additional effects, benefits, or utilities it delivers. This *incremental* approach to analysis of costs and consequences can be illustrated by reference to one of the examples cited in Chapter 2, namely strategies for the diagnosis of deep-vein thrombosis (DVT) (Hull *et al.* 1981).

Table 3.1 shows the costs and outcomes (in terms of correct diagnoses) generated by two alternative strategies: impedance plethysmography (IPG) alone versus IPG plus out-patient venography if impedance plethysmography is negative. (IPG is a non-invasive strategy, whereas venography, the diagnostic 'gold standard' for DVT, can cause pain and other unpleasant side effects.) Although one could compare the simple ratios of costs to outcomes for the two alternatives, the correct comparison is the one of incremental costs over incremental outcomes, since this tells us how much we are paying (for each extra correct diagnosis) in adding the extra diagnostic test. In this case the relevant figure is therefore $4781 per correct diagnosis, not the average figure for the second programme, $3003 per correct diagnosis. It may be decided that $4781 is still a price worth paying; however, it is important to be clear on the principle since earlier (in Chapter 2) we pointed out that, in the case of screening for cancer of the colon, there was a big difference between the average cost (per case detected) of a protocol of six sequential tests and the incremental cost of performing a sixth test, having already done five (Neuhauser and Lewicki 1975).

Similar incremental analyses could be performed if the effects were in years of life or healthy years. These can be illustrated graphically on a four quadrant diagram known as the *cost-effectiveness plane* (Black 1990). (See Box 3.2.)

Table 3.1.   Economic evaluation of alternative diagnostic strategies for 516 patients with clinically suspected deep-vein thrombosis*

Programme	Costs ($ US)	Outcomes (No. of correct diagnoses)	Ratio of cost to outcome ($ per correct diagnoses)
1. IPG (alone)	321 488	142	2264
2. IPG plus out-patient venography if IPG negative	603 552	201	3003
3. Increment (of Programme 2 over Programme 1)	282 064	59	4781

*Data drawn from Table 1, Hull *et al.* (1981), by permission.

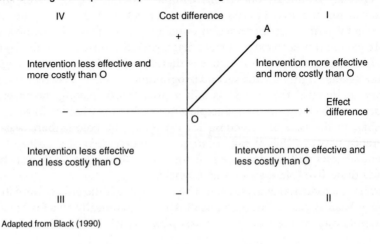

Box 3.2.   The cost-effectiveness plane

In the diagram the horizontal axis represents the difference in effect between the intervention of interest (A) and the relevant alternative (O), and the vertical axis represents the difference in cost. The alternative (O) could be the status quo or a competing programme.

If point A is in quadrants II or IV the choice between the programmes is clear. In quadrant II the intervention of interest is both more effective and less costly than the alternative. That is, it *dominates* the alternative. In quadrant IV the opposite is true. In quadrants I and III the choice depends on the maximum cost-effectiveness ratio one is willing to accept. The slope of the line OA gives the cost-effectiveness ratio.

IV   Cost difference   I
                                +   A

Intervention less effective and   Intervention more effective
more costly than O   and more costly than O

                                                                        Effect
  – ————————————————————————————   +   difference
                                O

Intervention less effective   Intervention more effective and
and less costly than O   less costly than O

        III   –   II

Adapted from Black (1990)

In practice the impact of most interventions falls in quadrant I. That is, they add to cost but increase effectiveness, certainly when compared with no intervention. Let us therefore plot the data given in Table 3.1 (see Fig. 3.2). Here we only show quadrant I and the slopes of the lines from the origin give the average cost-effectiveness ratios for the two programmes, which are $2264 and $3003 per case detected for A and B respectively. The incremental cost-effectiveness ratio ($4781 per case detected) is given by the slope of the line joining points A and B.

Figure 3.2. Average and incremental cost-effectiveness ratios

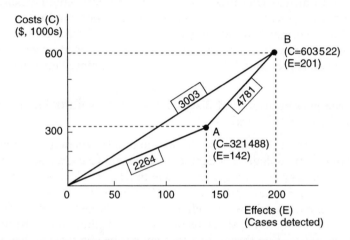

9. Was allowance made for uncertainty in the estimates of costs and consequences?

Every evaluation will contain some degree of uncertainty, imprecision, or methodological controversy. What if the compliance rate for influenza vaccination was 10 per cent higher than considered for the analysis? What if the *per diem* hospital cost still understated the true resource cost of a treatment programme by $100? What if a discount rate of six per cent had been used instead of two per cent? Or what if indirect costs and benefits had been excluded from the analysis? Users of efficiency studies will often ask these and similar questions; therefore, careful analysts will identify critical methodological assumptions or areas of uncertainty. Furthermore, they will often attempt to rework the analysis (qualitatively if not quantitatively), employing different assumptions or estimates in order to test the sensitivity of the results and conclusions to such changes. If large variations in the assumptions or estimates underlying an analysis do not produce significant alterations in the results then one would tend to have more confidence in the original results. If the converse occurs, more effort is then required to reduce the uncertainty and/or improve the accuracy of the critical variables. In either case, this *sensitivity analysis* is an important element of a sound economic evaluation. Sensitivity analysis is discussed further in Chapter 5.

Up until recently most of the data presented in economic evaluations have been deterministic (i.e. given as point estimates). Therefore, sensitivity analysis has been the primary method for allowing for uncertainty. However, today more economic evaluations are being conducted alongside clinical trials. Here the data are typically stochastic (i.e. having a mean and variance). For the stochastic clinical data it is customary to perform tests of statistical significance, or to present confidence intervals around the estimates of clinical effect. This would also be an option for the resource use or cost data; for example, statistical tests could be performed to determine whether or not the mean lengths of stay or total costs for two treatments were indeed different from one another.

Therefore, in principle uncertainty in the estimates of costs and consequences can be allowed for by sensitivity analysis, statistical inference, or some combination of the two approaches. This issue is explored in more detail in Chapter 8.

10. Did the presentation and discussion of study results include all issues of concern to users?

It will be clear from the foregoing discussion that the economic analyst has to make many methodological judgements when undertaking a study. Faced with users who may be mainly interested in the 'bottom line' – e.g. 'Should we buy a CT scanner' – how should the analyst present the results?

Decision indices such as cost-effectiveness and cost–benefit ratios are a useful way of summarizing study results. However, they should be used with care for, in interpreting them, the user may not be completely clear on what has gone into their construction. Some analysts give a range of results. For example, in their economic evaluation of neonatal intensive care for very-low-birth-weight infants, Boyle *et al.* (1983) compare the results for infants below 1000 g and from 1000-1500 g in terms of costs to hospital discharge, costs and consequences to age 15, and costs and consequences for lifetime (Table 3.2). They leave it to the users of the study to decide on which index (or indices) neonatal intensive care should be judged, since the different measures incorporate different value judgements and varying amounts of precision. (For example, the index of 'net economic benefit' includes production gains/losses, and the index of 'cost per quality-adjusted life-year' incorporates the preferences for health states of a sample of the local population.) This leads to another general point, namely it is important for analysts to be as explicit as possible about the various judgements they have made in carrying out the study. A good study should leave the user more (rather than less!) aware of the various technical and value judgements necessary to arrive at resource allocation decisions in health care.

Table 3.2. Measures of economic evaluation of neonatal intensive care according to birth-weight class (5 per cent discount rate)[a]

Period	Birth-weight class	
	1000–1499 g	500–999 g
	$	
To hospital discharge[b]		
Cost/additional survivor at hospital discharge	59 500	102 500
To age 15 (projected)		
Cost/life-year gained	6 100	12 200
Cost/QALY[c] gained	7 700	40 100
To death (projected)		
Cost/life-year gained	2 900	9 300
Cost/QALY[c] gained	3 200	22 400
Net economic benefit (loss)/live birth	(2 600)	(16 100)
Net economic cost/life-year gained	900	7 300
Net economic cost/QALY[c] gained	1 000	17 500

[a]Values are expressed in 1978 Canadian dollars. Multiply by 0.877 to calculate equivalent 1978 US dollars.
[b]All costs and effects occurred in year one.
[c]QALY denotes quality-adjusted life-year.
(From Boyle *et al.* (1983), by permission.)

Finally, a good study should begin to help the user interpret the results in the context of his or her own particular situation. This can be done by being explicit about the viewpoint for the analysis (an earlier point) and by indicating how particular costs and benefits might vary by location. For example, the costs of instituting day-care surgery may vary, depending on whether a purpose-built day-care unit already exists or whether wards have to be converted. Similarly, the benefits of day-care surgery may vary depending on whether, in a particular location, there is pressure on beds and whether beds will be closed or left empty (Russell *et al.* 1977). Obviously it is impossible for the analyst to anticipate every possibility in every location, but one limitation of economic evaluation techniques (discussed in Section 3.2) is that they assume that freed resources will be put to other beneficial uses. Evans and Robinson (1980) argue that in the case of day-care surgery the full economic pay-off may not have been obtained in at least one Canadian hospital.

The presentation, interpretation, and use of economic evaluation results raise a number of practical issues. For example, can the results (e.g. cost-effectiveness ratios) from different studies be meaningfully compared; can results of studies be generalized from one setting, or country, to another; can guidelines for good practice in the presentation of results be specified? These issues will be explored in Chapter 9.

3.2. LIMITATIONS OF ECONOMIC EVALUATION TECHNIQUES

Our main purpose in this chapter is to make the user of economic evaluation results more aware of the methodological judgements involved in undertaking an economic evaluation in the health care field. In Box 3.1 we have consolidated the points made in this chapter into a suggested check-list of questions to ask when critically assessing economic evaluation results. Some of these questions signal limitations of economic evaluation techniques. For example, economic evaluation techniques rely on the establishment of programme effectiveness. In addition, there are several other limitations of which users should be aware.

Of primary concern from a policy viewpoint is the fact that economic evaluations do not usually incorporate the importance of the distribution, of costs and consequences, among different patient or population groups, into the analysis. Yet, in some cases, the identity of the recipient group (e.g. the poor, the elderly, working mothers, or a geographically remote community) may be an important factor in assessing the social desirability of a service or programme. Indeed, it may be the motivation for the programme in the first place. Although it is sometimes suggested that differential weights be attached to the value of outcomes accruing to special recipient groups, this is not normally done within an economic evaluation. Rather, an equitable distribution of costs and consequences across socioeconomic or other defined groups in society is viewed as a competing dimension upon which decisions are made, in addition to that of efficient deployment of resources.

A more subtle, yet important, point is that the various forms of analysis discussed above embody different equity criteria. For example, cost–benefit analysis values health outcomes in terms of individuals' willingness-to-pay. Sometimes willingness-to-pay may be constrained by ability to pay and therefore valuations are dependent on the existing income distribution. On the other hand the simple aggregation of QALYs in a cost–utility analysis implies that QALY is being valued the same no matter to whom it accrues. Therefore, in reality it is difficult to divorce equity considerations from the economic evaluation and analysts should be aware of this when selecting a particular analytic technique.

It should also be noted that economic evaluation techniques assume that resources freed or saved by preferred programmes will not in fact be wasted but will be employed in alternative worthwhile programmes. This assumption warrants careful scrutiny, for if the freed resources are consumed by other ineffective or unevaluated programmes, then not only is there no saving, but overall health system costs will actually increase without any assurance of additional improvements in the health status of the population.

Finally, evaluation of any sort is in itself a costly activity. Bearing in mind that *even a cost–benefit analysis should be subject to a cost–benefit analysis*, it seems reasonable to suggest that economic evaluation techniques will prove most useful in situations where programme objectives require clarification, the competing alternatives are significantly different in nature, or large resource commitments are under consideration.

3.3. CONCLUSIONS

In these introductory chapters, we have tried to assist users of economic evaluations in interpreting evaluation studies and assessing their usefulness for health care decisions, or for planning further analyses. The rationale for economic evaluation, its fundamental characteristics, and the basic types of economic evaluation were described in Chapter 2. In Chapter 3 we have identified and discussed 10 questions which readers of economic evaluations can ask in order to critically assess a particular study; a check-list of these questions is given in Box 3.1.

Our intent in offering a check-list is not to create hypercritical users who will be satisfied only by superlative studies. It is important to realize, as emphasized at the outset, that for a variety of reasons it is unlikely that every study will satisfy all criteria. However, the use of these criteria as screening devices should help users of economic evaluations to identify quickly the strengths and weaknesses of studies. Moreover, in assessing any particular study, users should ask themselves one final question, '*How does this evaluation compare with our normal basis for decision-making?*' They may find that the method of organizing thoughts embodied in the evaluation compares well with alternative approaches, even bearing in mind the possible deficiencies in the study.

3.4. CRITICAL APPRAISAL OF A PUBLISHED ARTICLE

MARK, D. B. *et al.* **Cost-effectiveness of thrombolytic therapy with tissue plasminogen activator (t-PA) as compared with streptokinase (SK) for acute myocardial infarction (AMI)**

1. Was a well-defined question posed in an answerable form?

    __X__ YES   _____ NO   _____ CAN'T TELL

The authors explain the context of their study, which is that some observers have questioned whether the improved survival rates observed in the GUS-TO study (a multicentre, randomized clinical trial, comparing t-PA with SK) are worth the substantial additional cost (p.1418).

The authors state that they conducted a cost-effectiveness analysis to compare the value of t-PA treatment with that of streptokinase (p.1418).

They state that they used a social perspective to identify relevant costs, although indirect costs (e.g. time lost from work) and non-medical costs were not included (p. 1419). The reasons for exclusion of some relevant costs are not given. The reader would have to assess whether the exclusion of some costs biases the results.

2. Was a comprehensive description of the competing alternatives given (i.e. can you tell who, did what, to whom, where, and how often)?

    X   YES   _____ NO   _____ CAN'T TELL

Details are given of the GUSTO study which compared four different regimens: accelerated tissue plasminogen activator (t-PA), streptokinase with intravenous heparin, SK with subcutaneous heparin and a combination of t-PA and SK. Accelerated is defined as the administration of t-PA over a period of 1.5 hours, rather than the conventional period of three hours (p.1418). The alternatives for the economic study are accelerated t-PA and SK.

For further details the reader would have to consult the GUSTO clinical study. However, one can infer a hospital setting as SK can only be administered in hospital. One important factor is the period of time, post-AMI, before patients receive thrombolytic therapy. This has been shown to be important in previous studies, but no details are given here.

In addition, some subgroup analyses are performed, by age of patient and location of infarction. Implicitly these represent additional alternatives for economic analysis, although they are not the major alternatives being examined.

3. Was there evidence that the programmes effectiveness had been established?

    X   YES   _____ NO   _____ CAN'T TELL

The primary clinical endpoint, survival to one year, was estimated in the randomized controlled trial, representing the strongest form of evidence. One year after enrolment, patients who received t-PA had a higher survival rate (an increase of 1.1 per cent, or 11 per 1000 patients treated) than SK-treated patients.

However, in order to calculate the life-years gained, the denominator in the cost-effectiveness ratio, it was necessary to extrapolate beyond one year. This was done by; (i) a Cox proportional-hazards model based on the experience of 4379 patients in the Duke Cardiovascular Disease Database (giving an extrapolation from one to 15 years) and; (ii) a statistical extrapolation for the tail of the survival curve (beyond 15 years) (p.1419).

A number of assumptions were necessary for the extrapolation, the main one being that the hazard of death after one year did not depend on the thrombolytic agent received (i.e. that the survival curves of the two treatment groups were parallel).

4. Were all the important and relevant costs and consequences for each alternative identified?

_____ YES   _____ NO   __X__ CAN'T TELL

As mentioned above, changes in productive output and non-medical costs were excluded. This probably makes no substantial difference to the cost-effectiveness ratio, but it is hard to tell.

One area where these costs could be important is in disabling, non-fatal stroke. In the first 30 days after treatment in the GUSTO study, t-PA produced a net increase of one disabling non-fatal stroke per 1000 patients treated, as compared with the rate with SK. The authors investigate the impact of stroke on medical costs and overall reduction in the life expectancy for the t-PA group in a sensitivity analysis (see below). This has a modest impact on the cost-effectiveness ratio for t-PA. The impact could be greater if the excluded costs were considered.

5. Were costs and consequences measured accurately in appropriate physical units?

__X__ YES   _____ NO   _____ CAN'T TELL

The use of medical resources during the initial hospitalization was measured for all the US subjects (23,105) in the GUSTO study. Resource use up to one year was estimated for a random sample (2600) of the surviving members of the cohort. This was done by telephone survey. (These data are given in Table 2, p.1420.)

Many of the data presented in Table 2 are medians. This is appropriate for testing statistically, as the data are negatively skewed. However, for descriptive purposes, means are more informative, as in planning (say) hospital bed provision, it is important to know about the tail of the distribution. However, the resource consumption in the first year was generally similar for the two groups, so did not enter in the incremental cost-effectiveness ratio.

Resource use beyond one year was assumed to be the same for both groups. Although telephone surveys may not be the ideal method of determining resource use, practical considerations would seriously limit other methods. Overall, the authors provide an accurate measurement of resource use.

The main consquence of therapy (life years gained) was estimated by the methods described above.

6. Were costs and consequences valued credibly?

<table>
<tr><td>(for consequenses)</td><td></td><td>(for costs)</td></tr>
<tr><td>__X__ YES</td><td>_____ NO</td><td>__X__ CAN'T TELL</td></tr>
</table>

Health state preference values were measured in structured telephone interviews one year after treatment by the time trade-off method (p.1419). Thus, the quality of life impact of some morbidity, particularly that caused by strokes, may have been missed if these patients were unable to complete the interview. However, it would be unlikely to have a major impact on the result of the study.

The unit costs (prices) used in the analysis are given in Table 1 of the paper. These were a mixture of costs (from Duke University Hospital) and charges (Medicare DRG reimbursement rates). Two approaches were used to estimate the costs of the thrombolytic drugs, since these had a major impact on the results.

7. Were costs and consequences adjusted for differential timing?

__X__ YES   _____ NO   _____ CAN'T TELL

Both survival and costs were discounted at an annual rate of 5 per cent (p.1419). The authors state that this is consistent with conventional practice.

8. Was an incremental analysis of costs and consequences of alternatives performed?

__X__ YES   _____ NO   _____ CAN'T TELL

All the cost-effectiveness ratios presented in the paper are incremental of t-PA relative to SK. The primary analysis gave an incremental cost per year of life saved of $32,678.

9. Was allowance made for uncertainty in the estimates of costs and consequences?

___X___ YES   _____ NO   _____ CAN'T TELL

A number of one-way sensitivity analyses were performed. These included varying survival and costs in both the short and the long-term for the t-PA group, such as:

- taking the 95% confidence interval for the 1.1 per cent increase in one year survival, as estimated in the clinical trial;
- reducing life expectancy or assuming that the survival curves converge after one year;
- assuming that the (non-significant) increase in one year costs of t-PA (excluding the cost of the drug) did truly exist;
- assuming that the non-significant increase in costs was maintained beyond one year;
- assuming that the price for t-PA was much lower (e.g. the same as a typical European price).

In addition, sensitivity analyses were conducted on the impact of disabling strokes, and leaving costs and consequences undiscounted.

Finally, the quality-of-life adjustment is presented as a sensitivity analysis on the cost-effectiveness ratio. The incremental cost-effectiveness ratio changes from $32,678 per life-year gained to $36,402 per QALY.

In general, the authors highlight the changes in assumptions that would cause the incremental cost-effectiveness ratio to rise above a threshold of $50,000 per life-year gained.

10. Did the presentation and discussion of study results include all issues of concern to users?

___X___ YES   _____ NO   _____ CAN'T TELL

The authors include a fairly full discussion of the results. They introduce the notion that the upper limit for an acceptable cost-effectiveness ratio remains controversial, but values of more than $100,000 per year of life saved are generally considered too high (p.1422). Most estimates of the incremental ratio are less than $100,000.

The authors state that their subgroup analyses should be interpreted cautiously. A major finding, which perhaps may seem counter-intuitive, is that the incremental cost-effectiveness ratios for treatment by t-PA are more favourable for the older patients (especially those above 60 years old). This is because the younger patients have the lowest one-year mortality rates and the smallest increases in survival due to treatment with t-PA. The clinical and social implications of this finding are not explored.

Another issue, not explored in the paper, is whether the findings are generalizable beyond the trial and transferable to other settings. For example, the accelerated use of t-PA may not be achievable in some hospitals. In addition, other papers commenting on the GUSTO study have pointed out that the US patients (56% of total recruitment) were managed differently from the non-US patients in a number of ways, including greater use of invasive revascularization such as PTCA and CABG, and greater use of non-protocol medications (van der Verf *et al. 1995*).

This could lead to differences in costs and, in addition, the mortality reduction with t-PA was greater in the US (1.2% absolute decrease versus 0.7% elsewhere). However, the test for treatment-by-country interaction was not significant.

Finally, the costs of resources could vary from place to place, so overall, it may not be wise to assume that similar results would be found in other locations.

REFERENCES

Black, W. C. (1990). The cost-effectiveness plane: a graphic representation of cost-effectiveness. *Medical Decision Making,* **10**(3), 212–15.

Boyle, M. H., Torrance, G. W., Horwood, S. P., and Sinclair, J. C. (1982). *A cost analysis of providing neonatal intensive care to 500-1499-gram birth-weight infants,* Research Report No. 51, Programme for Quantitative Studies in Economics and Population. McMaster University, Hamilton, Ontario.

—, Torrance, G. W., Sinclair, J. C., and Horwood, S. P. (1983). Economic evaluation of neonatal intensive care of very-low-birth-weight infants. *N. Engl. J. Med.* **308**, 1330–7.

Drummond, M. F. (1981). Welfare economics and cost–benefit analysis in health care. *Scottish Political Economy,* **28**, 125–45.

Evans, R. G. and Robinson, G. C. (1980). Surgical day care: measurements of the economic pay-off. *Can. Med. Assoc. J.,* **123**, 873–80.

Hull, R., Hirsh, J., Sackett, D. L., and Stoddart, G. L. (1981). Cost-effectiveness of clinical diagnosis, venography and non-invasive testing in patients with symptomatic deep-vein thrombosis. *N. Engl. J. Med.,* **304**, 1561–7.

—, —, —, — (1982). Cost-effectiveness of primary and secondary prevention of pulmonary embolism in high-risk surgical patients. *Can. Med. Assoc. J.* **127**, 990–5.

Neuhauser, D. and Lewicki, A. M. (1975). What do we gain from the sixth stool guaiac? *N. Engl. J. Med.,* **293** (5), 226–8.

Russell, I. T., Devlin, H. B., Fell, M., Glass, N. J., and Newell, D. T. (1977). Day-case surgery for hernias and haemorrhoids: a clinical, social and economic evaluation. *Lancet,* i 844–7.

Sackett, D. L., Haynes, R. B., Guyatt, G. H., and Tugwell, P. (1991). *Clinical epidemiology: a basic science for clinical medicine.* (2nd edn). Little Brown and Co., Boston, MA.

Stason, W. B. and Weinstein, M. D. (1977). Allocation of resources to manage hypertension. *N. Engl. J. Med.*, **296**, 732–9.

Stoddart, G. L. (1982). Economic evaluation methods of health policy. *Evaluation and the Health Professions*, **5**, (4), 393-414.

Torrance, G. W. (1986). Measurement of health state utilities for economic appraisal. *Journal of Health Economics*, 5 1–30.

van der Werf, F., Topol, E. J., Lee, K. L., Woodlief, L. H., Granger, C. B. *et al.* (1995). Variations in patient management and outcomes for acute myocardial infarction in the United States and other countries. *J. Am. Med. Assoc.*, **273**, 1586–91.

Weinstein, M. C. (1981). Economic assessments of medical practices and technologies. *Medical Decision-Making*, **1** (4), 309–30.

and Stason, W. B. (1977). Foundations of cost-effectiveness analysis for health and medical practices. *N. Engl. J. Med.*, **296** 716–21.

Weisbrod, B. A., Test, M. A., and Stein, L. I. (1980). Alternatives to mental hospital treatment, II. Economic benefit-cost analysis. *Arch. General Psychiatry*, **37**, 400–5.

Williams, A. H. (1981). Welfare economics and health status measurement. In *Health, economics and health economics* (ed. J. van der Gaag and M. Perlman), pp. 271–81. North-Holland, Amsterdam.

4

Cost analysis

4.1. SOME BASICS

The analysis of the comparative costs of alternative treatments or health care programmes is common to all forms of economic evaluation and therefore most of the methodological issues discussed in this chapter are likely to be of relevance to all analyses (Luce and Elixhauser, 1990). Although many of the issues surrounding costing are context-specific and the analysts options are often limited by the availability of data, it is possible to give some general guidance. Two particularly thorny issues, the treatment of overhead costs (techniques for allocating shared overhead costs to individual projects) and allowance for differential timing of costs (the techniques of discounting and annuitization of capital expenditure), will be discussed in some detail. However, the chapter begins by covering some of the basic questions that an evaluator might have when embarking on a costing study in the health field.

4.1.1. Which costs should be considered?

The main categories of costs of health care programmes or treatments were identified in Fig. 3.1 of Chapter 3; these are the costs arising from the use of resources within the health sector, resource use by patients and their families, and resource use in other sectors. The particular range of costs included in a given study is likely to be decided upon as a result of considering the following four points.

1. What is the viewpoint for the analysis?

It is essential to specify the viewpoint since an item may be a cost from one point of view, but not a cost from another (see Box 4.1). For example, patients' travel costs are a cost from the patients' point of view and from the point of view of society, but not a cost from the Ministry of Health's point of view. Workers compensation payments are a cost to the paying government, a gain to the patient (recipient), and neither a cost nor a gain to society. (These money transfers, which do not reflect resource consumption, are called *transfer payments* by economists. Costs are involved in their administration, but these are not measured by the amounts themselves.)

Box 4.1. The influence of viewpoint on study results

The study by Weisbrod *et al.* (1980) shows how a different answer can be obtained depending upon the viewpoint adopted. It can be seen from the table that a community-oriented programme for mental illness patients looks expensive from the viewpoint of the agency providing the programme, compared with a traditional hospital-based programme (an extra $1700 per annum).

However, when costs falling on other health care agencies and those involved in law enforcement are considered, the cost difference is reduced. Finally, when broader societal costs and benefits are considered, such as the provision of food and shelter and the differences in productivity resulting from patients ability to work, the community-oriented programme has a lower net cost ($400 per annum lower).

Item	Community-oriented programme ($ per annum)	Hospital-based programme ($ per annum)	Difference in programmes ($ per annum)
COSTS (C)			
Primary treatment costs	4800	3100	1700
Other treatment costs (e.g. social services)	1800	2100	
Wider social costs (e.g. law enforcement, food, shelter)	1420	2020	
BENEFITS (B)			
Patient earnings	2400	1200	
NET ECONOMIC COST (B−C)	5620	6020	400

Adapted from Weisbrod *et al.* (1980)

Possible points of view include: society, Ministry of Health, other government ministries, the government in general, patient, employer, the agency providing the programme, etc. If the evaluation is being commissioned by a given body, this may give a clue to the relevant point(s) of view. However, when in doubt the analyst always adopts the societal point of view, which is the broadest one and is always relevant.

2. Is the comparison restricted to the two or more programmes immediately under study?

If the comparison is restricted to the programmes or treatments immediately under study, costs common to both need not be considered as they will not affect the choice between the given programmes. (Elimination of such costs can save the evaluator a considerable amount of work.) However, if it is thought that at some later stage a broader comparison may be contemplated, including other alternatives not yet specified, it might be prudent to consider all the costs of the programmes.

3. Are some costs merely likely to confirm a result that would be obtained by consideration of a narrower range of costs?

Sometimes the consideration of patients' costs merely confirm a result that might be obtained from, say, consideration of only operating costs within the health sector. Therefore, if consideration of patients' costs requires extra effort and the choice of programme is very unlikely to be changed, it may not be worthwhile to complicate the analysis unnecessarily. However, some justification for such an exclusion of a cost category should be given.

4. What is the relative order of magnitude of costs?

It is not worth investing a great deal of time and effort considering costs that, because they are small, are unlikely to make any difference to the study result. However, some justification should be given for the elimination of such costs, perhaps based on previous empirical work. It is still worthwhile identifying such cost categories in any event, although the estimation of them might not be pursued in any great detail.

Above all, the main point to remember when embarking on a costing study is that, to an economist, cost refers to the sacrifice (of benefits) made when a given resource is consumed in a programme or treatment. Therefore, it is important not to confine one's attention to expenditures, but to consider also other resources, the consumption of which is not adequately reflected in market prices, e.g. volunteer time, patients' leisure time, donated clinic space, etc.

4.1.2. How should costs be estimated?

Once the relevant range of costs has been identified the individual items must be measured and valued. That is, costing has two elements: measurement of the *quantities* of resource use (q) and the assignment of unit costs or *prices* (p). The measurement of resource quantities often depends on the context for the economic evaluation. For example, if an economic study is being conducted alongside a clinical trial, data on the resource quantities may be collected on the case report forms. On the other hand, if the economic study is free-standing, resource quantities may be estimated by a review of patients charts (case notes) or from routine data systems, such as hospital records. The quantities of some resources, such as domiciliary nursing visits, may only be estimated by asking patients, or by having them keep a diary.

Market prices will be available for many of the resource items. Although the theoretical proper price for a resource is its opportunity cost (i.e. the value of the forgone benefits because the resource is not available for its best alternative use), the pragmatic approach to costing is to take existing market prices unless there is some particular reason to do otherwise (e.g. the price of some resources may be subsidized by a third party such as a charitable institution). This is discussed further below.

Although the costing of most resource items is relatively unambiguous, the following issues commonly arise in costing studies.

1. How are values imputed for non-market items?

The major non-market resource inputs to health care programmes are volunteer time and patient/family leisure time. One approach to the valuation of these would be to use market wage rates (e.g. for volunteer time one might use unskilled wage rates). The market value of leisure time is harder to assess. One can argue for a value of lost leisure time of anything from zero, through average earnings, to average overtime earnings (time and a half or double time). The argument for the overtime rate is that this is the price that an employer must pay, at the margin, to buy some of the worker's leisure time. The most common practice is to value lost leisure time at zero in the base case (or primary) analysis, and to investigate the impact of the other assumptions through sensitivity analysis.

A slightly different approach is to identify and measure units of, say, volunteer input and to document these alongside the other costs when reporting results. This would enable the decision-maker to note those programmes relying heavily on volunteers. It would then be up to the programme director (or advocate of the programme or therapy) to demonstrate that such an input could be obtained without an opportunity cost to other programmes arising from the diversion of volunteers to the new programme.

2. When should existing market prices be adjusted?

It has long been recognized that, owing to the imperfections in health care markets, market prices may not reflect opportunity costs. For example, hospital charges may deviate from costs if a hospital has a local monopoly or seeks to cross-subsidize one activity from another (Finkler 1982). Physician fees may not accurately reflect the relative skill level and time required for different procedures. Drug prices may be set in negotiations between a pharmaceutical company and the government, where the company's commitment to research and provision of employment might be taken into account, as well as the costs of discovery, production, and distribution of the drug in question.

Having said that, it is by no means clear when an analyst should attempt to adjust observed market prices to reflect true opportunity costs. As mentioned above, most studies use market prices unadjusted and it has often been remarked that health economists recognize that market imperfections exist in health care, unless they are undertaking an economic evaluation!.

In order for analysts to attempt to adjust market prices, they should be convinced that:

(1) to leave prices unadjusted would introduce substantial biases into the study;
(2) there is a clear and objective way of making the adjustments.

These issues have been explored most extensively in the context of hospital charges in the USA. For example, Cohen *et al.* (1993) found that charges for cardiac procedures were substantially different from costs, although the relationships between the four procedures were largely unchanged (see Box 4.2). Of course, this is an empirical issue and the same may not be true for other procedures or programmes.

Box 4.2. Costs or charges: does it make a difference?

An analysis was undertaken by Cohen *et al.* of in-hospital charges from the itemized hospital accounts of 3000 patients at Boston's Beth Israel Hospital (1990 and 1991). Costs were then derived by adjusting for department-specific cost/charge ratios by using data on actual resource consumption. Comparison of estimates showed the following:

	Standard hospital charges (SD)	*Costs* (SD)
PTCA	$8369 ($3885)	$5396 ($2829)
Atherectomy	$8,301 ($2299)	$5726 ($2716)
Stent	$12670 ($5247)	$7828 ($3270)
CABG	$27739 ($7051)	$20927 ($6048)

It can be seen that whilst the ordering (in expense) of the procedures remains the same, the absolute differences change.

Source: Cohen. *et al.* (1993).

The methodology employed by Cohen *et al.*, and many other studies in the USA, was to derive costs by adjusting for department-specific cost-to-charge ratios. (These are generally in the public domain.) This is probably an improvement on the uncritical use of charges, but it is still dependent upon the quality of the accountancy study that generated the costs in the first place. Often this is difficult to assess. Nevertheless, adjustments by cost-to-charge ratios are becoming more commonplace in studies undertaken in the USA. However, there is probably no substitute for a well-conducted original costing study. In most countries, where hospital charges are not as detailed as in the USA, this is often the analyst's only alterative to using a general *per diem* or average hospital cost.

Finally, we should note that if the economic study is being undertaken from the viewpoint of the third party payer, the actual charges may be more relevant than the costs, although often the third party does not pay the full amount billed.

3. For how long should costs be tracked?

It can be seen from Fig 4.1 that not only does the analyst have a choice about whose costs to consider but also a choice of time period. In assessing how long costs should be tracked, the main objective should be to avoid misleading the decision maker or user. For example, a comparison of the costs of coronary artery bypass grafting (CABG) versus percutaneous transluminal coronary angioplasty (PTCA) to hospital discharge has shown CABG to be substantially more expensive ($9138 versus $22711) (Black *et al.* 1988). However, there is a possibility that patients receiving PTCA may require additional treatment subsequently, including CABG. In a costing study undertaken alongside a randomized controlled trial, Sculpher *et al.* (1991) showed that by 24 months post randomization, the cost difference between patients randomized to the alternative therapies had reduced substantially.

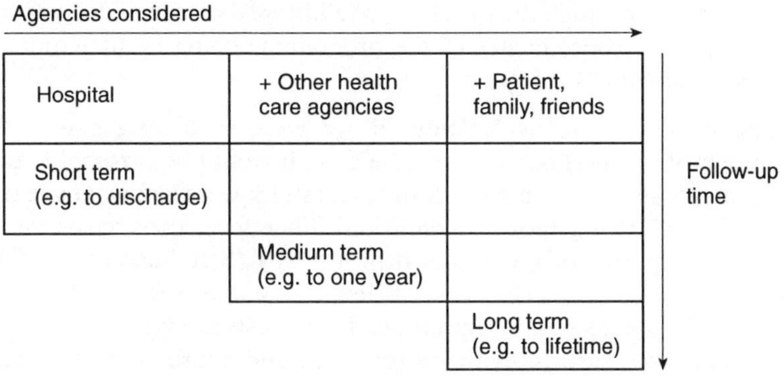

Figure 4.1. Choices in the consideration of costs

There is fairly broad agreement amongst analysis that in the case of *therapy-specific* or *disease-specific* costs, the choice of follow-up period should not bias the analysis in favour of one intervention over another. In some cases this may involve tracking costs for lifetime, although the quantitative impact of costs (on the analysis) far into the future will be reduced by discounting to present values (see Section 4.2 below).

4. Should health care costs unrelated to the programme or intervention under study be included?

The question of whether *unrelated* health care costs in the future should be included is much more open to debate. On the one hand, health care costs in later years of life are a clear consequence of keeping individuals alive. On the other hand, it does not seem totally fair to assign these costs to a prevention programme (e.g. hypertension screening), when they result from therapeutic decisions (e.g. to give cancer chemotherapy for advanced stages of disease) that should be considered on their own merits. Nevertheless, it is common in evaluations of prevention programmes to assign all the credit for life extension to the programme concerned. Therefore, it would make sense to assign all costs.

In considering this issue it has to be remembered that all the forms of economic evaluation discussed in this book are what economists call partial equilibrium analyses. That is, whilst it is recognized that any change in economic activity (such as investment in health programmes) includes many ripples throughout the economy, it is argued that such investments can be assessed against a background of all else remaining constant. Therefore, an artificial boundary is always being drawn around analyses.

There is no agreement amongst economic analysts about whether unrelated health care costs in later years of life should be included (Gold *et al.*, 1996). However, two considerations may guide our decision about the importance of trying to estimate them. These are:

(1) the extent to which the provision of additional care in added years of life is a necessary consequence of the programme being evaluated;
(2) the availability of data.

Taking the first consideration, if we were evaluating a new drug for treatment of septic shock in intensive care, it would be reasonable to assume that patients surviving an episode of septic shock were likely to have treatment for their underlying morbid condition. Therefore, these costs would be a direct consequence of giving the drug therapy (Schulman *et al*, 1991). The same would be true of the costs of diagnosing and treating cases of disease identified by a screening programme. These costs are very closely linked and it would make sense to evaluate the costs and consequences of screening, diagnosis, and treatment as a single package.

On the other hand, if we were evaluating a new drug for treatment of hypercholesterolaemia, the added years of life, through reduction in the incidence of coronary heart disease, may be in the distant future. Treatment of unrelated disease (e.g. cancer) is not a necessary consequence of treatment of hypercholesterolaemia and may be determined by protocols that have not yet been defined. Few analysts attempt to track all these costs and consequences, although it is clear that additional costs will be incurred if individuals live longer. However, the fact that such costs and consequences are more distant is not the only consideration that leads to their frequent exclusion from economic evaluations. (Indeed it could be argued that the costs of treating the coronary heart disease events are themselves distant, but most analysts would include these in an evaluation of drugs for hypercholesterolaemia.)

The other consideration relates to the availability of data. Ideally, in projecting to the future we would like data on the likely health care costs of those individuals whose lives would be extended by drug therapy for hypercholesterolaemia. Often it is very difficult to be more precise than an average annual per capita health expenditure, perhaps age-related. Therefore, one approach would be to include an estimate of age-related per capita health expenditure on the cost side of the equation for every year of life added by the intervention. This amount could either be included as a gross amount, or net of medical expenses that were already being included for treatment of the individuals main condition. Depending on the importance the analyst attaches to costs in added years of life, these could either be included in the primary analysis or a sensitivity analysis (see Chapter 5).

When estimates such as these have been included in economic evaluation of health care programmes they sometimes do not alter cost-effectiveness ratios by very much. For example, Drummond *et al.* (1993) found that adding an average expenditure figure for costs in added years of life only changed their estimate of the cost per life year gained from treatment for hypercholester-olaemia by 2 per cent.

The small quantitative impact in the example given is partly due to the fact that costs in added years of life are often heavily discounted and, in the words of one analyst, 'may amount to no more than a hill of beans' (Bush, 1973). Therefore, in many instances it may be that unrelated health care costs in added years of life can be ignored without seriously biasing the analysis. However, the quantitative importance of costs in added years of life may vary from one evaluation to another and requires more empirical investigation. In a recent paper Meltzer (1997) makes a strong case for including future costs (both health care and non-health care) in economic evaluations. In particular, he argues that their omission biases cost-effectiveness estimates in favour of those interventions that increase length of life, at the expense of those that increase quality of life. This effect is particularly pronounced in evaluations of interventions for the elderly. Therefore analysts would be wise to assess, through sensitivity analysis, whether the inclusion or exclusion of costs in added years of life greatly affects the results of their study.

5. *How should capital outlays (on equipment, buildings, and land) be handled?*

Capital costs are the costs to purchase the major capital assets required by the programme; generally equipment, buildings, and land. Capital costs differ from operating costs in a number of ways. First, they represent investments at a single point in time, often at the beginning of the programme, rather than annual sums like operating costs. Frequently, the capital costs are often not listed in the accounts or budgets of the organization because they have been funded in advance, perhaps by a one-time grant, while the budgets and accounts represent operating expenses only. Sometimes, the annual budgets and accounts contain an item called depreciation which relates to capital costs, as explained below.

Capital costs represent an investment in an asset which is used over time. Most assets, such as equipment and buildings, wear out or depreciate with time. On the other hand, land is a non-depreciable asset because it maintains its value. There are two components of capital cost. One is the opportunity cost of the funds tied up in the capital asset. This is clearly seen in the case of land. Although an investment in non-depreciable land will return the original capital sum when sold, there is still a 'cost'. This cost is the lost opportunity to invest the sum in some other venture yielding positive benefits. It is usually valued by applying an interest rate (equal to the discount rate used in the study) to the amount of capital invested. (Discounting is discussed below.)

The second component of a capital cost represents the depreciation over time of the asset itself. Various accounting procedures (straight line, declining balance, double declining balance, etc.) are available for use in the accounts of the organization. Often, accounting practices relate more to the company tax laws governing the depreciation of assets than to the real change in the value of the asset.

There are several methods of measuring and valuing capital costs in an economic evaluation. The best method is to annuitize the initial capital outlay over the useful life of the asset; that is, to calculate the 'equivalent annual cost'. This method and its advantages are discussed in more detail by Richardson and Gafni (1983). The method automatically incorporates both the depreciation aspect and the opportunity cost aspect of the capital cost. It is our preferred approach and is described in Section 4.2 below. An alternative but less exact method is to determine the depreciation cost each year using an accounting method and to determine the opportunity cost on the undepreciated balance for each year (see Levin 1975; Boyle *et al.* 1982). Where market rates exist for the rental of buildings or lease of equipment, these may be used to estimate capital costs. This method also incorporates both the depreciation and the opportunity components of the cost.

If capital outlays relate to resources that are used by more than one programme they may require allocation in a similar fashion to 'overhead' costs. See the discussion of this point below.

6. What is the significance of the average cost-marginal cost distinction?

Economists tend to emphasize this point, and the example of the sixth stool guaiac in Chapter 2 illustrated the pitfalls in making decisions based on average cost. In fact, marginal cost and average cost are but two concepts relating costs to quantity (Horngren 1994). (See Boxes 4.3 and 4.4.)

The major significance of the average-cost/marginal-cost distinction to the evaluator is as follows. First, when making a comparison of two or more programmes it is worth asking independently of each, 'What would be the costs (and consequences) of having a little more or a little less?' (e.g. Suppose Neuhauser and Lewicki (1975) had been comparing the six-stool protocol for detecting colonic cancer with another diagnostic test. Perhaps the question of six- versus five-tests may never have been asked!) Second, when examining the effects (on cost) of small changes in output, it is likely that these will differ from average costs. For example, the extra cost of keeping patients in hospital for another day at the end of their treatment might be less than the average daily cost for the whole stay. (In fact, this issue usually arises in the opposite sense – the savings from a reduction of one day's stay are usually lower than the average daily cost (see Box 4.5).)

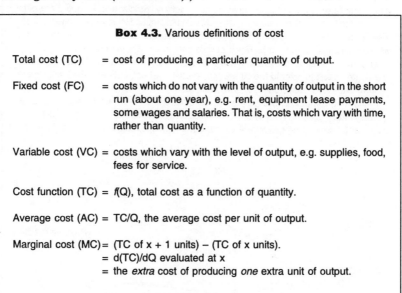

Box 4.3. Various definitions of cost

Total cost (TC) = cost of producing a particular quantity of output.

Fixed cost (FC) = costs which do not vary with the quantity of output in the short run (about one year), e.g. rent, equipment lease payments, some wages and salaries. That is, costs which vary with time, rather than quantity.

Variable cost (VC) = costs which vary with the level of output, e.g. supplies, food, fees for service.

Cost function (TC) = $f(Q)$, total cost as a function of quantity.

Average cost (AC) = TC/Q, the average cost per unit of output.

Marginal cost (MC)= (TC of x + 1 units) – (TC of x units).
= d(TC)/dQ evaluated at x
= the *extra* cost of producing *one* extra unit of output.

In practice, whereas it is important to acknowledge the difference between marginal and average costs (or savings), this issue can only really be explored in the context of specific locations or situations. For example, the extent to which costs can be saved when hospital stay is shortened depends on the flexibility available locally and the time period over which the change is made.

Therefore, in some studies analysts turn their attention to issues of marginal costs or savings in the discussion, after presenting average results as the primary analysis. For example, in a study investigating the costs and benefits of shortening time to discharge from a coronary intensive care unit by use of a more expensive sedative agent, Sherry *et al.* (1996) investigated the impact on nurse staffing requirements through fewer patients requiring intensive care during the night. It turned out that the hospital concerned had access to a bank of agency nurse staff that could be called in as required; so it was possible to realize potential savings from fewer patients requiring care. In another hospital, with different nurse staffing arrangements, the outcome could be quite different.

It was mentioned in Chapter 3 that economic evaluations tacitly assume that freed resources will be redeployed efficiently. Clearly this is not always the case and it is the responsibility of analysts to at least point this out, even if they do not explore the implications in great detail.

Box 4.4. Is it marginal or incremental?

The terms 'marginal' and 'incremental' are often used interchangeably in the literature. They both refer to a change in the scale of an activity. Strictly speaking, the *marginal cost* relates to the cost of producing *one extra* unit of output. However, it is often used to refer to the cost of producing the *next logical batch* of output, e.g. in expanding a screening programme from high risk people only to the whole population.

The term 'incremental' is sometimes also used to refer to such a change, but is more often used to refer to the difference, in cost or effect, between the two or more programmes being compared in the evaluation.

In the diagram below, MC_A, Q_1 is the marginal cost of programme A evaluated at quantity (scale of activity) Q_1. MC_B, Q_1 is the equivalent estimate for programme B. The incremental cost, of programme A over programme B, evaluated at Q_1, is IC_{A-B}, Q_1.

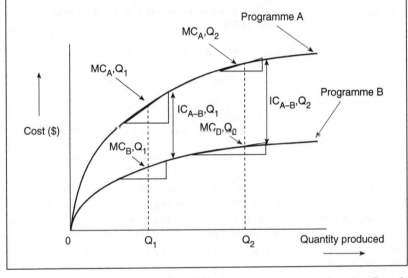

The recent report of the United States Public Health Service Panel on Cost-Effectiveness in Health and Medicine(Gold *et al.* 1996) recommends that when information on capacity utilization in hospitals or other health care facilities is not available, analysts should use the benchmark assumption that capacity is utilized at the rate of 80%, under a long run perspective. However, the prime motivation for this was to encourage some consistency in study reporting and the 80% figure is not etched in stone. It is very unlikely to apply in all settings or all health care systems.

7. How should shared (or overhead) costs be handled?

The term *'overhead costs'* is an accounting term for those resources that serve many different departments and programmes, e.g. general hospital administration, central laundry, medical records, cleaning, porters, power, etc. If individual programmes are to be costed, these shared costs may need to be attributed to programmes.

Box 4.5. Estimating the cost savings associated with reductions in hospital in-patient stay

Hospital cost can be considered to consist of two elements; the hotel cost, which is broadly constant over the length of stay, and the treatment cost, which may peak just after admission but then tail-off in the later days of the stay (see the figure below).

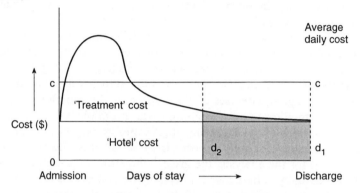

If the length of stay is reduced from d_1 to d_2, use of the average daily cost (c) would give an estimate of the saving of $c(d_1-d_2)$. However, this would overestimate the actual saving, the shaded area on the diagram. Saving in this case means the value of the resources freed for alternative uses. Whether they *will* be usefully redeployed, or actual expenditure saved, also needs to be investigated.

The main point to note at the outset is that there is no unambiguously *right* way to apportion such costs. The approach that is favoured by economists is to employ marginal analysis. That is, to see which (if any) of such costs would change if a given programme were added to, or subtracted from, the overall activity. Whilst this is fine up to a point, the most common situation is that the choice is not such an addition or subtraction, but one between two programmes, each of which would consume the given central services (perhaps because they are competitors for the same space in the hospital). For example, suppose the question concerned space in the hospital that could be used either for anticoagulant therapy for pulmonary embolism, or for renal dialysis. If the economic evaluation concerned a choice between these two programmes then there would be no methodological problem; the costs associated with use of the space would be common to both and could be excluded from the analysis. However, typically the comparison might be between the anticoagulant therapy and another programme in the same field. This could be a programme of more definitive diagnosis of pulmonary embolism, which would avert some hospitalization. In such an instance it would be relevant to obtain an estimate of the value of the freed resources (e.g. hospital floor space) that could be diverted to other uses.

A number of methods can be used to determine a more accurate cost of a programme in a hospital or other setting where shared (or overhead) costs are involved. The methods are illustrated below in terms of a hospital setting. The basic idea is to determine the quantities of service consumed by the patient (days of stay in ward A, B, or C, number of laboratory tests of each type, number of radiological procedures, number of operations, etc.), to determine a full cost (including the proper share of overhead, capital, etc.) for a unit of each type of service, and to multiply these together and sum up the results. The allocation methods described below are different ways to determine the cost per unit for each type of service. In these methods the overhead costs (e.g. housekeeping) are allocated to other departments (e.g. radiology) on the basis of some measure, called an *allocation basis*, judged to be related to usage of the overhead item (e.g. square feet of floor space in the radiology department might be used to allocate housekeeping costs to radiology).

In deciding which of the following approaches to use, the comments made in Section 4.1.1 above, should be borne in mind. That is, the more important the cost item is for the analysis, the greater the effort that should be made to estimate it accurately. There may conceivably be evaluations for which simple *per diem*, or average daily costs will suffice, since the result is unlikely to change irrespective of the figure assumed for the cost of hospital care. However, we suspect that such situations are in the minority, given the relative order of magnitude of hospital costs compared with other elements of health care expenditures.

Alternatively, the intermediate approach suggested by Hull *et al.* (1982) may suffice. Here the *per diem* cost is purged of any items relating to medical care costs, leaving just the 'hotel' component of hospital expenditure. It is then assumed that all patients are 'average' in respect of their hotel costs and that this expenditure can therefore be apportioned on the basis of patient days. Thus, the hotel cost can be calculated for the patients in the programme of interest and combined with the medical care costs attributable to those patients to give the total costs of the programme. (The medical care costs would be estimated separately, using data specifically relating to the patients in the programme.)

If a more detailed consideration of costs is required, various methods for allocating shared (or overhead) costs are available, namely:

(1) *Direct allocation* (ignores interaction of overhead departments). Each overhead cost (e.g. central administration, housekeeping) is allocated directly to final cost centres (e.g. programmes like day surgery; departments like wards or radiology). Programme X's allocated share of central administration is equal to central administration cost times Programme X's proportion is Programme X's paid hours divided by total paid hours of all final cost centres, not total paid hours for the whole organization. The latter method would underestimate the costs in all final cost centres;

(2) *Step down allocation* (partial adjustments for interaction of overhead departments). The overhead departments are allocated in a stepwise fashion to all of the remaining overhead departments and to the final cost centres;

(3) *Step down with iterations* (full adjustment for interaction of overhead departments). The overhead departments are allocated in a stepwise fashion to all of the other overhead departments and to the final cost centres. The procedure is repeated a number of times (about three) to eliminate residual unallocated amounts;

(4) *Simultaneous allocation* (full adjustment for interaction of overhead departments). This method uses the same data as (2) or (3) but it solves a set of simultaneous linear equations to give the allocations. It gives the same answer as method (3) but involves less work. (The method is shown diagrammatically in Fig 4.2.)

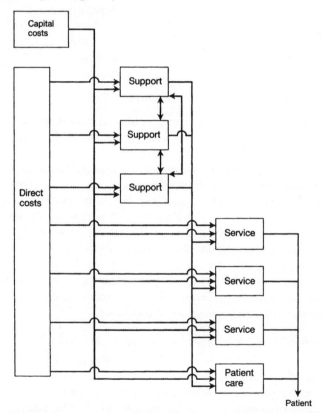

Figure 4.2. Schematic illustration of cost allocations (from Boyle *et al.* 1982)

An example showing the different approaches to the allocation of overhead costs is presented in Section 4.3. Further details are available in Horngren (1994), Clements (1974), Kaplan (1973), and Boyle *et al.* (1982).

The effort that one would put into overhead cost allocation would depend on the likely importance of overhead costs (in quantitative terms) for the whole analysis. A much simpler, but cruder, approach is to:

(1) identify those hospital costs unambiguously attributable to the treatment or programme in question (e.g. physicians' fees, laboratory tests, drugs). (These are known as the directly allocatable costs.) Allocate these directly and immediately to the programme, then;
(2) deduct, from total hospital operating expenses, the cost of departments already allocated above and departments known not to service the programme being costed, then;
(3) allocate the remainder of hospital operating expenses on the basis of number of patient days, e.g.:

$$
\begin{array}{l}
\text{Hospital cost} \\
\text{of the} \\
\text{programme}
\end{array}
=
\begin{array}{l}
\text{directly} \\
\text{allocatable} \\
\text{osts}
\end{array}
+
\frac{\text{net hospital expenditure}}{\text{total number of hospital patient-days}}
\times
\begin{array}{l}
\text{hospital} \\
\text{patient days} \\
\text{attributable} \\
\text{to the} \\
\text{programme}
\end{array}
$$

(4) finally, undertake a sensitivity analysis.

Whilst there is nothing to suppose that this method is anything but crude, if the choice between programmes is fairly insensitive to the value derived it may suffice.

There is now a growing literature on *activity-based costing* (ABC) for hospitals (Ramsey, 1994). This does not refer to a separate allocation methodology, but instead emphasizes the importance of identifying the activities/inputs that drive the final cost of a product or service. Activity based costing is implicitly shown in the allocation example in Section 4.3 below. In this example the costs of overhead departments (e.g. administration, housekeeping, laundry) are allocated to service departments based on the activities/inputs that drive them (e.g. paid hours for administration, square footage for housekeeping), instead of using a more generic allocation basis for all overhead departments, such as direct costs.

8. How should productivity changes be estimated?

As was mentioned in Chapter 3, this is a particularly contentious issue. The discussion of this point will be postponed until Chapter 5 since changes in productive output more often enter into the economic evaluation as a consequence of health care programmes; that is, the therapy often averts future production losses in that it enables the sick person to return to work or work until later in life. Productivity changes are less important on the cost side of the equation since the patient is already off work because of his or her condition. Therefore, the time taken to receive care rarely results in additional production losses. Exceptions here would include population screening or other preventive programmes and anyone considering an evaluation of these should consult the relevant section in Chapter 5.

4.1.3. Overall, how accurate does costing have to be?

Costing can take considerable time and effort and it is important not to make the perfect the enemy of the merely good. Therefore, analysts need to form a judgement on how accurate (or precise) cost estimates need to be within a given study.

Box 4.6 indicates the different levels of precision in costing for hospital costs. The least precise estimates are likely to be based on average *per diems* (or daily costs); the most precise estimates are likely to be based on micro-costing.

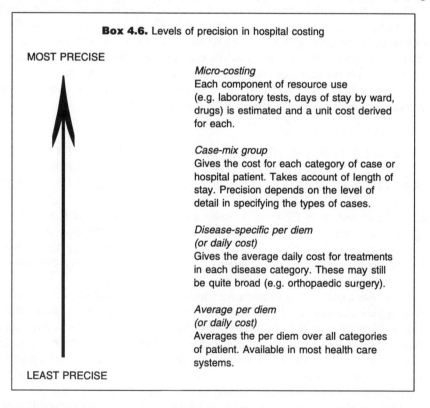

Box 4.6. Levels of precision in hospital costing

MOST PRECISE

Micro-costing
Each component of resource use (e.g. laboratory tests, days of stay by ward, drugs) is estimated and a unit cost derived for each.

Case-mix group
Gives the cost for each category of case or hospital patient. Takes account of length of stay. Precision depends on the level of detail in specifying the types of cases.

Disease-specific per diem
(or daily cost)
Gives the average daily cost for treatments in each disease category. These may still be quite broad (e.g. orthopaedic surgery).

Average per diem
(or daily cost)
Averages the per diem over all categories of patient. Available in most health care systems.

LEAST PRECISE

The guidance for deciding on the accuracy of costing is similar to that for deciding on the inclusion or exclusion of costs discussed earlier. Clearly a major factor is the likely quantitative importance of each cost category in the evaluation. For example, in an evaluation comparing two drug therapies it is likely that the study result will be sensitive to the costs of the drugs themselves. Therefore, it will be importance to record dosages and routes of administration carefully, to facilitate micro-costing. On the other hand, if the drugs concerned have side-effects which may infrequently cause hospitalizations, it may suffice to use a *per diem* or case-mix group cost for these, if one is available.

Similarly, even if it has been decided to follow a micro-costing approach, different levels of accuracy can be applied to different cost items. For example, it is well known that many laboratory tests cost only a few cents each. Therefore, it does not make sense to invest considerable effort in costing these accurately. An average laboratory charge may suffice. On the other hand, nursing costs are often a major component of overall hospital costs. Therefore, it may be important to record the numbers and grades of nursing staff in the ward where the patients of interest are being cared for.

Finally, it is worth bearing in mind that the calculation of total cost requires the quantities of resources to be multiplied by the prices (unit costs) of those resources. Therefore, when deciding on the level of precision in the estimation of resource quantities, it is worthwhile considering what degree of detail will be available on the costs, or vice versa. For example, it may not be worthwhile collecting considerable detail on the resource quantities if, for example, only average per diem costs are available in a given setting.

4.2. ALLOWANCE FOR DIFFERENTIAL TIMING OF COSTS (DISCOUNTING AND THE ANNUITIZATION OF CAPITAL EXPENDITURES)

As was mentioned in Chapter 3, some allowance needs to be made for the differential timing of costs and consequences. That is, even in a world with zero inflation and no bank interest, it would be an advantage to receive a benefit earlier or to incur a cost later – it gives you more options. Economists call this the notion of *time preference*.

There are a number of reasons why individuals may have a *positive rate of time preference*; that is, a preference for benefits today rather than in the future. First, they may have a short-term view of life; living for today rather than thinking about the future. Secondly, the future is uncertain so, as the saying goes, a bird in the hand is worth two in the bush. Thirdly, with positive economic growth, the long-term trend since the Second World War, individuals might expect to be more wealthy in the future. Therefore, a dollar today would be of higher value than one in the future when you are richer. Finally, since most individuals appear to have a positive rate of time preference, one can usually obtain a positive return when making a riskless investment.

However, it should be noted that the notion of preferring benefits today, or wanting to postpone costs, extends beyond money transactions and could extend to goods and services that could not easily be traded. It is of most significance for those economic evaluations that compare programmes or interventions with different time profiles. For example, if two options for dealing with heart disease were; (a) expanding funding for coronary artery bypass grafting, and (b) a health education campaign to influence diet and lifestyle; we might expect option (a) to deliver benefits earlier. Therefore, if a positive rate of time preference were acknowledged, it would look more attractive, compared with the preventive option, than would otherwise be the case.

Typically, economic evaluation texts discuss the situation where the costs of the alternative programmes A and B can be identified by the year in which they occur:

Year	Cost of Programme A ($000s)	Cost of Programme B ($000s)
1	5	15
2	10	10
3	15	4

In this example, B might be a preventive programme which requires more outlay in Year 1 with the promise of lower cost in Year 3. The crude addition of the two cost streams shows B to be of lower cost (29,000 versus 30,000), but the outlays under A occur more in the later years.

A comparison of A and B (adjusted for the differential timing of resource outlays) would be made by discounting future costs to present values. The calculation is performed as follows. If P = present value; F_n = future cost at year n; and r = annual interest (discount) rate (e.g. 0.05 or 5 per cent), then

$$P = \sum_{n=1}^{3} F_n (1+r)^{-n}$$

$$= \frac{F_1}{(1+r)} + \frac{F_2}{(1+r)^2} + \frac{F_3}{(1+r)^3}$$

$$= \frac{F_1}{(1.05)} + \frac{F_2}{(1.05)^2} + \frac{F_3}{(1.05)^3}$$

In our example this gives: present value of cost of A = 26.79; present value of cost of B = 26.81.

This assumes that the costs all occur at the end of each year. An alternative assumption which is commonly used is to assume that the costs all occur at the beginning of each year. Then, Year 1 costs need not be discounted, Year 2 costs should be discounted by one year, etc. Calculated in this way, the previous example is:

$$P = \sum_{n=0}^{2} F_n (1+r)^{-n}$$

$$= F_0 + \frac{F_1}{(1+r)} + \frac{F_2}{(1+r)^2}$$

Present value of A $=$ 28.13; present value of B $=$ 28.15.

The factor $(1+r)^{-n}$ is known as the *discount factor* and can be obtained for a given n and r from Table 1 in Annex 4.2. For example, the discount factor for three periods (years) at a discount rate of 5 per cent is 0.8638.

While this approach is the most convenient for many programme comparisons, a more common situation is that where most of the costs are easily expressed on an annual recurring basis and it is only capital costs which differ from year to year (typically these will be at the beginning of the programme, or Year O). Here it might be more convenient to express all the costs on an annual basis, obtaining an *equivalent annual cost* (E) for the capital outlay by an amortization or annuitization procedure. This works as follows:

If the capital outlay is K, we need to find the annual sum E which over a period of n years (the life of the facility) , at an interest rate of r, will be equivalent to K.

This is expressed by the following formula:

$$K = \frac{E_1}{(1+r)} + \frac{E}{(1+r)^2} + ... + \frac{E}{(1+r)^n}$$

$$K = E \frac{1 - (1+r)^{-n}}{r}$$

$K = E$ [Annuity factor, n period, interest r]

As before, the annuity factor is easily obtainable from Table 2 in Annex 4.2. For example, in the cost analysis of providing long-term oxygen therapy, Lowson *et al.* (1981) found the total capital (set up) costs (K) to be £2153. Therefore, applying the formula given above:

$$2153 = \frac{E}{(1+r)} + \frac{E}{(1+r)^2} + \frac{E}{(1+r)^3} + \frac{E}{(1+r)^4} + \frac{E}{(1+r)^5}$$

2153 = E [Annuity factor, 5 years, interest rate 7 per cent]
2153 = E [4.1002] (from Table 2 in Annex 4.2)
E = £525 (as shown in Table III of Lowson *et al.* (1981).

Note that Lowson *et al.* (1981) assumed that the annuity was in arrears, that is, due at the end of the year. It might be argued that a more realistic assumption would be that it were payable in advance. This is equivalent to the formula:

$$2153 = E + \frac{E}{(1+r)} + \frac{E}{(1+r)^2} + \frac{E}{(1+r)^3} + \frac{E}{(1+r)^4}$$

The value for E can still be obtained from Table 2 by taking one less period and adding 1.000. This gives a lower value for $E = £491$. This is logical since the repayments are being made earlier (at the beginning of each year) rather than in arrears.

This approach can be generalized to handle the situation where the equipment or buildings have a resale value at the end of the programme. If:

$S =$ the resale value;
$n =$ the useful life of the equipment;
$r =$ discount (interest rate);
$A(n,r) =$ the annuity factor (n years at interest rate r);
$K =$ Purchase price/ initial outlay;
$E =$ equivalent annual cost;

then:

$$E = \frac{K - \dfrac{S}{(1+r)^n}}{A(n,r)}$$

The method described above is unambiguous for new equipment. For old equipment, there are two choices:

Choice 1 – use the replacement cost of the equipment or the original cost indexed to current dollars and a full life;
Choice 2 – Use the current market value of the old machine and its remaining useful life.

Choice 1 is usually better as the results are more generalizable – less situational. Note that using the undepreciated balance from the accounts of the organization is never a method of choice.

It can be seen that the equivalent annual cost of buildings or equipment to a given programme depends on the values of *n*, *r*, and *S*, all of which must be assumed at the time of evaluation. Practical points that evaluators might care to note are:

1. Useful life and resale value (n and S)

It is important to make a distinction between the physical life of a piece of equipment and its useful clinical life. The latter is highly dependent on technological change. Obviously one can undertake a sensitivity analysis using different values for n, but in general it is best to be conservative and assume short lives (say, around five years) for clinical equipment.

2. Choice of discount rate (r)

Traditionally there have been *two competing theories* regarding the proper measure for the discount rate for public projects (the social discount rate):

(a) r = the real rate of return (to society) forgone in the private sector (known as the social opportunity cost approach). This can be estimated empirically, although not without controversy;

(b) r = the social rate of time preference.

The basic notion behind the social opportunity cost approach is that public investments can displace or crowd out private investments or consumption.

The social rate of time preference is a measure of society's willingness collectively, to forgo consumption (gratification) today in order to have greater consumption (gratification) tomorrow. Frequently it is argued that the interest rate on a risk-free investment (e.g. long-term government bonds) represents the individual investor's willingness to forgo the present for the future, and that this rate is the individual's rate of time preference. Then if society's collective rate of time preference is simply the aggregate of the individual rates (a controversial assumption), the required rate is simply given by the real (adjusted for inflation) rate of return on long-term government bonds.

Another approach, termed the shadow price of capital approach (Gold *et al.* 1996), uses the social rate of time preference to discount costs and benefits, once they have been transformed. The stream of programme costs are transformed into the corresponding stream of consumption losses that would be induced by the forgone investment and consumption opportunities. The stream of programme benefits are transformed into the corresponding stream of consumption gains. The basic premise is that the ultimate purpose of all private investment (and economic activity in general) is consumption; thus, the proper measure of the opportunity cost of a public programme, in terms of forgone private activities, is the present value of the consumption that would be given up.

In practice, analysts have followed one of two conventions in choosing a discount rate. First, in jurisdictions (like the United Kingdom); where the government announces a common discount rate for all public sector projects, the advised rate is used. Alternatively, where there is no announced rate, the convention has been to use a rate consistent with the existing literature. A 5 per cent rate was used by a number of analysts publishing articles in the *New England Journal of Medicine* in the late 1970s and early 1980s, and this became the *de facto* convention for economic evaluations in the health care field.

The prevalence of a 5 per cent rate in the existing literature has the advantage that different studies are comparable, at least on this methodological dimension. However, Krahn and Gafni (1993) point out that the conventional practice of discounting all health care programmes at a rate of 5 per cent may not consistently reflect societal or individuals' preferences. They recommend, among other things, that a consensus approach, with political participation, offers a flexible, pragmatic, and explicit way of synthesizing the empirical, normative, and ethical considerations that underlie choice of a discount rate.

In the United Kingdom the choice of a public sector discount rate had its origins in the social opportunity cost approach, but it has increasingly been viewed as a general statement about social time preference. That is, the discount rate is a societal value judgement about intergenerational equity; namely to what extent should we, as a community, postpone our own gratification for the sake of future generations?

The US Public Health Service Panel on Cost-Effectiveness in Health and Medicine (Gold *et al.* 1996) has recently revisited the issue of the discount rate for health programmes. They argue that costs and consequences should be discounted at a rate consistent with the shadow-price-of-capital approach to evaluating public investments. Currently they estimate that 3 per cent would be the most appropriate real (riskless) discount rate for economic evaluations. However, they recognize that, given the large pool of studies using 5 per cent, it would also be useful to continue using this rate for a number of years.

Therefore, the best current advice would be the following:

(a) to present costs and consequences in their undiscounted form, so that others can investigate the implications, for the evaluation, of employing different discount rates;
(b) to undertake a base case analysis using either the announced rate in the jurisdiction concerned, or the rates of 3 per cent and 5 per cent currently recommended by analysts;
(c) to undertake a sensitivity analysis, making sure that this includes 0 per cent, 3 per cent and 5 per cent;
(d) to alert decision makers to the importance of the choice of discount rate, in those situations where it has a substantial impact on the study result. (Given that the choice of discount rate is a value judgement, as opposed to a technical judgement, this is probably the most important point.)

Finally, we should note that the discussion here has focused primarily on the discounting of costs. The discounting of consequences raises additional issues, which will be discussed further in Chapter 5.

3. How to handle inflation

If it is assumed that all the items of cost in the programme will inflate at the same rate and that this will be the same rate as inflation in general, there are two equivalent choices:

(a) inflate all future costs by this predicted inflation rate and then use a larger discount rate that allows for the effect of general inflation (the inflation adjusted discount rate*); or
(b) do not inflate any future costs (i.e. use constant dollars) and use a smaller discount rate that does not allow for inflation (the real discount rate). (All the announced rates, and the rates recommended by analysts, are real rates.)

Method (b) is the simpler and preferred approach.

If it is assumed that different items of cost in the programme will inflate at different rates, there are also two equivalent choices:

(a) inflate all future costs by their particular predicted inflation rates and then use a larger discount rate that allows for the effect of general inflation (the inflation adjusted discount rate*); or
(b) do not inflate any future costs (i.e. use constant dollars) and use a smaller discount rate that does not allow for inflation (the real discount rate), but adjust the discount rate for each item to account for the differential inflation rate between this item and the 'general' rate of inflation, e.g. if general inflation is 8 per cent, this item is expected to inflate 10 per cent, and the real r is equal to 4 per cent, then r adjusted for this item is

$$r = 1.04 \times \frac{1.08}{1.10} = 1.021, \text{ i.e. } 2.1 \text{ per cent}$$

Method (b) is again the preferred approach. In general, however, most studies perform the whole analysis in constant price terms and use a single discount rate. (See Annex 4.1 for a tutorial on methods of measuring and valuing capital costs.)

4.3. ALLOCATION OF OVERHEAD COSTS: EXAMPLE

The following example demonstrates the various methods of handling overhead costs discussed in Section 4.1.2(6). Suppose we wish to determine the cost of neonatal intensive care (NIC) for a specific group of patients. For each patient we have data on the length of stay in the neonatal intensive care unit

---

*Calculation of inflation-adjusted discount rate: if the real discount rate is 5 per cent and general inflation is 8 per cent, then the inflation-adjusted $r = (1.05)(1.08) = 1.134$ or 13.4 per cent.

Table 4.1. Cost allocation data

	Annual direct cost[a] $	Annual units of output[b]	Direct cost per unit $	Allocation basis	Annual pd-hrs	Ft^2	Annual lbs laundry
Overhead departments							
Administration	2,000,000			pd-hrs	200 000	30 000	0
Housekeeping	1,500,000			ft^2	300 000	4 000	80 000
Laundry	1,300,000			lbs	200 000	8 000	0
Other	10,200,000				300 000	158 000	120 000
Subtotal	*15,000,000*				*1 000 000*	*200 000*	*200 000*
Final departments (Pt. service)							
Laboratory	4,000,000	8 000 000	0.50/WMU	250 000	30 000	25 000	1 200 000
NICU	500,000	5 000	100/pt.–day	50 000	8 000	75 000	
Other	30,500,000				1 700 000	562 000	1 300 000
Subtotal	*35,000,000*				*2 000 000*	*600 000*	*1 300 000*
Hospital total	**50,000,000**				**3 000 000**	**800 000**	**1 500 000**

[a] Direct cost consists of salaries plus supplies. [b] Lab output is in workload measurement units (WMUs) and NICU output is in patient-days.

(NICU) and data on the number and type of laboratory tests performed. For simplicity, let us assume that these were the only services received by the patients – that is, the patients had no operations, no radiological or nuclear medicine investigations, no social work, etc. Furthermore, let us assume that there are only three overhead departments that serve the laboratory and the NICU: administration, housekeeping and laundry. (In principle it would be possible to consider other overhead departments, like plant operations and maintenance, bioengineering, and materials management.)

The first task is to determine a unit of output for those departments that directly serve patients. We will be determining a cost per unit of output, and multiplying this cost by the usage of each patient to determine the cost per patient. Thus, the unit of output must be as homogeneous as possible with respect to cost, and yet be available in the data for each patient. We have selected a *patient-day* as the unit of output of the NICU, and a *workload measurement unit* for the laboratory. Each lab test is assigned a predetermined number of workload measurement units (WMUs) according to the amount of work needed to perform the test.

Table 4.2. Method 1 – ignore overhead

Lab cost/WMU = \$4 000 000/8 000 000 = \$0.50/WMU
NICU cost/pt-day = \$500 000/5000 = \$100/pt-day

Table 4.3. Method 2 – direct allocation of overhead
(Note: Allocation denominator = sum of 'final' department.)

Lab cost = direct cost + lab's share of admin + lab's share of housekeeping + lab's share of laundry

$$= 4\,000\,000 + \frac{250\,000}{2\,000\,000}\,(2\,000\,000) + \frac{30\,000}{6\,000\,000}\,(1\,500\,000) + \frac{25\,000}{1\,300\,000}(1\,300\,000)$$

$$= 4\,000\,000 + 250\,000 + 75\,000 + 25\,000 = 4\,350\,000$$

Lab cost/WMU = 4 350 000/8 000 000 = \$0.54/WMU

NICU cost = direct cost + share of admin + share of housekeeping + share of laundry

$$= 4\,000\,000 + \frac{50\,000}{2\,000\,000}\,(2\,000\,000) + \frac{8\,000}{6\,00\,000}\,(1\,500\,000) + \frac{75\,000}{1\,300\,000}\,(1\,300\,000)$$

$$= 5\,00\,000 + 50\,000 + 20\,000 + 75\,000 = \$645,000$$

NICU cost/pt-day = 645 000/5000 = \$129/pt-day

Table 4.4. Method 3 – Step down allocation of overhead

(Note: Allocation denominator = sum of remaining departments in the step down sequence.)

	Admin	Housekeeping	Laundry	Other	Lab	NICU	Other
Direct cost	2 000 000	1 500 000	1 300 000	10 200 000	4 000 000	500 000	30 500 000 50m
Allocate admin	2 000 000 →	$\frac{3}{28}=214\,286$	$\frac{2}{28}=142\,857$	$\frac{3}{28}=214\,286$	$\frac{2.5}{28}=178\,571$	$\frac{0.5}{28}=35\,174$	$\frac{17}{28}=1\,214\,286$
Allocate housekeeping		1 714 286 →	$\frac{8}{766}=17\,904$	$\frac{158}{766}=353\,599$	$\frac{30}{766}=67\,139$	$\frac{8}{766}=17\,904$	$\frac{562}{766}=1\,257\,740$
Allocate laundry			1 460 761 →	$\frac{120}{1420}=123\,445$	$\frac{25}{1420}=25\,718$	$\frac{75}{1420}=77\,153$	$\frac{1200}{1420}=1\,234\,446$
Total cost				10 891 330	4 271 428	630 771	34 206 472 50m
Units					÷ 8 000 000	÷ 5 000	
Cost/unit					$0.53/WMU	$126.15/pt-day	

Cost analysis

Table 4.5. Method 4 – Step down with iterations

(Note: Allocation denominator = sum of all departments except the one being allocated.)

	Admin	Housekeeping	Laundry	Other	Lab	NICU	Other	
Iteration 1								
Direct cost	2 000 000	1 500 000	1 300 000	10 200 000	4 000 000	500 000	30 500 000	50m
Allocate admin	2 000 000	→ $= \frac{2}{28}$ 214 286	$\frac{2}{28} = 142\,857$	$\frac{3}{28} = 214\,286$	$\frac{2.5}{28} = 178\,571$	$\frac{0.5}{28} = 35\,714$	$\frac{17}{28} = 1\,214\,286$	
Allocate housekeeping	$\frac{30}{796}$ $= 64\,609$	← 1 714 286	$\frac{8}{796} = 17\,229$	$\frac{158}{796} = 340\,273$	$\frac{30}{796} = 64\,609$	$\frac{8}{796} = 17\,229$	$\frac{562}{796} = 1\,210\,338$	
Allocate laundry	$\frac{0}{1500} = 0$	$\frac{80}{1500} = 77\,871$	↓ 1 460 086	$\frac{120}{1500} = 116\,807$	$\frac{25}{1500} = 24\,335$	$\frac{75}{1500} = 73\,004$	$\frac{1200}{1500} = 1\,168\,069$	
New totals	64 609	77 871	0	10 871 366	4 267 515	625 947	34 092 693	50m
Iteration 2								
Allocate Admin	64 609	$\frac{3}{28} = 6\,922$	$\frac{2}{28} = 4\,615$	$\frac{3}{28} = 6\,922$	$\frac{2.5}{28} = 5\,769$	$\frac{0.5}{28} = 1\,154$	$\frac{17}{28} = 39\,227$	
Allocate HK	$\frac{30}{796} = 3\,196$	84 793	$\frac{8}{796} = 852$	$\frac{158}{796} = 16\,831$	$\frac{30}{796} = 3\,196$	$\frac{8}{796} = 852$	$\frac{562}{796} = 59\,866$	
Allocate Laundry	$\frac{0}{14500} = 0$	$\frac{80}{541500} = 292$	5 467	$\frac{120}{1500} = 437$	$= 91$	$\frac{75}{1500} = 273$	$\frac{1200}{41500} = 4\,374$	
New totals	3 196	292	0	10 895 556	4 276 571	628 226	34 195 160	50m

Table 4.5. (*Continued*)

	Admin	Housekeeping	Laundry	Other	Lab	NICU	Other
Iteration 3							
Allocate admin	3 196 →	$\frac{2}{28}$ = 342	= 228	$\frac{3}{28}$ = 342	$\frac{2.5}{28}$ = 285	$\frac{0.5}{28}$ = 57	$\frac{17}{28}$ = 1 940
Allocate housekeeping	$\frac{30}{796}$ = 24	634 $\frac{8}{796}$	= 6	$\frac{158}{796}$ = 126	$\frac{30}{796}$ = 24	$\frac{8}{796}$ = 6	$\frac{562}{796}$ = 448
Allocate laundry	$\frac{0}{1500}$ = 0	$\frac{80}{1500}$ = 12	234	$\frac{120}{1500}$ = 19	$\frac{25}{1500}$ = 4	$\frac{75}{1500}$ = 12	$\frac{1200}{1500}$ = 187
New totals	24	12	0	10 896 043	4 276 884	628 301	34 198 735 50m
Final direct allocations	24→			$\frac{3}{23}$ = 3	$\frac{2.5}{23}$ = 3	$\frac{0.5}{23}$ = 1	$\frac{17}{23}$ = 18
		12		$\frac{158}{758}$ = 3	$\frac{30}{758}$ = 0	$\frac{8}{758}$ = 0	$\frac{562}{758}$ = 9
Final totals	0	0	0	10 896 049	4 276 887	628 302	34 198 762 50m
Units					÷8 000 000	÷5 000	
Cost/unit					$0.53/WMU	$125.66/pt-day	

Table 4.6. Method 5 – simultaneous allocation (reciprocal method)
(Note: Allocation denominator = sum of all departments.)

Admin $\qquad C_1 = 2\,000\,000 + \dfrac{2\,C_1}{30} + \dfrac{30\,C_2}{3800}$

Housekeeping $C_2 = 1\,500\,000 + \dfrac{3\,C_1}{30} + \dfrac{4\,C_2}{800} + \dfrac{80\,C_3}{1500}$

Laundry $\qquad C_3 = 1\,300\,000 + \dfrac{2\,C_1}{30} + \dfrac{8\,C_2}{800}$

Lab $\qquad C_4 = 4\,000\,000 + \dfrac{2.5\,C_1}{30} + \dfrac{30\,C_2}{800} + \dfrac{25\,C_3}{1500}$

NICU $\qquad C_5 = 500\,000 + \dfrac{0.5\,C_1}{30} + \dfrac{8\,C_2}{800} + \dfrac{75\,C_3}{1500}$

$$\dfrac{28\,C_1}{30} - \dfrac{30\,C_2}{800} \qquad\qquad\qquad = 2\,000\,000$$

$$-\dfrac{3\,C_1}{30} + \dfrac{796\,C_2}{800} - \dfrac{80\,C_3}{1500} \qquad = 1\,500\,000$$

$$-\dfrac{2\,C_1}{30} - \dfrac{0\,C_2}{800} + C_3 \qquad\qquad = 1\,300\,000$$

$$-\dfrac{2.5\,C_1}{30} - \dfrac{30\,C_2}{800} - \dfrac{25\,C_3}{1500} + C_4 = 4\,000\,000$$

$$-\dfrac{0.5\,C_1}{30} - \dfrac{8\,C_2}{800} - \dfrac{75\,C_3}{1500} + C_5 = 500\,000$$

The solution of this set of equations is:

$C_1 = 2\,215\,531$

$C_2 = 1\,808\,772$

$C_3 = 1\,465\,790$

$C_4 = 4\,276\,886$

$C_5 = 628\,303$

Therefore, the cost/unit of output is:

Lab: $\$4\,276\,886/8\,000\,000 = \underline{\$0.53/\text{WMU}}$

NICU: $\$628\,303/5\,000 = \underline{\$125.66/\text{pt-day}}$

An allocation basis must be determined for each overhead department. For example, square feet of floor space has been selected for housekeeping. This means that housekeeping costs will be allocated to departments receiving housekeeping services in proportion to the square footage of floor space in the department. Similarly, paid hours has been selected as the allocation basis for administration costs, and pounds of laundry for the laundry costs.

The data for this simplified example are given in Table 4.1. The calculations, as performed by the different methods, are given in Tables 4.2 to 4.7.

Table 4.7. Method 6 – Patient-day allocation of overhead

This is the simple method described earlier. It may be useful in some cases.

Laboratory costs would be charged without overhead: $0.50/WMU.

NICU costs would be the direct costs of $500000 plus a share of all relevant other departments (2.0m + 1.5m + 1.3m = 4.8m) in proportion to patient-days (5000/500000 where the denominator is total annual hospital patient-days). Thus,

NICU cost = $500000 + $4800000 (5000/500000) = $548000.

NICU cost/pt-day = $548000/5000 = $110/pt-day.

4.4. EXERCISE: COSTING ALTERNATIVE RADIOTHERAPY TREATMENTS

Task

A clinical trial is being carried out comparing two forms of radiotherapy for patients with head and neck cancer and carcinoma of the bronchus. Patients receiving *conventional therapy* are treated once per day, five days per week, for about six weeks. They would normally travel on a daily basis to a hospital-based radiotherapy centre to receive care. Patients receiving *continuous hyperfractionated accelerated radiotherapy (CHART)* are treated three times on each of 12 consecutive days, including the weekend. Because of the intensity and frequency of treatment, patients would normally stay in hospital during therapy, either in a regular hospital ward or in a hostel owned by the hospital.

The different treatment regimens obviously give rise to different costs. However, in addition, there may be differences in the period following treatment for the following reasons:

(1) the higher intensity of the CHART regimen might give rise to more side effects, and hence a greater need for community care after hospital discharge.
(2) the CHART regimen might give better tumour control, thereby slowing down the progression of the disease;
(3) CHART might reduce the extent of late radiation changes, and a lower incidence of necrosis may also reduce the need for salvage surgery.

The clinical trial will provide an opportunity to gather data on the use of resources by patients in the two treatment groups. You are asked to:

(1) *identify* which categories of resource you feel it would be important to assess.
(2) indicate how you might *measure* the use of these resources in physical units.
(3) Say how you might *value* the resource consumption in money terms.

1 Identification of resource categories

Resource use can he considered under the three broad headings outlined in Chapters 2 and 3.

Health care resource use

Hospital resources	– radiotherapy, bed days, out-patient attendances, overheads
Community care resources	– general practitioner (family physician) visits, nurse visits (types of nurse will vary by country or setting), ambulance or hospital car

Patient and family resource use

	– patients' time, time of relatives, out-of-pocket expenses for transport (e.g. car, train, taxi)

Resource use in other sectors

	– social worker visits, home help (homemaker) visits

2 Measurement of resource use

The fact that a clinical trial is taking place greatly increases the opportunity for accurate data collection as case report forms are completed for patients enrolled in the trial. Normally these record data on clinical events, but they can be modified to include resource use, such as number and type of investigations, date of hospital admission and discharge. Also, the fact that patients are enrolled in a trial provides the opportunity to interview them about resource use in community care, time taken to travel to hospital, and personal expenditure. They can also be given diary cards to record expenditure or time spent by relatives in home nursing.

In the absence of a trial the two major sources of data on resource use are routine statistics kept at the hospital or by other agencies, and patients' case notes (charts). The quality of these records varies by agency and data are usually more comprehensive at the main place (clinic) where the patient is being treated. In addition, there are no routine records for patient and family resource use.

Turning to the specific resource items identified above, we might expect to record quantities used as follows:

Item	*Possible Measurements*
(a) HOSPITAL CARE	
Radiotherapy	– The number of treatment sessions could be recorded, possibly differentiating by length of session and time of day (e.g. normal working hours, after-hours, weekends).
Bed days	– The number of bed days could be recorded, differentiating by type of hospital ward.
Outpatient attendances	– The number of attendances could be recorded.
Overheads	– These would probably be related to the number of bed-days or other suitable resource item (see valuation below).
(b) COMMUNITY CARE	
General practitioner visits	– The number could be ascertained, either by asking patients, or by consulting the general practitioners. It may make sense to differentiate between home visits and visits to the practitioners office.
Nurse visits	– The number could be recorded as for GP visits above. The purpose of the nurse visit and type of nurse (e.g. general nurse, specialist cancer nurse) would be recorded.

Item	*Possible Measurements*
Ambulance	– The number and length of trips could be recorded. Length of trip could be ascertained from the patients place of residence.

(c) PATIENT AND FAMILY RESOURCES

Patients' time	– The time taken in seeking and receiving care could be estimated by asking the patient. Time off work could be estimated separately.
Relatives' time	– Relatives could spend time in home nursing and in accompanying patients to hospital. It could be estimated as for patients time above.
Out-of-pocket expenses	– Some may be estimated directly in money terms (e.g. bus fares). Others may be estimated by asking patients (e.g. distance travelled in private car).

(d) RESOURCES IN OTHER SECTORS

Social worker and home help visits	– These would be estimated in a similar way to nurse visits above.

3 Valuation of resource items

It is extremely difficult to give general advice on this since it is so dependent on the availability of local financial data. In some settings, like the USA, there may be data on hospital billings or charges. In other settings, detailed costing studies would be necessary. As mentioned elsewhere in this chapter, when using charge data it is important to:

(a) investigate the relationship between charges and costs;
(b) record physical quantities as well as charges, so as to facilitate generalization of study results to other settings.

The general strategies for costing, ranging from the use of average costs (or per diems) to micro-costing, were outlined in Box 4.6. The skill in costing is to match the level of precision (and effort) to the importance (in quantitative terms) of the cost item. Turning to the specific resource items measured above, we might expect to value them as follows:

(a) HOSPITAL CARE

Radiotherapy treatment sessions

In some settings there may be charge data, or average cost figures, for radiotherapy sessions. However, even if these exist, which is unlikely in many locations, they may not differentiate by type of session (e.g. normal hours, out-of-hours, weekend). This distinction is critical to understanding the relative costs of conventional radiotherapy and CHART. Therefore, it is likely that micro-costing would be required.

In micro-costing the approach would be to derive the cost of a treatment session from its component parts, namely: consultant (medical) time, radiographer time, medical physics time, consumables, equipment, buildings and departmental overheads. Some survey work may be required, plus data from the hospital finance department on staff salaries, overtime allowances and equipment prices. Costing of equipment and buildings will require assumptions to be made about useful life and re-sale value. It would be necessary to express these costs first as *equivalent annual costs* (see the methods outlined on pp. 70–71) and then to apportion them to individual treatment sessions. Judgements would also need to be made about which components of hospital overheads (e.g. cleaning, building maintenance, administration) are most appropriately allocated to departments and the allocation basis (e.g. square metres, cubic metres, number of staff, etc.). Some elements of overhead may be better allocated on the basis of in-patient days or number of patients.

Bed days

It may be possible to use the average daily costs (or per diems) for different types of wards, including hostel wards. However, these may be considered too imprecise, in which case micro-costing might be undertaken. This would derive a daily cost for a particular category of ward by considering nurse staffing levels, medical (consultant) input, and overheads.

Since hostel wards may not feature in the standard hospital accounts, micro-costing may be required for these, e.g. they may be slightly off-site or rely partly on staffing by volunteers. An opportunity cost for volunteer time may have to be inputed. In costing hospital beds it may be decided to make an allowance for the fact that there is usually less than 100% occupancy.

Out-patient attendances

There may be an average cost or charge available for an out-patient visit, although this may not differentiate between oncology and other clinical specialties. Depending on the quantitative importance of this item, micro-costing may be undertaken.

Overheads
As mentioned above, these could be allocated to the radiotherapy treatments, to out-patient attendances, or to hospital bed days, depending on the overhead item.

(b) COMMUNITY CARE

General practitioner visits
There may be data available on physician fees for various types of visit (e.g. general assessment, home visit, etc.). Alternatively, there may be nationally available data on the average costs of various general practitioner services. Failing this, micro-costing may be required. This would calculate the cost of practitioners' time (per minute or per hour) and add the cost of travel for home visits. Drug costs would also need to be considered.

Nurse visits
The agencies providing the nurses may have data on the average cost of a visit. This may even distinguish between various types of visit. Failing this, micro-costing would have to be employed, taking into account nursing salaries, length of visits, travel time, and nurses time spent in general administration. There may also be some consumables to be accounted for in the cost of nurse visits.

Ambulance and hospital car
Estimates may be available for the average cost per mile travelled. This could be combined with data on the distances involved to generate total costs.

(c) PATIENT AND FAMILY RESOURCES

Patients' time
If the time was taken from worktime, the gross salary (including employment benefits) could be used. Different assumptions could be made about the opportunity cost of leisure time.

Relatives' time
In general the valuation of this raises the same issues as the valuation of patients' time. The valuation of time spent in informal nursing care is complicated since the relative may also be able to carry out other tasks at the same time.

Out-of-pocket expenses
In general, the financial expenditures made (e.g. bus fares) would suffice. However, for some items, such as use of onprivate car, the expenditures

(say) on fuel would underestimate the true cost. Here, motoring organizations can often provide data on the cost (per mile or kilometre) of running a car.

Finally, a few rare events, such as hospital admission for particular types of surgery, may be handled separately. Depending on how quantitatively important they seem, case-mix group costs or disease-specific per diems may suffice. Alternatively, micro-costing may be undertaken.

Final comment

This exercise was based on an actual costing study, undertaken in the United Kingdom. If you want to see how it was tackled in practice, see Coyle and Drummond (1997).

REFERENCES

Black, A. J. *et al.* (1988). Comparative costs of percutaneous transluminal coronary angioplasty and coronary bypass grafting in mutivessel coronary artery disease *Am. J. Cardiol.*, **62** (10 part 1), 809–11.

Boyle, M. H., Torrance, G. W., Horwood, S. P., and Sinclair, J. C. (1982). *A cost analysis of providing neonatal intensive care to 500-1499-gram birth-weight infants.* Research Report no 51, Programme for Quantitative Studies in Economics and Population, McMaster University, Hamilton, Canada.

Bush, J. W. (1973). Discussion. In *Health status indexes* (ed. R. L. Berg). Hospital Research and Educational Trust, Chicago, IL.

Clements, R. M. (1974). *The Canadian hospital accounting manual supplement.* Livingston Printing. Toronto.

Cohen, D. J., Breall, J. A., Kalon, K. L. H., Weintraub, R. M., Kuntz, R. E., Weinstein, M. C., *et tal.*, D. S. (1993). Economics of elective coronary revascularization: comparison of costs and charges for conventional angioplasty, directional atherectomy, stenting and bypass surgery. *J. Am. Coll. Cardiol.*, 22(4), 1052-59.

Coyle and Drummond, M. F. (1997). Costs of conventional radical radiotherapy versus continuous hyperfractionated accelerated radiotherapy (CHART) in the treatment of patients with head and neck cancer and carcinoma of the bronchus. Centre for Health Economics, University of York (*mimeo*).

Drummond, M. F., McGuire, A. L., and Fletcher, A. (1993). *Economic evaluation of drug therapy for hypercholesterolaemia in the United Kingdom.* Centre for Health Economics Discussion Paper 104. University of York, York.

Finkler, S. A. (1982). The distinction between costs and charges. *Annals of Internal Medicine*, 102-109.

Gold, M. R., Siegel, J. E., Russell, L. B., and Weinstein, M. C. (ed.) (1996). *Cost-effectiveness in health and medicine.* Oxford University Press, New York.

Horngren, C. T. (1994). *Cost accounting: a managerial emphasis* (5th ed.). Prentice Hall, Englewood Cliffs, N.J.

Hull, R., Hirsh, J., Sackett, D. L. and Stoddart, G. L. (1982). Cost-effectiveness of primary and secondary prevention of fatal pulmonary embolism in high-risk surgical patients. *Can. Med. Assoc. J.*, 127, 990-5.

Kaplan, R. S. (1973). Variable and self-service costs in reciprocal allocation models. *The Accounting Review* **XLVIII**, 738-48.

Krahn, M. and Gafni, A. (1993). Discounting in the economic evaluation of health care interventions. *Medical Care* 31, 403-18.

Levin, H. M. (1975). Cost-effectiveness analysis in evaluation research. In *Handbook of evaluation research*, Vol. 2 (ed. M. Guttentag and E. L. Struening) (eds) *Handbook of evaluation research*, Vol. 2, pp.89-122. Sage, London.

Lowson, K. V., Drummond, M. F., and Bishop, J. M. (1981). Costing new services: Long-term domiciliary oxygen therapy. *Lancet*, i, 1146-9.

Luce, B. R., andElixhauser, A. (1990). Estimating costs in economic evaluation of medical technologies. *Int J Technology Assessment in Health Care*, 6, 57-75.

Neuhauser, D. and Lewicki, A. M. (1975). What do we gain from the sixth stool guaiac? *N Eng J Medi*, 293(5), 226-8.

Meltzer, D. (1997). Accounting for future costs in medical cost-effectiveness analysis. *J Health Economics*. 16(1), 33–64.

Ramsey, R. H. (1994). Activity-based costing for hospitals. *Hospital and Health Services Administration*, 39, 385-96.

Richardson, A. W. and Gafni, A. (1983). Treatment of capital costs in evaluating health care programmes. *Cost and Management*, Nov-Dec, 26-30.

Schulman, K. A., Glick, H. A., Rubin, H., and Eisenberg, J. M. (1991). Cost-effectiveness of HA-1A monoclonal antibody for gram-negative sepsis. *J. Am. Med. Associ.*, 266, 3466-71.

Sculpher, M. J., Seed, P., Henderson, R. A., Buxton, M. J., Pocock, and S., Parker, J. (1993). Health service costs of coronary angioplasty and coronary artery bypass surgery: the randomized intervention treatment of angina (RITA) trial. *Lancet*, 244, 927-30.

Sherry, K. M., McNamara, J., Brown, J. S., and Drummond, M. F. (1996). An economic evaluation of propofol/fentanyl compared with midazolam/fentanyl on recovery of the ICU following cardiac surgery. *Anaesthesia*, 51(4), 312-17.

Weisbrod, B. A., Test, M. A., and Stein, L. I. (1980). Alternative to mental hospital treatment. II Economic benefit – cost analysis. *Arc General Psychiatry*, 37, 400-5.

ANNEX 4.1. TUTORIAL ON METHODS OF MEASURING AND VALUING CAPITAL COSTS

We are indebted to Morris Barer of the University of British Columbia for producing these examples, which should clarify the treatment of capital costs.

As a first note, we need to distinguish two classes of 'capital' – land and equipment. This is an important consideration, because in costing exercises we assume land does not depreciate, while of course capital equipment does. You can think of there being a continuum along which materials and supplies 'depreciate' or are used up instantaneously and so are costed fully in the year of use; capital equipment depreciates more slowly and may be handled in a variety of ways; land does not depreciate at all.

As a second note, recall that capital equipment costs have three components – depreciation, opportunity cost, and actual operating costs. We will ignore the last of these here.

First consider *equipment*, and let us use an example of a machine costing $200 000 that, at the end of five years, has a resale value of $20 000. Assume straight-line depreciation and a discount rate of 4 per cent. There are, then, four approaches to costing:

(1) one can assume all costs accrue at time 0. This amounts to treating the equipment as one would less durable materials and supplies:

Time	0	1	2	3	4	5
Depreciation	200 000	0	0	0	0	(20 000)
Undepreciated balance at beginning of period		0	0	0	0	0
Opportunity cost		0	0	0	0	0
Dep'n. + opp cost	200 000	0	0	0	0	(20 000)
Present value (PV)	200 000	0	0	0	0	(16 439)

Net present value (NPV) of equipment cost = $183 561

Alternatively, but equivalently, one can treat the machine as instantaneously depreciating, except for the $20 000 resale value, which then is maintained through the 5 years:

Time	0	1	2	3	4	5
Depreciation	180 000	–	–	–	–	–
Undepreciated balance at beginning of period		20 000	20 000	20 000	20 000	20 000
Opportunity cost		800	800	800	800	800
Dep'n. + opp cost		800	800	800	800	800
PV	180 000	769	740	711	684	658

NPV of equipment cost = $183 562

(ii) One can compute depreciation and opportunity costs separately. They are related in that the opportunity cost of equipment refers to the use of the resources embodied in the equipment, in their next best use – this is 'approximated' by calculating the return on the funds implicit in the undepreciated value of the equipment at each point in time. Hence, the higher the rate of depreciation, the lower the opportunity cost, all else equal. Again, one has the choice of building the $20 000 resale in at the end, or just depreciating less of the machine. It works out the same.

Time	1	2	3	4	5
Depreciation	36 000	36 000	36 000	36 000	36 000
Undepreciated balance at beginning of period	200 000	164 000	128 000	92 000	56 000
Opportunity cost	8 000	6 560	5 120	3 680	2 240
Dep'n. + opp cost	44 000	42 560	41 120	39 680	38 240
PV	42 308	39 349	36 556	33 919	31 430

NPV of equipment cost = $183 562

Time	1	2	3	4	5
Depreciation	40 000	40 000	40 000	40 000	20 000
Undepreciated balance at beginning of period	200 000	160 000	120 000	80 000	40 000
Opportunity cost	8 000	6 400	4 800	3 200	1 600
Dep'n. + opp cost	48 000	46 400	44 800	43 200	21 600
PV	46 154	42 899	39 827	36 928	17 754

NPV of equipment cost = $183 562

(iii) One can compute an equivalent annual cost. This may be useful in a situation where other operating costs are the same each year, making necessary the comparison of only a single year of cost data for each alternative in the economic evaluation:

$$NPV = E \cdot AF_{5,4\%}$$ (where $AF_{5,4\%}$ is the annuity factor for 5 years at an interest rate of 4 per cent. See Table 2 in Annex 4.2)

$$183 562 = E \cdot 4.4518 \rightarrow E = \$41 233$$

In other words, an *equal* stream of costs amounting to $41 233 in *each* of the five years of the programme has a present value equivalent to any of the *unequal* cost streams in (i) or (ii) above. Note, therefore, that the equivalent annual cost embodies both depreciation and opportunity cost.

(iv) One can use equivalent or actual rental costs, if available or estimable. Note that because the renter will need to recover not only depreciation of the rental equipment but also a rate of return at least as good as that from the next best use of the resource, one can take rental cost to embody both depreciation and opportunity cost.

Second, the treatment of *land* is quite different because of the lack of depreciation. A land purchase of $200 000 at time 0 would generate the following cost time stream:

Time	1	2	3	4	5
Depreciation	–	–	–	–	–
Undepreciated balance at beginning of period	200 000	200 000	200 000	200 000	200 000
Opportunity cost	8 000	8 000	8 000	8 000	8 000
Dep'n + opp cost	8 000	8 000	8 000	8 000	8 000
PV	7 692	7 396	7 112	6 838	6 575
NPV = $35 613					

Converted to an equivalent annual cost.

$$NPV = E \cdot AF_{5,4\%}$$

$$\$35\ 613 = E \cdot 4.4518$$

It comes as no particular surprise that E = $8000!

Annex 4.2.   Discount Table 1

Present value of $1

N	1%	2%	3%	4%	5%	6%	7%	8%	9%	10%	11%	12%	13%	14%	15%
1	0.9901	0.9804	0.9709	0.9615	0.9524	0.9434	0.9346	0.9259	0.9174	0.9091	0.9009	0.8929	0.8850	0.8772	0.8696
2	0.9803	0.9612	0.9426	0.9246	0.9070	0.8900	0.8734	0.8573	0.8417	0.8264	0.8116	0.7972	0.7831	0.7695	0.7561
3	0.9706	0.9423	0.9151	0.8890	0.8638	0.8396	0.8163	0.7938	0.7722	0.7513	0.7312	0.7118	0.6931	0.6750	0.6575
4	0.9610	0.9238	0.8885	0.8548	0.8227	0.7921	0.7629	0.7350	0.7084	0.6830	0.6587	0.6355	0.6133	0.5921	0.5718
5	0.9515	0.9057	0.8626	0.8219	0.7835	0.7473	0.7130	0.6806	0.6499	0.6209	0.5935	0.5674	0.5428	0.5194	0.4972
6	0.9420	0.8880	0.8375	0.7903	0.7462	0.7050	0.6663	0.6302	0.5963	0.5645	0.5346	0.5066	0.4803	0.4556	0.4323
7	0.9327	0.8706	0.8131	0.7599	0.7107	0.6651	0.6227	0.5835	0.5470	0.5132	0.4817	0.4523	0.4251	0.3996	0.3759
8	0.9235	0.8535	0.7894	0.7307	0.6768	0.6274	0.5820	0.5403	0.5019	0.4665	0.4339	0.4039	0.3762	0.3506	0.3269
9	0.9143	0.8368	0.7664	0.7026	0.6446	0.5919	0.5439	0.5002	0.4604	0.4241	0.3909	0.3606	0.3329	0.3075	0.2843
10	0.9053	0.8203	0.7441	0.6756	0.6139	0.5584	0.5083	0.4632	0.4224	0.3855	0.3522	0.3220	0.2946	0.2697	0.2472
11	0.8963	0.8043	0.7224	0.6496	0.5847	0.5268	0.4751	0.4289	0.3875	0.3505	0.3173	0.2875	0.2607	0.2366	0.2149
12	0.8874	0.7885	0.7014	0.6246	0.5568	0.4970	0.4440	0.3971	0.3555	0.3186	0.2858	0.2567	0.2307	0.2076	0.1869
13	0.8787	0.7730	0.6810	0.6006	0.5303	0.4688	0.4150	0.3677	0.3262	0.2897	0.2575	0.2292	0.2042	0.1821	0.1625
14	0.8700	0.7579	0.6611	0.5775	0.5051	0.4423	0.3878	0.3405	0.2992	0.2633	0.2320	0.2046	0.1807	0.1597	0.1413
15	0.8613	0.7430	0.6419	0.5553	0.4810	0.4173	0.3624	0.3152	0.2745	0.2394	0.2090	0.1827	0.1599	0.1401	0.1229
16	0.8528	0.7284	0.6232	0.5339	0.4581	0.3936	0.3387	0.2919	0.2519	0.2176	0.1883	0.1631	0.1415	0.1229	0.1069
17	0.8444	0.7142	0.6050	0.5134	0.4363	0.3714	0.3166	0.2703	0.2311	0.1978	0.1696	0.1456	0.1252	0.1078	0.0929
18	0.8360	0.7002	0.5874	0.4936	0.4155	0.3503	0.2959	0.2502	0.2120	0.1799	0.1528	0.1300	0.1108	0.0946	0.0808
19	0.8277	0.6864	0.5703	0.4746	0.3957	0.3305	0.2765	0.2317	0.1945	0.1635	0.1377	0.1161	0.0981	0.0829	0.0703
20	0.8195	0.6730	0.5537	0.4564	0.3769	0.3118	0.2584	0.2145	0.1784	0.1486	0.1240	0.1037	0.0868	0.0728	0.0611

Annex 4.2. Discount Table 1 *(contd)*

N	1%	2%	3%	4%	5%	6%	7%	8%	9%	10%	11%	12%	13%	14%	15%
21	0.8114	0.6598	0.5375	0.4388	0.3589	0.2942	0.2415	0.1987	0.1637	0.1351	0.1117	0.0926	0.0768	0.0638	0.0531
22	0.8034	0.6468	0.5219	0.4220	0.3418	0.2775	0.2257	0.1839	0.1502	0.1228	0.1007	0.0826	0.0680	0.0560	0.0462
23	0.7954	0.6342	0.5067	0.4057	0.3256	0.2618	0.2109	0.1703	0.1378	0.1117	0.0907	0.0738	0.0601	0.0491	0.0402
24	0.7876	0.6217	0.4919	0.3901	0.3101	0.2470	0.1971	0.1577	0.1264	0.1015	0.0817	0.0659	0.0532	0.0431	0.0349
25	0.7798	0.6095	0.4776	0.3751	0.2953	0.2330	0.1842	0.1460	0.1160	0.0923	0.0736	0.0588	0.0471	0.0378	0.0304
26	0.7720	0.5976	0.4637	0.3607	0.2812	0.2198	0.1722	0.1352	0.1064	0.0839	0.0663	0.0525	0.0417	0.0331	0.0264
27	0.7644	0.5859	0.4502	0.3468	0.2678	0.2074	0.1609	0.1252	0.0976	0.0763	0.0597	0.0469	0.0369	0.0291	0.0230
28	0.7568	0.5744	0.4371	0.3335	0.2551	0.1956	0.1504	0.1159	0.0895	0.0693	0.0538	0.0419	0.0326	0.0255	0.0200
29	0.7493	0.5631	0.4243	0.3207	0.2429	0.1846	0.1406	0.1073	0.0822	0.0630	0.0485	0.0374	0.0289	0.0224	0.0174
30	0.7419	0.5521	0.4120	0.3083	0.2314	0.1741	0.1314	0.0994	0.0754	0.0573	0.0437	0.0334	0.0256	0.0196	0.0151
35	0.7059	0.5000	0.3554	0.2534	0.1813	0.1301	0.0937	0.0676	0.0490	0.0356	0.0259	0.0189	0.0139	0.0102	0.0075
40	0.6717	0.4529	0.3066	0.2083	0.1420	0.0972	0.0668	0.0460	0.0318	0.0221	0.0154	0.0107	0.0075	0.0053	0.0037
45	0.6391	0.4102	0.2644	0.1712	0.1113	0.0727	0.0476	0.0313	0.0207	0.0137	0.0091	0.0061	0.0041	0.0027	0.0019
50	0.6080	0.3715	0.2281	0.1407	0.0872	0.0543	0.0339	0.0213	0.0134	0.0085	0.0054	0.0035	0.0022	0.0014	0.0009

Annex 4.2. Discount Table 2

Present value of annuity of $1 in arrears

N	1%	2%	3%	4%	5%	6%	7%	8%	9%	10%	11%	12%	13%	14%	15%
1	0.9901	0.9804	0.9709	0.9615	0.9524	0.9434	0.9346	0.9259	0.9174	0.9091	0.9009	0.8929	0.8850	0.8772	0.8696
2	1.9704	1.9416	1.9135	1.8861	1.8594	1.8334	1.8080	1.7833	1.7591	1.7335	1.7125	1.6901	1.6681	1.6467	1.6257
3	2.9410	2.8839	2.8286	2.7751	2.7232	2.6730	2.6243	2.5771	2.5313	2.4869	2.4437	2.4018	2.3612	2.3216	2.2832
4	3.9020	3.8077	3.7171	3.6299	3.5460	3.4651	3.3872	3.3121	3.2397	3.1699	3.1024	3.0373	2.9745	2.9137	2.8550
5	4.8534	4.7135	4.5797	4.4518	4.3295	4.2124	4.1002	3.9927	3.8897	3.7908	3.6959	3.6048	3.5172	3.4331	3.3522
6	5.7955	5.6014	5.4172	5.2421	5.0757	4.9173	4.7665	4.6229	4.4859	4.3553	4.2305	4.1114	3.9975	3.8887	3.7845
7	6.7282	6.4720	6.2303	6.0021	5.7864	5.5824	5.3893	5.2064	5.0330	4.8684	4.7122	4.5638	4.4226	4.2883	4.1604
8	7.6517	7.3255	7.0197	6.7327	6.4632	6.2098	5.9713	5.7466	5.5348	5.3349	5.1461	4.9676	4.7988	4.6389	4.4873
9	8.5660	8.1622	7.7861	7.4353	7.1078	6.8017	6.5152	6.2469	5.9952	5.7590	5.5370	5.3282	5.1317	4.9464	4.7716
10	9.4713	8.9826	8.5302	8.1109	7.7217	7.3601	7.0236	6.7101	6.4177	6.1446	5.8892	5.6502	5.4262	5.2161	5.0188
11	10.3676	9.7868	9.2526	8.7605	8.3064	7.8869	7.4987	7.1390	6.8052	6.4951	6.2065	5.9377	5.6869	5.4527	5.2337
12	11.2551	10.5753	9.9540	9.3851	8.8633	8.3838	7.9427	7.5361	7.1607	6.8137	6.4924	6.1944	5.9176	5.6603	5.4206
13	12.1337	11.3484	10.6350	9.9856	9.3936	8.8527	8.3577	7.9038	7.4869	7.1034	6.7499	6.4235	6.1218	5.8424	5.5831
14	13.0037	12.1062	11.2961	10.5631	9.8986	9.2950	8.7455	8.2442	7.7862	7.3667	6.9819	6.6282	6.3025	6.0021	5.7245
15	13.8651	12.8493	11.9379	11.1184	10.3797	9.7122	9.1079	8.5595	8.0607	7.6061	7.1909	6.8109	6.4624	6.1422	5.8474
16	14.7179	13.5777	12.5611	11.6523	10.8378	10.1059	9.4466	8.8514	8.3126	7.8237	7.3792	6.9740	6.6039	6.2651	5.9542
17	15.5623	14.2919	13.1661	12.1657	11.2741	10.4773	9.7632	9.1216	8.5436	8.0216	7.5488	7.1196	6.7291	6.3729	6.0472
18	16.3983	14.9920	13.7535	12.6593	11.6896	10.8276	10.0591	9.3719	8.7556	8.2014	7.7016	7.2497	6.8399	6.4674	6.1280
19	17.2260	15.6785	14.3238	13.1339	12.0853	11.1581	10.3356	9.6036	8.9501	8.3649	7.8393	7.3658	6.9380	6.5504	6.1982
20	18.0456	16.3514	14.8775	13.5903	12.4622	11.4699	10.5940	9.8181	9.1285	8.5136	7.9633	7.4694	7.0248	6.6231	6.2593

Annex 4.2. Discount Table 2 (*contd*)

N	1%	2%	3%	4%	5%	6%	7%	8%	9%	10%	11%	12%	13%	14%	15%
21	18.8570	17.0112	15.4150	14.0292	12.8212	11.7641	10.8355	10.0168	9.2922	8.6487	8.0751	7.5620	7.1016	6.6870	6.3125
22	19.6604	17.6580	15.9369	14.4511	13.1630	12.0416	11.0612	10.2007	9.4424	8.7715	8.1757	7.6446	7.1695	6.7429	6.3587
23	20.4558	18.2922	16.4436	14.8565	13.4886	12.3034	11.2722	10.3711	9.5802	8.8832	8.2664	7.7184	7.2297	6.7921	6.3988
24	21.2434	18.9139	16.9355	15.2470	13.7986	12.5504	11.4693	10.5288	9.7066	8.9847	8.3481	7.7843	7.2829	6.8351	6.4338
25	22.0232	19.5235	17.4131	15.6221	14.0939	12.7834	11.6536	10.6748	9.8226	9.0770	8.4217	7.8431	7.3300	6.8729	6.4641
26	22.7952	20.1210	17.8768	15.9828	14.3752	13.0032	11.8258	10.8100	9.9290	9.1609	8.4881	7.8957	7.3717	6.9061	6.4906
27	23.5596	20.7069	18.3270	16.3296	14.6430	13.2105	11.9867	10.9352	10.0266	9.2372	8.5478	7.9426	7.4086	6.9352	6.5135
28	24.3164	21.2813	18.7641	16.6631	14.8981	13.4062	12.1371	11.0511	10.1161	9.3066	8.6016	7.9844	7.4412	6.9607	6.5335
29	25.0658	21.8444	19.1885	16.9837	15.1411	13.5907	12.2777	11.1584	10.1983	9.3696	8.6501	8.0218	7.4701	6.9830	6.5509
30	25.8077	22.3965	19.6004	17.2920	15.3725	13.7648	12.4090	11.2578	10.2737	9.4269	8.6938	8.0552	7.4957	7.0027	6.5660
35	29.4086	24.9986	21.4872	18.6646	16.3742	14.4982	12.9477	11.6546	10.5668	9.6442	8.8552	8.1755	7.5856	7.0700	6.6166
40	32.8347	27.3555	23.1148	19.7928	17.1591	15.0463	13.3317	11.9246	10.7574	9.7791	8.9511	8.2438	7.6344	7.1050	6.6418
45	36.0945	29.4902	24.5187	20.7200	17.7741	15.4558	13.6055	12.1084	10.8812	9.8628	9.0079	8.2825	7.6690	7.1232	6.6543
50	39.1961	31.4236	25.7298	21.4822	18.2559	15.7619	13.8007	12.2335	10.9617	9.9148	9.0417	8.3045	7.6752	7.1327	6.6605

5

Cost-effectiveness analysis

5.1 SOME BASICS

Cost-effectiveness analysis (CEA) is one form of full economic evaluation where both the costs and consequences of health programmes or treatments are examined. Therefore, all the points discussed in Chapter 4 on cost analysis apply here also. This chapter introduces some additional issues that need to be confronted when undertaking a CEA; in addition to the general introduction, it contains a study design exercise in Section 5.2, followed by a critical appraisal exercise in Section 5.3. Then, in Section 5.4, the use of quality of life scales in CEA is discussed. Finally, in Section 5.5, the interpretation of incremental cost-effectiveness ratios is discussed. As before, the chapter progresses by attempting to answer some of the questions that analysts might need to consider when undertaking a CEA.

5.1.1 What will be the chosen measure of effectiveness?

In general terms the answer to this question lies in the objectives of the programmes or treatments being evaluated, and it is always worthwhile taking time to clarify what these are. Sometimes the objectives will be unclear, often there will be multiple objectives. In order to carry out a CEA, one or other of the following conditions must hold:

(1) that there is one unambiguous objective of the intervention(s) and therefore a clear dimension along which effectiveness can be assessed; or
(2) that there are many objectives, but that the alternative interventions are thought to achieve these to the same extent.

An example of the first case would be where two therapies could be compared in terms of their cost per year of life gained, or, say, two screening procedures could be compared in terms of the cost per case found. As was mentioned in Chapter 2, comparisons can be made across a broad range of disparate programmes (e.g. treatments for chronic renal disease or seatbelt legislation) if there is a common effect of interest (e.g. lives saved).

An example of the second case would be where, say, two surgical interventions gave similar results in terms of complications and recurrences. A cost-effectiveness study in such an instance would, in the terminology of Chapter 2, be called a cost-minimization analysis. (If it were merely a costing study, carried out on the assumption that the effectiveness of the alternatives was equivalent, but without active consideration of that evidence, it would be termed a cost analysis.)

A cost-minimization analysis can only be carried out without ambiguity if it is based on existing (medical) evidence of effectiveness. However, if the effectiveness evidence were to be generated at the same time as the costs, one would not know in advance whether equivalence in effects would be obtained (Although the null hypothesis of the associated clinical trial might give some clues). Therefore, the *ex ante* design for these studies is usually CEA. On some occasions the study may require a more sophisticated approach. For example, multiple dimensions of effectiveness may need to be assessed relative to one another. (Those faced with this problem should consult Chapter 6 on cost–utility analysis.) Similarly, it might be thought in the early stages of a cost-effectiveness analysis that just one dimension of effectiveness were important, only to find that unforeseen effects are also relevant to the assessment. (For example, two diagnostic tests might be compared in terms of cost per case found, only to discover that the approach with the higher effectiveness in case finding resulted in minor clinical complications.)

Therefore, when beginning a study one can never be completely sure of its final form, particularly if the effectiveness evidence is to be generated at the same time as the costs. As was mentioned in Chapter 2, the distinction between cost-effectiveness analysis and cost–utility analysis often becomes blurred. However, since it is important to specify the form of evaluation and to outline an analysis plan in advance, the following rules of thumb should be of some help:

1. Always take time to clarify the objectives of the programme or treatment.
2. If one major dimension for the measurement of success is apparent, perform a cost-effectiveness analysis based on this dimension. (Or perform a cost-minimization analysis if it turns out that the alternatives have equivalent effectiveness on the chosen dimension.)
3. Be on the lookout for other attributes of the alternatives being assessed, even if the medical research design does not consider these formally. Where possible, record the effectiveness of the alternatives as judged on these extra dimensions and be prepared to mount *ad hoc* surveys to obtain more information (e.g. in a study of day care surgery, where the main clinical endpoint might be *number of complications*, it may also be relevant to undertake a patient satisfaction survey).

4. Keep open the possibility of employing more sophisticated forms of analysis if it turns out that there is more than one appropriate dimension for judging effectiveness. The utility assessments (to be discussed in Chapter 6) can always be undertaken separately. Alternatively, it might be necessary only to present an array of the differential achievements, by dimension, of the alternative programmes. These can then be given to the decision-makers, at the programmatic or clinical level, so that they can make their own trade-off between effects. We called this form of evaluation a cost-consequences analysis in Chapter 1.

There is one further important methodological issue to be addressed in the choice of effectiveness measure; namely, should this always relate to a *final* health output such as *life-years gained*, or can it relate to an *intermediate* output such as *cases found* or *patients appropriately treated*. Table 5.1 gives examples of effectiveness measures used in CEAs. Intermediate outputs are admissible, although care must be taken to establish a link between these and a final health output, or to show that the intermediate outputs themselves have some value. For example, correct diagnosis of cases and the consequent confirmation of true negatives can provide reassurance both to the patient and to the doctor, and therefore may have a value in their own right quite apart from the health effects resulting from subsequent treatment. In general though, one should choose an effectiveness measure relating to a final output. (This is discussed further below and in Chapter 8.)

Table 5.1   Examples of effectiveness measures used in
cost-effectiveness analyses

Study reference	Clinical field	Effectiveness measure
Logan *et al.* (1981)	Treatment of hypertension	mmHg blood pressure reduction
Schulman *et al.* (1990)	Treatment of hypercholesterolaemia	% serum cholesterol reduction
Hull *et al.* (1981)	Diagnosis of deep-vein thrombosis	Cases of DVT detected
Sculpher and Buxton (1993)	Asthma	Episode-free days
Mark *et al.* (1995)	Thrombolysis	Years of life gained

5.1.2 How are the effectiveness data to be obtained?

Although primarily an epidemiological issue, the availability of data on the effectiveness of the programmes or treatments being assessed is crucial to the cost-effectiveness analyst. (In fact CEAs are more often criticized for the quality of the medical evidence on which they are based, rather than for the subsequent economics.)

A major source of effectiveness data is the existing medical literature. Use of such data raises two issues: quality and relevance. Appraisal of the *quality* of medical evidence is beyond the scope of this book and the reader should consult the users guides to the medical literature produced by the Department of Clinical Epidemiology and Biostatistics, McMaster University (1981). These papers set out a checklist of questions to ask of any published study of diagnostic or therapeutic interventions. Although there are a number of important methodological features of a well-designed clinical study, probably the most important aspect is the random allocation of patients to treatment groups (including a control group). Application of this single test would lead one to have serious reservations about the clinical evidence used in many published economic evaluations.

In general, economists support the quality criteria laid down by clinical epidemiologists for clinicians seeking evidence to support clinical recommendations. One example is the relationship between levels of evidence and grades of recommendation proposed by Cook *et al.* (1992) (see Table 5.2).

Table 5.2 The relationship between levels of evidence and grades of recommendation

Level of evidence		Grade of recommendation
Level I	Large randomized trials with clear-cut results (and low risk of error)	Grade A
Level II	Small randomized trials with uncertain results (and moderate to high risk of error)	Grade B
Level III	Non-randomized, contemporaneous controls	Grade C
Level IV	Non-randomized, historical controls	Grade D
Level V	No controls, case series only	Grade E

In judging the *relevance* of results published in the literature, one would have to consider how close one's own situation is to those where the published clinical studies were conducted. Important factors to consider are the patient case-load, the expertize of medical and other staff, and the existence of backup facilities.

Potentially, the criteria laid down to judge quality of evidence may conflict with those for judging relevance. This is because many randomized controlled trials are undertaken under atypical conditions. For example, the case-load may be highly selective, patient and doctor may be blind to the treatment assignment, a comparison may be made with placebo rather than another active agent, the trial protocol may require additional tests or procedures to be performed, patients may be closely monitored to ensure compliance with therapy, and patients and physicians may be more highly motivated than the average. These conditions make sense when one is seeking to assess the therapy's ability to do more good than harm. (We called this *efficacy* in Chapter 2.) However, assessments made under these conditions may not tell us much about the therapy's performance in actual clinical use. (We called this *effectiveness* in Chapter 2.)

Ideally, economic evaluations should incorporate clinical data on effectiveness (rather than efficacy) but these may not be available, at least from controlled trials. This is particularly true in the case of pharmaceuticals, where the bulk of the clinical research before the medicine's launch concentrates on establishing efficacy and safety for licensing purposes. Economic analysts are consequently often in a dilemma. Do they argue for additional randomized controlled trials, with more naturalistic designs, to accommodate economic evaluation, or alternatively do they adjust or supplement the data from controlled trials in an economic model?

Undertaking economic analysis alongside clinical trials raises a number of practical and methodological challenges which have been widely discussed (Drummond and Stoddart, 1984; Drummond and Davies, 1991; Adams *et al*, 1992). These challenges relate both to the suitability of particular trials as vehicles for economic analysis and the additional burdens in data capture. (We discuss this further in Chapter 8.)

In using the existing published literature for estimates of effectiveness, the economic analyst can either use data from a single trial or, where they exist, data from an overview or meta-analysis of a group of trials. To date very few published economic studies have used data from overviews, although Mugford (1989) used data from a systematic overview of 58 controlled trials to estimate the cost-effectiveness of giving prophylactic antibiotics routinely to reduce the incidence of wound infection after caesarian section. Also, Jefferson and Demicheli (1994) undertook a systematic overview of both the epidemiological and economic variables pertaining to vaccination against hepatitis B.

Those who undertake systematic overviews have a series of methodological principles covering issues such as the description of the literature search techniques, inclusion/exclusion criteria for individual studies, choice of (clinical) endpoints, records of individual study characteristics (e.g. patient characteristics), details about the therapy (e.g. drug dose), tests of statistical homogeneity, statistical pooling procedures and sensitivity analysis (LAbbe *et al*. 1987; Detsky 1995).

In general, one might expect economic analysts to be in agreement with these principles. Any concerns are more likely to relate to the design of the original controlled trials included in the overview rather than the process of combining the data. However, as more economic evaluations are undertaken using data from systematic overviews, it will be interesting to see whether economists have a different perspective on issues like inclusion/exclusion criteria and the reliability or relevance of particular clinical endpoints.

The question of whether any adjustments should be made to published clinical data for use in an economic evaluation is much more complicated. For example, should adjustments be made for the likelihood of lower compliance in actual clinical use, or for the possibility that clinical practices or conventions vary from place to place? Also, should adjustments be made for the possibility that the trial protocol itself affects costs or benefits? For example, should data from trials of ulcer medications, where patients are endoscoped every month, be adjusted for the fact that many ulcers would not come to the notice of the patient or clinician in regular practice (Hillman and Bloom 1989; O'Brien *et al.* 1995). (See Box 5.1.)

Box 5.1. Adjustments to trial-based data in a study of ulcer therapy

O'Brien *et al.* (1995) wanted to assess the cost-effectiveness of *H. Pylori* eradication relative to alternative pharmacologic strategies in the long-term management of persons with confirmed duodenal ulcer. A key factor in the calculation was the probability of ulcer recurrence (at six months and 12 months) under the various regimens.

Given the large number of randomized trials, they obtained the probabilities by undertaking a meta-analysis (systematic overview). However, in most ulcer trials the rates of recurrence are estimated by endoscopic examination. This is problematic for the economic analysis as this seeks to estimate costs and consequences *as they would occur in normal clinical practice.* In normal practice patients would not be endoscoped unless they had bothersome symptoms and consulted their physicians.

Therefore, it is likely that some of the ulcers detected by endoscopy would be asymptomatic, or silent. In order to account for this O'Brien *et al.* reviewed the trials that reported symptomatic and asymptomatic recurrence separately and estimated that about 75% of recurrences determined by endoscopy are symptomatic. The *adjusted* rates of ulcer recurrence were used in their cost-effectiveness model. Since the adjustment was made for all regimens, it did not change the ranking of programmes (in cost-effectiveness) in this study, but it does affect the *absolute value* of *H. Pylori* eradication or maintenance therapy for ulcer.

Ulcer Recurrences Per 1000 Patients

Strategy	Total	Symptomatic	Expected one-year cost per patient ($)
1. Heal and wait; treat DU recurrence with:			
(a) ranitidine	108	81	329
(b) omeprazole	108	81	341
2. Heal and H. Pylori eradication immediately with:			
(a) omeprazole and amoxicillin	20	15	272
(b) triple therapy	20	15	253

Adapted from O'Brien *et al.* (1995).

The choice of approach for integrating clinical and resource use data in economic evaluations is one of the main methodological issues facing economic analysts. It is discussed further in Chapter 8, on *Collecting and analysing data*. Also, issues of generalising and interpreting economic data from one location to another are discussed further in Chapter 9 on *Presenting and using evaluation results*. Although raised here first in the context of CEA, these issues apply equally to all four forms of full economic evaluation.

Finally, in situations where no good clinical evidence exists, the cost-effectiveness analyst may proceed by making assumptions about the clinical evidence and then undertaking a sensitivity analysis of the economic results to different assumptions. (The basic notion of sensitivity analysis was introduced in Chapter 3. The underlying logic is that if the final result is not sensitive to the estimate used for a given variable, then it is not worth much effort to obtain a more accurate estimate.) It may be that in some cases a CEA based on existing medical evidence, with an appropriate sensitivity analysis, can obviate the need for a costly and time consuming clinical trial. This might be the case in extreme situations where a very small improvement in effectiveness (much smaller than that expected to be observed) would make the new programme or treatment cost-effective, or where even high effectiveness of the new programme (much higher than that observed before in similar programmes) would not make the new programme cost-effective (Sculpher *et al.* 1996).

At any rate, sensitivity analysis can be used to estimate the minimum level of effectiveness required to make the given programme or treatment more cost-effective than the alternative. Given the importance of sensitivity analysis in all economic evaluations, it is discussed in more detail in Section 5.1.6.

5.1.3 How does one link intermediate and final outcomes?

We mentioned earlier that, although intermediate outcomes may themselves have some value (or clinical meaning), the economic analyst should choose an effectiveness measure relating to a final outcome.

Sometimes the final outcomes may be obtained directly from clinical trials, but often the clinical data require some additional interpolation or adjustment. This is true even of trials seemingly reporting final endpoints such as survival. For example, in the study by Mark *et al.* (1995) of thrombolytic therapy following acute myocardial infarction, the economic analysts wanted to calculate the life years gained. (See the critical appraisal of this study in Chapter 3.) The clinical study reported survival at one year. Extrapolation beyond one year was accomplished by; (i) using a Cox proportional-hazards model based on the experience of 4379 patients in the Duke Cardiovascular Disease Database (giving an extrapolation from one to 15 years), and (ii) a statistical extrapolation for the tail of the survival curve (beyond 15 years).

The extrapolation of data beyond the period observed in a clinical study is not straightforward. Many of the issues are discussed in Gold *et al.* (1996) and later in Chapter 8. However, in some cases the available clinical literature may report only intermediate endpoints. This is often true of the literature on prevention, mainly because studies to estimate an improvement in final endpoints are costly and time-consuming to conduct. Here, apart from conducting the cost-effectiveness analysis using the intermediate endpoint, the only option for the economic analyst is to establish a link with a final outcome. For example, Oster *and Epstein*. (1987) used an epidemiological model, based on the risk equations from the Framingham Heart Study, to link reduction in total serum cholesterol with coronary heart disease risk and survival. The success of this approach depends on the extent to which the link between intermediate and final outcome has been established.

In some cases, where the size of the relative risk (e.g. of death) comparing individuals with and without the risk factor is large, it may be possible to establish the link through observational or case control studies. An example here is the link between smoking and lung cancer. However, in many situations it might be necessary to establish the link through studies of stronger methodology, such as intervention studies with random assignment of subjects to treatment groups. For example, the Framingham Heart Study shows that individuals who have lived their lives with cholesterol levels towards the lower end of the distribution have a lower incidence of coronary heart disease. This is different from saying that lowering serum cholesterol by drug therapy increases survival. Accordingly, until the recent publication of large, long term, intervention studies (e.g. the Scandinavian Simvastatin Survival Study Group, 1994), there was scepticism in some quarters over whether lowering cholesterol by drugs did indeed increase overall survival. Therefore, economic evaluations based on models have, in such circumstances, been viewed with suspicion.

We give more examples of the use of modelling in economic evaluation in Chapter 8. However, when undertaking a CEA using effectiveness data relating to an intermediate endpoint the economic analyst should either:

(1) make a case for the intermediate endpoint having value or clinical relevance in its own right, or;
(2) be confident that the link between intermediate and final outcomes has been adequately established by previous research.

5.1.4 Should productivity changes be included?

As was indicated earlier, the relevance of this depends on the viewpoint for the analysis. For example, if an evaluation is being undertaken from a government budget perspective, there may be interest in estimating the financial flows relating to employment (e.g. the impact on tax receipts and sickness benefit payments). (We called these *transfer payments* earlier.) However, when a societal viewpoint is being adopted, the inclusion of productivity changes, either as costs or consequences, is contentious. In CEA this issue might arise as follows. Suppose one were evaluating two programmes in the field of mental health. One programme requires institutionalization of the patient for a given period; the other, being a community-based programme using community psychiatric nurses in association with out-patient hospital visits, mean that patients can remain in their own homes. (For simplicity, let us assume that the programmes turn out to be equivalent in their medical effectiveness, as assessed by some agreed measure of clinical symptomatology. Furthermore, assume that a survey of patients shows them to be indifferent to the treatment modes, providing they are cured.)

Suppose it turns out that the community care programme has higher costs to the health care system, but that the number of workdays lost by the cohort of patients on the community regimen is lower, as many more of them can remain at work. Would it be right to deduct these production gains from the higher health care costs of the community care programme? If so, how would the production gains be valued?

One might take the view that the production gains should be included in the analysis, since in principle there is no difference between these resource savings and any of the other labour inputs included in the health care cost estimates. Many analysts would follow this approach. The productivity changes would be estimated by using the extra earnings of patients on the community care regimen, gross of taxes and benefits (i.e. gross earnings before deductions, plus employer-paid benefits). The logic here is that the gross wage reflects the value of the production at the margin.

Whilst the approach followed above is quite defensible, it gives rise to a number of wider considerations that should be noted. First, the approach assumes that the community loses production if the institutional-based programme removes patients from employment. However, it may be that, given a pool of unemployed labour, the jobs vacated by patients admitted to institutional care would be filled by other members of the community. If this were the case there may be few overall production gains from adopting the community care programme. Second, it may be that, at some later stage, the cost-effectiveness estimates obtained in this study are compared with those obtained in other fields of health care, say a community care programme for people with learning difficulties or for the elderly. Since the patients benefiting from these programmes are unlikely to be in employment, there is less potential for production gains. This would make the community care programme for mental illness patients seem relatively inexpensive in terms of net cost, particularly if it were for workers earning high incomes, such as business executives, psychiatrists or, dare we say, economists! Thus, in making a choice on the basis of net cost-effectiveness estimates, decision-makers may be tacitly accepting priorities different from their stated ones – if these are for the care of the elderly or people with learning difficulties.

There are at least four concerns about the inclusion of productivity changes in evaluations undertaken from the societal perspective. The first concern is related to *measurement* of changes in productivity. As mentioned above, these are typically estimates using the gross earnings (including employment overheads and benefits) of those in employment. Also, some studies impute an equivalent value for those not in paid employment (e.g. homemakers) by one of a number of methods. These include the use of average wages, the cost of replacing the role fulfilled by the individual, or the opportunity cost of the production they could have contributed were they not at home.

However, it is frequently argued that these valuations overestimate the true cost to society if individuals were to be taken out of the workforce, either through illness or to receive health care. For example, for short-term absences, losses in production could be compensated for by the worker on his or her return to work, or by colleagues. Also, for many categories of worker the value of the productivity lost at the margin is likely to be lower than the average wage, on the grounds that all jobs contain tasks that are more or less important, and it is the less important ones that are usually forgone as a result of a short period of absence. Finally, for long-term absences the employer is likely to hire a replacement worker. Therefore, the amount of productivity lost depends on the time and cost of organizing the replacement, and the resulting adjustments in the economy more generally. That is, if the President gets sick, sooner or later one person will be removed from the ranks of the unemployed!

We should note that many of these points arose in the context of the valuation of health care costs in Chapter 4. Namely, it was argued that costs or savings at the margin may not be reflected by average costs, and that there are frequently costs or inefficiencies associated with changes in resource allocation. For example, the closure of a large mental illness institution cannot take place overnight and there may be times, during the closure process, where wards are underoccupied.

In the context of productivity losses, Koopmanschap *et al.* (1995) have proposed that these should be estimated by the *friction cost method*. The basic idea is that the amount of production lost due to disease depends on the time-span organizations need to restore the initial production level. This friction period is likely to differ by location , industry, firm and category of worker. The challenge is therefore to estimate the relevant friction periods and some calculations have been made for the Netherlands (Koopmonschap and Rutten 1996). These give estimates of lost production much lower than those obtained from traditional methods. Questionnaires are now being developed to estimate productivity changes more precisely (Van Roijen *et al.* 1996).

The second concern relates to *double-counting*, especially in relation to productivity gains. If the value of improved health estimated in a given study already includes the value of the increased productivity that would result, then it would not be appropriate to include an additional estimate of the value of this item. This is most likely to be a problem in the case of the two forms of evaluation yet to be discussed, cost–utility and cost–benefit analysis. Here health state scenarios are presented to individuals for valuation, either in utility or monetary terms. Unless specifically told to ignore the impact that return to work would have on their income, respondents may factor this into their response. In the case of CEA specifically, double counting seems less of a problem and an estimate of productivity gains (e.g. in workdays gained) could be one of the effectiveness measures considered. (We discussed this point earlier in Chapter 3.)

The third concern relates to the issue of *objectives and perspective* in the use of economic evaluation. For example, Gerard and Mooney (1993) argue that when the measure of benefit in an economic evaluation is health-specific (e.g. life years gained, or quality-adjusted life-years gained), the opportunity cost of scarce health care resources is defined in terms only of health forgone. It then follows that the opportunity cost of interest in the context of CEA or CUA is determined by the best alternative use of small increases to total health care budgets and not opportunity costs elsewhere in the economy. It would thus be confusing to include productivity changes, or indeed other non-health care costs such as patients' time, volunteer time and costs falling on other agencies.

We take the view that, whilst the benefit measure in the denominator of many economic evaluations in health care is indeed often health-specific, it is not helpful for economic analysis to reinforce artificial budgetary boundaries by limiting consideration to health care costs only. One way forward would be to present health care and non-health care costs and benefits separately in the analysis, so that the opportunity cost on the health care budget is clearly identified. This would be consistent with Gerard and Mooney's position and the notion, introduced in Chapter 2, that analyses can be undertaken from different viewpoints, including the societal viewpoint. In short, we believe that economic evaluations in health care should, where feasible, consider the societal viewpoint, although on occasions analytical difficulties will preclude the full measurement and valuation of all costs and consequences in monetary terms.

The fourth concern is the one hinted at in the discussion of the mental health programmes above; namely that the inclusion of productivity changes in an evaluation raises *equity* considerations. This problem might be alleviated by either:

(1) expressing productivity changes as the number of days of work or normal activity lost or gained, rather than the dollar amount, or
(2) using a general wage rate to value productivity changes, rather than the actual wages of individuals affected by the health programme being evaluated.

Given the controversy surrounding the inclusion and estimation of productivity changes, we would suggest the following:

(1) report productivity changes separately so that the decision maker can make a decision on whether or not to include them;
(2) report the quantities (in days of work, or normal activity lost or gained) separately from the prices (e.g. earnings) used to value the quantities. (This mirrors the recommendation made for costing in Chapter 4.);
(3) consider whether earnings adequately reflect the value of lost production at the margin and whether an approach based on the adjustments necessary to restore productivity (e.g the friction approach) would be more valid;
(4) pay attention to the equity implications of the inclusion of productivity changes, and, where equity concerns are important, continue to conduct the base case analysis using the actual estimates of the impact of the programme; but also consider a sensitivity analysis to explore the impact of using more equitable estimates, for example, a general wage rate rather than age, gender, or disease-specific rates;
(5) consider whether the inclusion of productivity changes represents double counting. (As indicated above, this is particularly pertinent when undertaking a cost–utility or cost–benefit analysis, but less likely when the effectiveness measure does not incorporate any *valuation* of the health consequences.)

For a more theoretical discussion of some of the issues surrounding the inclusion and measurement of productivity changes in economic evaluation see Olsen (1994) and Posnett and Jan (1996).

5.1.5 Should effects occurring in the future be discounted?

In Chapter 4, the logic and procedures for discounting costs to present values were outlined. Since cost-effectiveness analysis also considers effects, should these be discounted too? This issue has aroused controversy, although it should be pointed out that in many CEAs it does not arise because the effects occur in a short period of time. (Capital costs may have to be converted to an annual amount using the annuitization procedure outlined in Chapter 4, however.) Nevertheless, the discounting of effects does have major practical consequences for the economic evaluation of preventive programmes. It is often argued that these are penalized by discounting.

The reasons often given for not discounting effects are that:

(1) unlike resources, it is difficult to conceive of individuals investing in health or trading flows of healthy years through time;
(2) discounting years of life gained in the future gives less weight to future generations in favour of the present one. Whereas this may make sense in the context of resources, where one would expect future generations to be

wealthier, it might not make sense in the context of health. (On the other hand, it might, if one expects future generations to have better therapeutic technologies available.)

(3) empirical evidence suggests that individuals discount health at a different rate from monetary benefits (see Cairns 1992; Parsonage and Neuburger (1992); (Gold *et al.* (1996); Viscusi (1995) for a fuller discussion of these issues).

However, there are some fairly powerful arguments in favour of discounting effects as well as costs. These are:

(1) it can be shown, by the use of simple numerical examples, that leaving effects undiscounted while discounting costs, or discounting costs and effects at different rates, can lead to inconsistencies in reasoning. For a simple numerical example see Weinstein and Stason (1977); for a theoretical treatment see Keeler and Cretin (1983);

(2) leaving effects undiscounted leads to quite impossible conclusions. For example, a health programme giving rise to $1 of health benefits each and every year stretching into the future would be worthwhile whatever the size of the initial capital sum;

(3) contrary to the argument set out above, one *can* conceive of investments in health and the trading of health through time (Grossman 1972). Although it is not possible to give up a year now in return for a year at the end of one's life, individuals can trade reductions in health status or other goods and services now, in return for healthy time in the future (and *vice versa*). If this were not the case, people would not abstain from pleasurable but potentially unhealthy (in the long term) pursuits;

(4) whereas one of the arguments for not discounting effects is to avoid the problem of giving less weight to future generations, it may lead one to defer decisions *whenever* they are considered, this generation or next! This is because, with discounting of costs, the present value of a stream of expenditure starting next year is always lower than the present value of the same stream starting today. Therefore, it will be better to build the hospital next year; until we get to next year, when it will then be better to build the hospital the year after that!

(5) treating health care projects differently from those in other sectors of the economy may lead to inconsistencies in the overall allocation of resources. That is, health care projects would get an inside track.

Therefore, the weight of the argument is for discounting health effects occurring in the future, although both theoretical and empirical research is currently being carried out into the rate at which individuals discount health. Nevertheless, the current state of the art would suggest that effects should be treated in the same way as costs, and discounted at the same rate (Viscusi 1995; Gold *et al.*, 1996). However, as mentioned in Chapter 4, it is advisable to set out all the costs and consequences in the years in which they occur and to present them undiscounted, so that others can apply different discount rates if they wish. Also, in those jurisdictions such as the UK, where the government requests an analysis with health benefits undiscounted (Parsonage and Neuburger, 1992) this should be one of the results presented.

5.1.6. What are the main points to consider when undertaking a sensitivity analysis?

It was mentioned in Chapter 3 that sensitivity analysis has, until recently, been the main method by which analysts have allowed for uncertainty in economic evaluations. Now that more stochastic data are available to economists, through the increasing practice of collecting economic data alongside clinical trials, classical statistical approaches may be used instead. (We discuss this further in Chapter 8.) However, it is unlikely that the need for sensitivity analysis will disappear altogether because some data (e.g. the discount rate) will still be deterministic (i.e. known only as a point estimate).

There are a number of sources of uncertainty in economic evaluation. First, no data may be available and informed guesses are required. This may be the case for estimates of the effectiveness of new, unproven, medical technologies. Secondly, estimates may be available but they may be known to be imprecise. This may be the case for estimates of hospital costs where only the average cost per day, or per admission, is known. Thirdly, there may be methodological controversy, or value judgements may be incorporated in the study. This may be the case for analytic decisions such as the choice of discount rate, whether or not productivity changes should be included, or the source of values for health state preferences.

Finally, the analyst may use sensitivity analysis to explore the generalizability of study results to other settings. This is often an issue even where the estimates within a given study are known to be precise. (Issues relating to the generalizability of economic evaluations are discussed further in Chapters 8 and 9.).

In each of these situations the analyst may wish to explore how sensitive the results of the study are to the estimates used for particular variables, or the assumptions made. In general, sensitivity analysis involves three steps:

(1) identify the uncertain parameters for which sensitivity analysis is required;
(2) specify the plausible range over which uncertain factors are thought to vary;
(3) calculate study results based on combinations of the best guess, most conservative, and least conservative estimates.

Identifying the uncertain parameters

It is difficult to specify firm guidelines for this step, beyond the fact that, in principle, all variables in the analysis are potential candidates for sensitivity analysis. One approach might be for the analyst to give the reasons why particular variables had *not* been included. Possible reasons for exclusion could be that parameter estimates are known with absolute certainty, or that a preliminary analysis shows that, even if the variable is allowed to vary over a wide range, this has a minimal impact on the overall study results.

Specifying the plausible range

A frequent weakness in published economic evaluations is that, while they include a sensitivity analysis, the reasons for specifying the plausible ranges for the variables are not given. Frequently estimates are doubled or halved with no justification. A plausible range could be determined by:

- reviewing the literature;
- consulting expert opinion
- using a specified confidence interval around the mean (for stochastic data).

When judging published studies the user should assess the justification given for plausible ranges, in conjunction with the statements authors make about their analyses. Sometimes the author's conclusion is that the result is very robust, although the ranges chosen for varying key estimates are unjustifiably small. The moral appears to be that if you do not shake your study too hard it is unlikely to fall apart!

Instead of taking point estimates for the base case (best guess) estimate and the upper and lower bound, an alternative approach is to undertake a *probabilistic sensitivity analysis*. This considers the relative likelihood that particular values (e.g the extremes) will occur. It applies distributions to the specified ranges and samples at random from these distributions to simulate uncertainty, thereby generating an empirical distribution of the cost-effectiveness ratio (see Doubilet *et al.*, 1985).

Many computer packages for economic evaluation and decision analysis (see section 5.2 below) offer this facility. The main problem surrounds whether the analyst has sufficient information to specify the range and distribution for the particular variables. If this information is lacking, a probabilistic sensitivity analysis may be misleading because it gives an aura of sophistication to the statements of precision, when in fact the analysis is too heavily dependent on a few crude assumptions.

Calculating study results

The simplest form of sensitivity analysis is to undertake a *one-way analysis*. Here estimates for each parameter are varied one at a time in order to investigate the impact on study results. To date this is the most common form of sensitivity analysis found in the literature and is often performed before some of the more advanced approaches discussed below.

A more sophisticated approach is to undertake a *multi-way analysis*. This recognizes that more than one parameter is uncertain and that each could vary within its specified range. Overall, this approach is more realistic but, unless there are only a few uncertain parameters, the number of potential combinations becomes very large. In this case the principles of experimental design can be applied to select the particular combinations to be included (Goldsmith *et al.*, 1987). Alternatively, a multi-way probabilistic sensitivity analysis partly overcomes this problem but may be difficult for the reader to interpret.

Another approach is to use *scenario analysis*. Here a series of scenarios is constructed representing a subset of the potential multi-way analysis. Typically, the scenarios will include a base case (best guess) scenario and the most optimistic (best case) and most pessimistic (worst case) scenarios. Alternatively they may include scenarios that the analyst or user of the study feel could probably apply.

Finally, yet another approach is to undertake a *threshold analysis*. Here the critical value(s) of a parameter or parameters central to the decision are identified. For example, a decision maker might specify an increase in cost, or an incremental cost-effectiveness ratio, above which the programme would not be acceptable. Then the analyst could assess which combinations of parameter estimates could cause the threshold to be exceeded. Alternatively, the threshold values for key parameters that would cause the programme to be too costly or not cost-effective could be defined. The decision makers could then make a judgement about whether particular thresholds were likely to be breached or not.

An extensive review of the methodology and practice of sensitivity analysis has recently been carried out by Briggs *et al.* (1994) and Briggs and Sculpher (1995). They conclude that the current state of the art is disappointing overall, although there are a number of good examples. (Box 5.2 summarizes some of the samples they identify.)

Box 5.2. Examples of sensitivity analysis found in the literature

Briggs and Sculpher (1995) undertook a structured methodological review of journal articles published in 1992 in order to assess how well they dealt with the issue of uncertainty (through sensitivity analysis). Out of 93 studies sampled, 13 (14%) were judged to have provided a good account of uncertainty. Of these 13 studies, the following four employed a variety of different approaches and also justified the ranges over which estimates were varied.

Author(s)	Disease Area	Types of Sensitivity Analysis
Brown M. L.	Breast cancer screening	One-way, multi-way
Davey *et al.*	Antibiotic prophylaxis in surgery	One-way, threshold, probabilistic
Hillner *et al.*	Bone marrow transplantation in metastatic breast cancer	One-way
Majid *et al.*	Prevention of lyme disease after tick bites	One-way, multi-way, threshold, extreme scenario

Adapted from Briggs and Sculpher (1995).

A key point to remember about sensitivity analysis is that, in contrast to classical statistical analysis, it is rarely data driven and allows considerable analyst discretion. Over time clearer guidelines for undertaking sensitivity analysis may emerge. Briggs (1996) has developed guidelines for presenting sensitivity analysis, depending on whether the health care programme of interest is dominant over the alternative using baseline assumptions, or whether it is more costly yet more effective (implying an incremental cost-effectiveness ratio). Guidelines also need to be developed for interpreting the results of sensitivity analysis. At what point does the result change from being robust to sensitive?

5.2 EXERCISE: DESIGNING A COST-EFFECTIVENESS STUDY

Imagine that you have been consulted on the following issue. Try to apply the knowledge you have gained so far.

5.2.1. Description of situation

Occasionally patients die from pulmonary embolism (i.e. clots in the blood vessels leading to the lung) following general surgery. Although death is relatively rare, the incidence is higher in patients over the age of 40 years who have undergone surgery lasting at least 30 minutes under general anaesthetic. Existing studies suggest that about eight in 1000 patients will die.

The current approach is to treat postoperatively as and when venous thromboembolism becomes clinically apparent. The clinical signs might include (for pulmonary embolism) pleuritic chest pain, shortness of breath or coughing up blood, or (for deep-vein thrombosis, a related condition) pain and tenderness in the thigh or calf. Once the signs occur, the diagnosis is confirmed by lung scanning (for pulmonary embolism) or by venography (for deep-vein thrombosis). The treatment for both types of venous thromboembolism is the same – full-dose anticoagulant therapy consisting of heparin given intravenously for 7-10 days, followed by out-patient treatment with sodium warfarin for 12 weeks. Anticoagulant therapy prolongs hospital stay following surgery and some patients will have major bleeding complications.

Recently there has been an interest in prophylaxis. The options include the following:

1. Primary prophylaxis

(a) *Subcutaneous administration of heparin in low doses.* In this approach all patients would be given heparin subcutaneously for two hours preoperatively and then every eight hours for seven days postoperatively. If clinically suspected deep-vein thrombosis or pulmonary embolism were to develop, venography or lung scanning would be performed. If this confirmed the diagnosis, full-dose anticoagulant therapy (with heparin) would be given. The low dose prophylaxis is not associated with significant bleeding.

(b) *Intravenous administration of dextran.* In this approach all patients would be given dextran intravenously for four days postoperatively. If clinically suspected deep-vein thrombosis or pulmonary embolism develops, venography or lung scanning would be performed. If this confirms the diagnosis, full-dose anticoagulant therapy would be given, as in (a). Dextran prophylaxis carries slight risks of complications but these can be reduced to less than 2 per cent by careful administration.

(c) *Intermittent pneumatic compression of legs.* In this approach, an inflatable cuff is strapped to the patient's leg, enabling gentle pressure to be applied to the calf in a regular cycle. The procedure typically begins during the operation and is continued until the patient is considered no longer at risk, e.g. when the patient is ambulant. The cuff is worn continuously but is removed once per nursing shift. The modern devices that provide intermittent pneumatic compression are free of clinically significant side effects; in particular, there is no risk of bleeding. As in (b), if clinically suspected deep-vein thrombosis or pulmonary embolism developed, venography or lung scanning would be performed. If this confirmed the diagnosis, full-dose anticoagulant therapy (with heparin) would be given.

2. Secondary prevention

The approach here would be to perform leg scanning using iodine-125-labelled fibrinogen daily for three days following surgery and then on alternate days for up to five days, or up to the time of discharge if the patient was not ambulant. Leg scanning is free of complications.

If a positive scan was obtained, venography would be performed to confirm that diagnosis. Also, lung scanning would be performed on patients showing clinical signs of pulmonary embolism. If the diagnosis was confirmed, patients would undergo full-dose anticoagulant therapy, as in the case of primary prophylaxis above.

5.2.2. Tasks

(A) Set out the five alternatives in a clear form, showing the sequence of diagnostic and therapeutic actions arising under each. (You may find that a diagrammatic representation helps.)

(B) Consider the following methodological issues, important in designing the cost-effectiveness study:

1. What should be the viewpoint for the study? (In particular, whose costs should be considered?)

2. What broad categories of cost should be considered for each alternative?
3. What would you choose as the main measure of effectiveness of the alternatives?
4. Are there any other attributes of the alternatives that should also be considered in addition to the main effectiveness measure?
5. What kind of medical evidence will be required for the cost-effectiveness study?
6. What are likely to be the main uncertain factors for which a sensitivity analysis might be required?

Do not turn to Task (C) until Task (B) has been completed.

(C) Assume that the following data have been made available. Use them to calculate the cost-effectiveness of the alternatives. Also, indicate the major points you would make in a discussion of the cost-effectiveness results.

Costs ($)
1. *Prophylactic procedures (per patient)*

Intermittent pneumatic compression of the legs	33
Leg scanning with iodine-125-labelled fibrinogen	85
Intravenous administration of dextran	103
Subcutaneous administration of heparin in low doses	20

2. *Diagnostic procedures (per patient)*

Venography	88
Lung scanning	117

3. *Full-dose anticoagulant therapy (per patient)*

Hospitalization costs (for seven extra days at $290 per day)	2030
Intravenous heparin therapy	30
Laboratory tests	104
Warfarin therapy	10
Physician fees	35
Total:	2209

Outcomes (obtained from controlled clinical trials and given for a cohort of 1000 patients receiving each regimen)

1. *Current (no programme) approach*

Number of patients with clinically suspected deep-vein thrombosis	40
Number of patients with clinically suspected pulmonary embolism	30
Number of positive venograms	19
Number of positive lung scans	14
Deaths	8

2. *Subcutaneous administration of heparin*
Number of patients with suspected deep-vein thrombosis 10
Number of patients with suspected pulmonary embolism 10
Number of positive venograms 4
Number of positive lung scans 4
Deaths 1

3. *Intravenous administration of dextran*
Number of patients with suspected deep-vein thrombosis 20
Number of patients with suspected pulmonary embolism 10
Number of positive venograms 9
Number of positive lung scans 4
Deaths 1

4. *Intermittent pneumatic compression of legs*
Outcomes as for subcutaneous administration of heparin, except that number of deaths not known. However, it is known that the approach is effective in preventing deep-vein thrombosis.

5. *Leg scanning*
Number of positive scans 135
Number of patients with suspected pulmonary embolism 15
Number of positive venograms 107
Number of positive lung scans 7
Deaths (not known, although it is thought that leg scanning is effective in preventing fatal pulmonary embolism).

5.2.3. Solutions

1. Description of the alternatives
An algorithm of the clinical alternatives is given in Fig 5.1. This diagrammatic representation is useful in getting a feel for those clinical options involving not just one action, but a sequence of interrelated actions. In this example, the number of objective tests performed (i.e. venography and lung scanning) depends on the number of patients developing clinically suspected deep-vein thrombosis or pulmonary embolism under each approach. The number of patients receiving full-dose anticoagulant therapy will then depend on the results of the diagnostic tests.

The option involving leg scanning is somewhat different from the others in that it employs a further objective diagnostic test in order to identify possible cases at an early stage. It can be seen from the diagram that the cost of this strategy for 1000 patients will be crucially dependent on the number of positive leg scans and the number of these which are subsequently ruled out (as cases of DVT) by venography (the gold standard test for DVT).

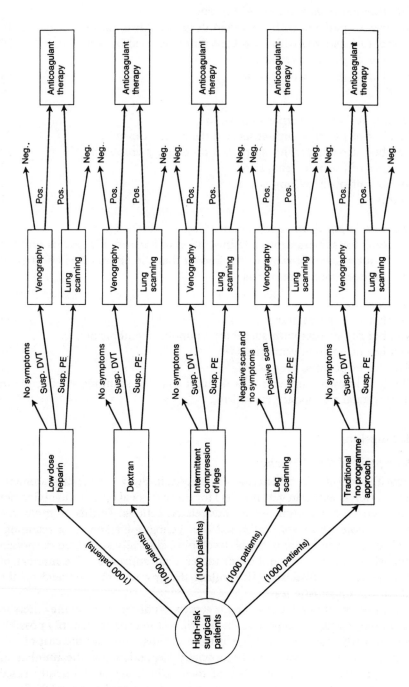

Figure 5.1. Algorithm of clinical alternatives

A slightly more advanced method of setting out complex sequences of clinical alternatives is the *decision tree*. This approach has gained considerable popularity as a vehicle for undertaking economic evaluations and is described in Fineberg (1980) and Weinstein and Fineberg (1980). A decision tree flows from left to right beginning with an initial clinical choice or decision (indicated by a box) on a defined category of patient (or cohort of patients). As a result of the decision made there will be outcomes of given prior probabilities, depicted in the decision tree at a chance node (indicated by a circle). The sum of prior probabilities at each chance node (e.g. $P_1 + P_2 + P_3$) is equal to unity. Our example is redrawn in decision tree format in Figure 5.2.

2. Methodological issues in study design

(a) *Viewpoint for the study.* One viewpoint from which to undertake the analysis would be that of the third party payer. Therefore, it would be most relevant to compare the health care costs of the alternative regimens (including physician charges). Then the issue would be one of whether alternative (or broader) viewpoints would change the kind of results that merely a health care cost comparison would give. For example:

From the patient's viewpoint:

- is length of hospital stay the same?
- is recovery time the same?
- are health outcomes the same; death, complications?
- will expenditure be the same under all options, e.g. out-patient visits?

From the society's viewpoint:

- are there any spillover costs or savings to other public or private sector agencies?

In this case, apart from the patient's interest in outcome there does not seem to be much conflict between the third party payer (e.g. Ministry of Health) and other viewpoints.

(b) *Categories of cost to be considered.* Obviously these depend on viewpoint, but one would definitely want to consider:

- hospital hotel costs;
- prophylaxis costs (for the three preventive measures);
- treatment costs (i.e. full-dose anticoagulant therapy).

The main issues are:

- do we consider costs common to all the alternatives as well as the differences? (This affects mainly the costing of hospital in-patient stay.)
- how accurate are the hospital *per diem* costs?

Cost-effectiveness analysis

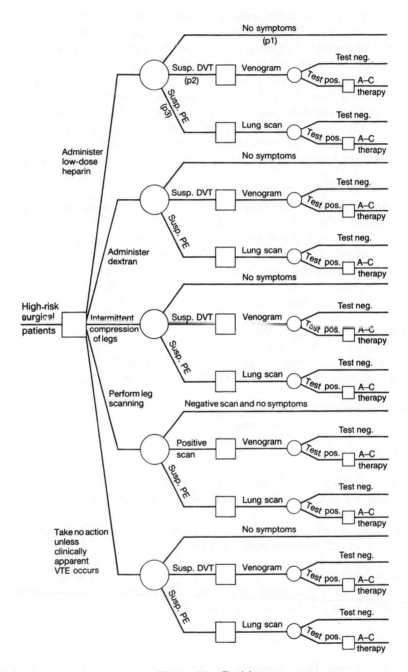

Figure 5.2. Decision tree

(c) *Measure of effectiveness and other attributes of the regimens.* The most obvious choice for the main measure of effectiveness would be deaths averted or life-years gained. Life-years gained would be preferable but would require some assumptions to be made about the likely life expectancy of patients undergoing this type of surgery. Other relevant attributes of the regimens include:

- unpleasantness of the diagnostic approaches, particularly venography;
- complications (e.g. bleeding) either from the prophylaxis or, more importantly, from the full-dose anticoagulant therapy
- prolongation of hospital stay by anticoagulant therapy.

An alternative approach would be to use an intermediate effectiveness measure, such as cases of venous thromboembolism averted. Although less generic than life-years gained, one might argue that a case of venous thromboembolism is a clinically and economically relevant event in its own right. Certainly it is a surrogate for the other relevant attributes mentioned above. An advantage of choosing this endpoint is that it would be much easier to design and execute a clinical study to determine any difference between the alternative strategies. Since deaths are rare for all options, a study powered to detect a difference in deaths would be very large.

Perhaps the cost-effectiveness study should use both endpoints, with cases of venous thromboembolism being estimated directly from a clinical trial and the number of deaths and life-years gained being obtained by extrapolation, using assumptions and the existing literature.

(d) *Source of medical evidence.* Ideally one would like evidence on the outcomes for each alternative, generated by controlled clinical trials. The variables that would be important to estimate include:

- the number of patients developing clinically suspected pulmonary embolism or deep-vein thrombosis
- the number of positive venograms or lung scans (for those patients tested) and hence the number of patients receiving full-dose anticoagulant therapy
- the number of complications from therapy
- the number of deaths from pulmonary embolism.

As mentioned above, it would be much easier to design a controlled clinical trial to detect a difference in cases of venous thromboembolism, rather than a difference in deaths.

(e) *Factors requiring a sensitivity analysis.* This will depend on which of the medical parameters can be established by randomized controlled trials – either in conjunction with this study or drawn from other sources.

Obviously, cost-effectiveness of the regimens would be highly sensitive to the number of deaths resulting from the no programme approach, the number of deaths averted by prophylaxis and the sensitivity and specificity of the leg scanning, venography, and lung scanning procedures. Also, as primary prophylaxis involves giving everyone the low-dose therapy, the cost-effectiveness results would be highly sensitive to the cost of this. Finally, hospitalization costs are a large part of the total cost. Therefore, it would be important to explore the sensitivity of results to variations in these costs and it would be worthwhile varying both the daily rate and the prolongation of hospital stay assumed.

3. Calculations of cost-effectiveness of the alternatives

The data on the flow of patients under each regimen are added to the algorithm of clinical alternatives in Fig. 5.3. Of particular note is the fact that leg scanning identifies a large number of cases of possible DVT, few of which are ruled out by venography. This means that many more patients are given full anticoagulant therapy under this approach with consequent high costs.

The number treated is much greater than the cases of suspected DVT under the no programme approach. This signifies that leg scanning is detecting a number of cases that would otherwise not become clinically apparent.

These data can then be combined with the cost data to give the total cost (per 1000 patients) for the five options. This cost is shown in Table 5.3, along with the effects, in terms of deaths. Table 5.3 also shows the incremental analysis in terms of costs and lives saved. It can be seen that the most cost-effective option is subcutaneous administration of heparin, which has the lowest costs yet saves seven lives. That is, it is dominant over the no programme approach.

Points that might be raised in a discussion of the results are:

1. How sensitive is this result to the assumptions made about the cost of prophylaxis and the cost of hospitalization?
2. Is the effectiveness of intermittent pneumatic compression worth evaluating through a randomized controlled trial? (This approach is almost as inexpensive as subcutaneous administration of heparin, yet does not carry any risk of bleeding or wound complications due to prophylaxis.)

The same data are presented in decision tree form in Fig 5.4. Rather than presenting flows of patients, the decision tree includes the probabilities of events occurring at each chance node. For example, if low-dose heparin is given to 1000 patients, 980 will have no symptoms, 10 will develop suspected DVT, and 10 will develop suspected PE. On the tree these translate to probabilities of 0.980, 0.010, and 0.010 respectively.

5.2.4. A published study

The situation upon which this exercise is based was, in fact, real. A group of Canadian researchers designed and undertook a cost-effectiveness study to address the issue concerned and this was published in the *Canadian Medical*

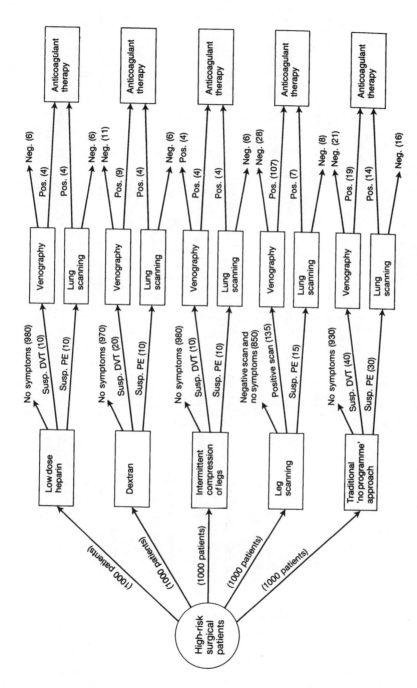

Figure 5.3. Algorithm indicating the flows of patients under regimen

Table 5.3. Alternative strategies for prevention of fatal pulmonary embolism in high-risk surgical patients

Strategy	Data		Incremental comparison		
	Cost/1000 $	Deaths/1000	Cost	Lives saved	C/E ratio (cost/ per life saved)
No programme	80 000	8			
Intravenous dextran	135 000	1	55 000	7	7 900
Low-dose subcutaneous heparin	40 000	1	−40 000	7	<0
Intermittent pneumatic compression of legs	53 000	?	−27 000	?	?
Leg scanning with ^{125}I-fibrinogen	350 000	?	270 000	?	?

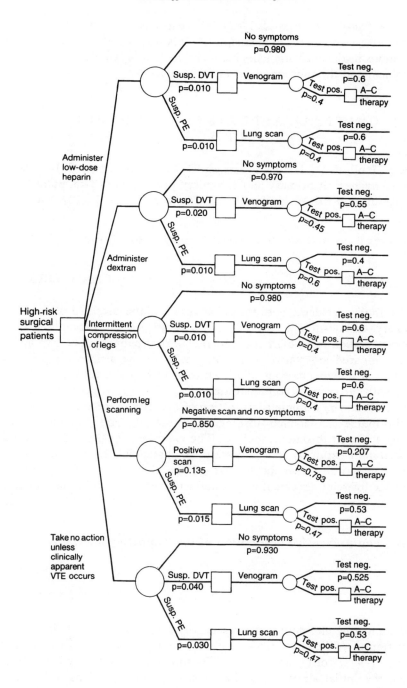

Figure 5.4. Decision tree

Association Journal (Hull *et al.* 1982). The paper is assessed in Section 5.3 using the 10 questions set out in Chapter 3. It is suggested that you locate the article and consider the comments below in the light of your own attempt at the problem and the solution given in Section 5.2.3.

5.3. CRITICAL APPRAISAL OF A PUBLISHED ARTICLE

Reference: Hull, R. D., Hirsh, J., Sackett, D. L., and Stoddart, G. L. (1982). Cost-effectiveness of primary and secondary prevention of fatal pulmonary embolism in high-risk surgical patients. *Can. Med. Assoc. J.*, 127, 990-5.

1. Was a well-defined question posed in answerable form?

___X___ YES   _____ NO   _____ CAN'T TELL

The authors considered both the dollar costs and the effects (deaths due to pulmonary embolism averted) of several strategies for preventing fatal pulmonary embolism in high-risk general surgical patients. The five alternatives compared are stated on p.990, col. 2, of the article; (1) primary prevention with subcutaneous administration of heparin; (2) primary prevention with intravenous administration of dextran; (3) primary prevention with intermittent pneumatic compression of the legs; (4) secondary prevention with iodine 125-labelled fibrinogen leg scanning, and (5) treatment of clinically apparent thromboembolism. The viewpoint for the analysis could have been more explicitly stated. From p.991, paragraph 2, col. 1, it appears that the analytical viewpoint is that of the third-party paying agency responsible for reimbursement of hospital and medical costs in the province of Ontario.

2. Was a comprehensive description of the competing alternatives given?

___X___ YES   _____ NO   _____ CAN'T TELL

The competing alternatives are reasonably well described. Details on the administration of heparin (p.991, col. 1), dextran (p.992, col.1) and leg scanning (p.992, col.1), are provided in subsections of the article which describe the initial strategy and its subsequent investigations. (Unfortunately, the layout of the article headings might confuse a reader, since it appears that this information is being provided under a section entitled Costs of the strategies.) Intermittent pneumatic compression of the legs (p.992, col.1) and treatment of clinically apparent thromboembolism, called traditional (no programme) approach (p.992, col.2), are dealt with similarly though in less detail; however, the authors have provided references for all clinical protocols used. The list of competing alternatives appears complete and, as the authors have stated, option (5) is, in essence, the *do-nothing* alternative. In complex comparisons such as this, it is useful to visualize the comparison in terms of a flow chart of patients or in a decision tree form. It might have been helpful for readers if the authors had done so in this case. An example of such a chart, showing the clinical options and the distribution of patients among the various pathways, was presented earlier in Fig. 5.3. The chart is based on the authors use of an illustrative cohort of 1000 patients in each alternative.

3. Was there evidence that the programmes effectiveness had been established?

   __X__ YES   _____ NO   _____ CAN'T TELL

The authors have addressed the clinical evidence directly (p.992, col.2). Most of the evidence is drawn from well-referenced randomized controlled trials, some from the authors' own setting. It is noted that evidence on the effectiveness of leg scanning and intermittent compression was inferred from knowledge of venous thrombosis and its relationship to fatal pulmonary embolism, since no RCTs with fatal pulmonary embolism as an endpoint exist for these two alternatives. This lack of evidence is taken into account in subsequent analyses. However, it would make the analyses problematic only if either leg scanning or intermittent compression were likely to be *more effective* prophylactic strategies than heparin.

4. Were all important and relevant costs and consequences for each alternative identified?

   __X__ YES   _____ NO   _____ CAN'T TELL

This may be a debatable assessment because the identification of consequences appears to be handled more clearly than that of costs. Deaths due to pulmonary embolism averted are clearly indicated as the effect of interest. Clinical complications of the alternative strategies also are identified, especially the risk of bleeding with heparin and the risk of anaphylactoid reaction and fluid overload with dextran (p993, col.2). Whilst detailed discussion of potential clinical complications is not provided, the authors have referenced their view that more explicit consideration of such complications would not change the basic results of the analysis.

With respect to the range of costs identified, the cost of each strategy is defined as the direct cost of the prophylactic procedure plus the diagnostic and treatment costs of non-fatal venous thromboembolism (p991, col.1). Although further detail is provided in Tables I and II of the article, the description of individual cost components could perhaps be clearer and more comprehensive. For example, it is not possible to ascertain whether capital costs are considered.

Other categories of costs and consequences, such as out-of-pocket costs, indirect costs and indirect benefits to patients, are excluded from the analysis because it has not been performed from a societal viewpoint. However, these would only be of significance if they were higher for primary prophylaxis (especially heparin) than for the traditional approach of waiting to treat clinically apparent venous thromboembolism.

5. Were costs and consequences measured accurately in appropriate physical units?

___X__ YES   _____ NO   _____ CAN'T TELL

The measurement of deaths due to pulmonary embolism averted is straightforward. With respect to costs, the ideal presentation would give both the quantities of all resources used and the unit costs of each resource, prior to multiplying the two and summing across all resources or cost items in order to derive the total cost for any alternative. The authors have attempted to summarize the quantities of resources used in a textual description (p.991-2) and in Tables I and II. Whilst this could perhaps be more thorough, it may be unreasonable to expect journal editors to be interested in a more detailed presentation! The authors have dealt with the issue of shared costs (especially overheads) by separating items used differentially by patients with venous thromboembolism from other hospital cost items, and by measuring the former separately while implicitly accepting average per diem measurements (and values) for the latter. Whilst more sophisticated methods exist for handling this problem, there does not appear to be a compelling case for their use in this instance.

6. Were costs and consequences valued credibly?

_____ YES   _____ NO   __X__ CAN'T TELL

Since the analysis deals (appropriately for the specific clinical focus) with effects measured in natural units, the progression to valuation of these effects in terms of their dollar benefit or utility is not applicable. The reporting of the valuation of costs is handled less adequately than readers might expect, however.

The only statement which deals directly with the issue suggests that costs are derived from the third party and operating costs incurred in a university teaching hospital in Ontario (p.991, col.1). This leaves readers to make at least two assumptions, both of which may be warranted, but which should have been made explicit. They are that; (1) the unit costs of specific items were based upon market values as represented by entries on hospital budgets, reimbursement schedules for specific procedures, or prevailing market prices for the prophylactic agents, and; (2) no significant imputations or adjustments to these values were required for any reason. While possible variations in these values are handled partially in the following sensitivity analysis, more explicit reporting of the valuation procedures would seem appropriate.

7. Were costs and consequences adjusted for differential timing?

_____ YES   __X__ NO   _____ CAN'T TELL

Costs and consequences are not discounted to present values. However, discounting to present values is inappropriate in the context of this study, since all costs and effects relevant to the analysis, as framed by the comparison statement and viewpoint, occur in the present. That is, the analysis is conducted at one point in time, and the analytic horizon, from the beginning of the interventions to their resolution in outcomes of interest, is well inside one year.

8. Was an incremental analysis of costs and consequences of alternatives performed?

__X__ YES   _____ NO   _____ CAN'T TELL

The presentation of the results provided at the bottom of p.992 and top of p.993 does this implicitly. However, the explicit presentation of the incremental analysis could be significantly improved. The increment in effectiveness associated with primary and secondary prophylaxis strategies is the number of deaths due to pulmonary embolism averted. This is found in the text. The increment in cost associated with primary and secondary prophylaxis is the difference in the total cost per 1000 patients between each alternative and the traditional (no-programme) approach. Incremental cost is rather tersely reported in the text at the top of p.993: The traditional approach costs twice as much as subcutaneous heparin prophylaxis and about half as much as intravenous dextran prophylaxis. The incremental analysis probably warrants a separate table, space permitting. An example of such a table was given earlier (Table 5.3). The use of a hypothetical cohort of 1000 patients managed by each of the clinical strategies facilitates considerably the presentation of the results.

9. Was allowance made for uncertainty in the estimates of costs and consequences?

   __ X __ YES   _____ NO   _____ CAN'T TELL

Sensitivity analysis is performed on several variables, as reported in Table III and IV, p.993. No specific justification is provided for the ranges of variables employed. The quite wide variation in cost values does, however, seem to deflect some of the criticism made above, since the study result is relatively robust. Of particular note is the joint possibility that the costs of prophylaxis have been underestimated and hospitalization costs overestimated in the initial analysis, since this would bias the analysis against the traditional (no-programme) approach. Sensitivity analysis on these assumptions simultaneously (Table IV, last column), rather than one-at-a-time as is typically done, showed that heparin became only slightly more costly than the traditional approach, while still saving seven lives.

10. Did the presentation and discussion of study results include all issues of concern to users?

   __ X __ YES   _____ NO   _____ CAN'T TELL

The analysis does not explicitly provide cost-effectiveness ratios for the alternatives; rather, it discusses directly the large incremental effectiveness of heparin and the likely cost saving that would accompany its use. The results are not compared with those of other investigators since this is the initial cost-effectiveness analysis of these methods. Based on the limited task of this analysis and the nature of the recommended strategy of subcutaneous heparin prophylaxis, further issues of generalizability, ethics, distributional considerations such as equity, and implementation would not appear problematic and are, therefore, not addressed in any detail by the authors.

5.4. USE OF QUALITY-OF-LIFE SCALES IN ECONOMIC EVALUATION

In recent years there has been increasing interest in assessing the health consequences of interventions in terms of their impact on quality of life. Indeed, for some conditions, such as arthritis, impact on quality of life might be the primary measure of the effectiveness of therapy. In other conditions, such as cancer, one might be interested in the quality of life during any increased survival from therapy, since many therapies are known to have toxic side effects.

Since improvement in health-related quality of life is one of the main *economic* benefits of treatment, it clearly needs to be incorporated in economic evaluation. In cost-effectiveness analysis the relative costs of treatments are compared with their relative consequences, measured in natural units. Therefore, the question arises as to whether health-related, quality-of-life scales can be used in the denominator of cost-effectiveness analyses, either alone or alongside other measures of the success of therapy, such as life years gained (O'Brien 1994).

5.4.1 Types of health-related, quality of life scales

The different types of quality of life scale have been reviewed by Guyatt *et al.* (1993). There are three main types:

(1) specific measures (e.g. disease-specific, age-specific, etc.),
(2) general health profiles; and
(3) preference-based measures.

Preference-based (or utility measures) are extensively used in cost–utility analysis and will therefore be discussed in Chapter 6. Our interest here is in the potential and problems of using specific measures or general health profiles in economic evaluation. These descriptive measures often do not generate a single index measure, which limits their usefulness to economic analysts.

Specific measures, as the name implies, focus on health outcomes specific to an individual disease, medical condition, or patient population. They usually concentrate on the dimensions (or domains) of quality of life that are most relevant to the disease in question. For example, a disease-specific measure in arthritis is likely to include assessments of pain and mobility.

The main advantages of such measures are that; (1) being focused, they are more likely to be responsive to changes in the patients condition and that; (2) they are likely to be seen as most relevant to patients and physicians and therefore more accepted (for inclusion in a study). Their main disadvantage, from the economist's viewpoint, is that they do not give comprehensive measures of quality of life and therefore cannot be used to compare the cost-effectiveness of programmes in different disease areas. Also, on occasions their focus may be too narrow even to capture fully the relevant dimensions of quality of life in a given disease area. For example, in a comparison of two drugs (say) for arthritis, a specific scale focusing on physical functioning and pain may miss some of the impacts on quality of life caused by side-effects of the medications (e.g. rashes).

General health profiles, on the other hand, *are* comprehensive measures of health-related quality of life. Typically, they include consideration of physical functioning, ability for self-care, psychological status, level of pain or distress, and amount of social integration. Therefore, in principle they can be applied across different patient populations and in different disease areas.

There are now several well-known general health profiles, the most widespread being the Short Form (SF)36, the Nottingham Health Profile, and the Sickness Impact Profile (Brazier 1993). The main advantage of using these scales are that they have been widely applied and have established reliability and validity. However, in some situations they may exhibit a lower responsiveness to change than disease-specific measures.

These instruments are useful in an economic evaluation as supplementary information, but there are several disadvantages from the economist's viewpoint to their use as an outcome measure. First, except for the Sickness Impact Profile, the instruments do not produce a single quality of life score, but rather produce a profile of scores across the different domains of the instrument. (Indeed, some of the developers of general health profiles would regard such aggregation as counter-productive.) This means it is not possible to compare directly an improvement in one dimension with another, or to compare across different programmes that produce outcomes of different types. Secondly, because the scoring for the instruments is not, in general, based on preferences of individuals for the various possible outcomes, it is not clear that higher scores are necessarily associated with outcomes that are more preferred. Thirdly, because the scores for these instruments are not calibrated onto a scale where dead = 0 and healthy = 1, they cannot be used to combine quality of life with quantity of life, as for example, in the quality-adjusted life year (QALY) calculation.

5.4.2 Problems and potential of using quality-of-life scales

Economic evaluations using either specific measures or general health profiles are best regarded as sophisticated examples of cost-effectiveness or cost-consequences analyses. Therefore, they suffer from the limitation, mentioned in Chapter 2, of telling us nothing about the *value* of the health consequences produced, and are most suited to answering more restrictive questions such as Is treatment A or treatment B better for a given category of patients? Even then, some judgements are likely to be required on the part of the decision maker, unless one treatment is superior to the other on all dimensions of quality of life.

When using specific or health profile measures in an economic evaluation the economic analyst should consider the following issues:

(1) is the measure recognised as being clinically relevant in the disease area concerned?
(2) has the measure been validated for use in this disease or on a similar patient population?

(3) is there a widely agreed interpretation of what would constitute a quantitatively important change in the dimension(s) of health-related quality of life being measured?

Finally, whilst specific and health-profile measures may have limited use as effectiveness measures in cost-effectiveness analysis, the information produced may be indirectly relevant to cost–utility analysis (discussed in Chapter 6 below). That is, it may be possible to convert the descriptive quality of life information to a utility or preference-based measure, either by:

(1) mapping health states from a specific or health profile measure onto an established preference-weighted classification (Chancellor *et al.* 1997); or

(2) using the quality of life information gained from the scales to construct scenarios for health state preference valuation.

This potential has been explored by Brazier and Dixon (1995). They concluded that, whilst potential exists, much more research is required. Therefore, in the short term specific or health profile measures are likely to be used alongside the preference-based measures discussed in Chapter 6.

5.5 INTERPRETING INCREMENTAL COST-EFFECTIVENESS RATIOS

In Chapter 3 we pointed out that the appropriate comparison between two health care programmes or interventions was in terms of the *incremental* cost-effectiveness ratio (see Fig 3.2). We also discussed the notion of *dominance*, where one programme could be said to dominate another if its effectiveness were higher and its costs lower.

In this section we discuss the same concepts, but in the context of a more complicated situation, where there are three competing programmes, each of which can be delivered with varying degrees of intensity. For example, suppose we are comparing three treatment programmes for three different groups of 1000 patients each. All three programmes are for life-threatening conditions (e.g. different types of cancer, end stage renal disease, or myocardial infarction), so a simple effectiveness measure, such as life-years saved, can be used for purposes of comparison. Also, more intensive programmes of treatment are more effective in each case, but at increased cost. How would we decide on an efficient allocation of resources among the three programmes if saving life years was our objective?

Tables 5.4 and 5.5, adapted from the paper by Karlsson and Johannesson (1996), give the data on costs, effects and incremental cost-effectiveness ratios for the three programmes. In essence there are 11 alternatives (A-M) to be considered, with the additional alternative (O) of doing nothing. (For simplicity this is assumed to have zero costs and zero effects, although often this is *not* the case.) Also, the various alternatives within each programme are assumed to be mutually exclusive, in that if a patient receives one of the treatments in the programme, they will not receive the others. Additionally, the treatment used in one patient group is assumed to be independent of the treatments used in other groups. That is, the costs and health effects of a treatment in one patient group are not affected by the treatment alternative chosen in any other patient group.

Table 5.4. Cost per patient (C), effectiveness per patient (E) for the available alternatives in each of three treatment strategies. (There are 1000 patients to be treated in each group.)

Treatment strategy I			Treatment strategy II			Treatment strategy III		
Alternative	*C*	*E*	Alternative	*C*	*E*	Alternative	*C*	*E*
A	100	10	F	200	12	K	100	5
B	200	14	G	400	16	L	200	8
C	300	16	H	550	18	M	300	12
D	400	19						
E	500	20						

Adapted from Karlsson and Johannesson (1996)

In Table 5.5 the incremental cost-effectiveness ratios are calculated for each successive alternative, from the least costly to the most. The same data are presented in Fig 5.5. Here the incremental cost-effectiveness ratios are given by the slope of the line joining any two points (alternatives). (This is a development of the idea first presented in Fig 3.2.)

The figure enables us to explore another notion of dominance, called *extended dominance* (Weinstein, 1990). This is where the incremental cost-effectiveness ratio for a given treatment alternative is higher than that of the next, more effective, alternative. There are two cases of extended dominance in Fig 5.5; alternatives C and L. For example, if all 1000 patients were given alternative C, this would cost 300,000 and 16,000 life years would be gained. However, if 500 patients were given alternative B and 500 alternative D, the total cost would still be 300,000 but 16,500 life-years would be gained in total.

Graphically, we can see that points B and D can be connected with a line of lower slope (i.e. lower cost-effectiveness ratio), in essence missing out point C. This is the same as saying that alternative C should be excluded from consideration as it is dominated. The same applies to alternative L. However, it should be noted that this analysis requires two simplifying assump-

Table 5.5. Incremental cost (ΔC), incremental effectiveness (ΔE) and incremental cost-effectiveness ratio ($\Delta C / \Delta E$) per patient for the different treatment alternatives shown in Table 5.4. There are 1000 patients in each patient group

	Treatment strategy I				Treatment strategy II				Treatment strategy III		
Alternative	ΔC	ΔE	$\Delta C/\Delta E$	Alternative	ΔC	ΔE	$\Delta C/\Delta E$	Alternative	ΔC	ΔE	$\Delta C/\Delta E$
A	100	10	10	F	200	12	17	K	100	5	20
B	100	4	25	G	200	4	50	L	100	3	33
C	100	2	50	H	150	2	75	M	100	4	25
D	100	3	33								
E	100	1	100								

Adapted from Karlsson and Johannesson (1996).

tions: (1) that the treatments are perfectly divisible; and (2) that there are constant returns to scale. In other words, it has to be possible to deliver alternatives B and D to smaller numbers of patients without any reduction in cost-effectiveness. In real life this may not be possible and more complicated approaches are needed. (This is discussed further in Chapter 9.)

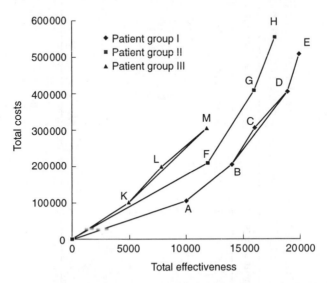

Figure 5.5. Total costs and effectiveness of alternative treatment options (A-M) for the three treatment strategies (each has 1000 patients). (Source: Karlsson and Johannesson 1996)

Finally, this example can be used to determine how a fixed budget could be spent, if the objective is to maximize the number of life years gained. With the budget as the decision making constraint, the choice of treatments depends on the size of the budget. In order to maximize the life years gained for a given budget, we order all the treatments in terms of their incremental cost-effectiveness ratios, starting with the do nothing or status quo option. We then begin by implementing the treatment with the lowest incremental ratio and then add independent treatments or replace mutually exclusive treatments until the budget is exhausted.

Figure 5.6 shows the alternatives that would be adopted, given increased sizes of budget. The steps in the curve indicate the increases in the incremental cost of producing life-years ($\Delta C / \Delta E$) as successive alternatives are added, beginning with A, which has an incremental ratio (over doing nothing) of 10.

Each budgetary limit defines a shadow price of life years gained. For example, if the budget enabled us to adopt alternatives of successively higher incremental cost-effectiveness ratio up to and including G, the implied shadow price would be 50. That is, the implication of setting a budget of this size is that we are not willing to pay more than 50 for a unit of effectiveness. The alternative approach would be to state what we are willing to pay for a unit of effectiveness and to see what size of budget this implies. This approach is sometimes advocated as a decision rule for adoption or rejection of health technologies (Laupacis *et al.*, 1992). However, it raises a number of practical and conceptual issues, which we discuss further in Chapter 9.

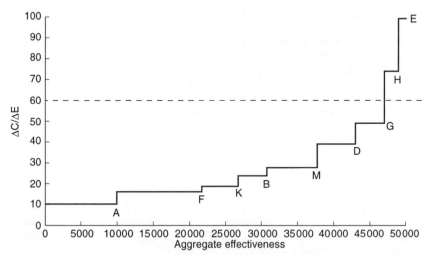

Figure 5.6.   The marginal cost of producing effectiveness (hypothetical treatments A to M) (Source: Karlsson and Johannesson 1996)

5.6 CONCLUDING REMARKS

Cost-effectiveness analysis is a form of full economic evaluation where both costs and consequences are considered. Many of the issues raised in this chapter, such as allowing for uncertainty, discounting of health effects and the ways of combining clinical and resource data, are also pertinent to the other forms of economic evaluation discussed below.

CEA has been very popular to date and is a very useful approach where there is a single unambiguous objective of therapy. However, many health care programmes have multiple objectives or outcomes and the issue of assigning preferences or values to these outcomes becomes central to the evaluation. This issue is tackled in the chapters to follow.

REFERENCES

Adams, M. E., McCall, N. T., Gray, D. T. *et al.* (1992). Economic analysis in randomized control trials. *Medical Care*, **30**, 231–43.
Brazier, J. (1993). The SF-36 Health Survey Questionnaire – a tool for economists. *Health Economics*, **2**(3), 213–15.

— and Dixon, S. (1995). The use of condition specific outcome measures in economic appraisal. *Health Economics*, 4(4), 255–64.

Briggs, A. H. (1995). Handling uncertainty in the results of economic evaluation. OHE Briefing No. 32. Office of Health Economics, September 1995, London.

—, Sculpher, M. J., and Buxton, M. J. (1994). Uncertainty in the economic evaluation of health care technologies: the role of sensitivity analysis. *Health Economics*, 3, 95–104.

—, and Sculpher, M. J. (1995). Sensitivity analysis in economic evaluation: a review of published studies. *Health Economics*, 4(5), 355–71.

Brown, M. L. (1992). Sensitivity analysis in the cost-effectiveness of breast cancer screening. *Cancer* 69 (Suppl. 7), 1963–7.

Bush, J. W. (1973). Discussion. *In Health status indexes* (ed. R. L. Berg). Hospital Research and Educational trust, Chicago.

Cairns, J. (1992). Discounting and health effects for medical decisions. In *Valuing health care: costs, benefits and effectiveness of pharmaceuticals and medical technologies* (ed F. A. Sloan), pp. 123–45. Cambridge University Press, New York.

Chancellor, J., Coyle, D., and Drummond, M. F. (1997). Constructing health state preference values from descriptive quality of life data: mission impossible? *Quality of Life Research*. (In press.)

Cook, D. J., Guyatt, G. H., Laupacis, A., Sackett, D. L. (1992). Rules of evidence and clinical recommendations on the use of antithrombitic agents. *Chest*, 102 (suppl.4), 305S–11S.

Davey, P., Lynch, B., Malek, M., Byrne, D., and Thomas, P. (1992). Cost-effectiveness of single dose cefotaxime plus metronidazole compared with three doses each of cefuroxime plus metronidazole for the prevention of wound infection after colorectal surgery. *J Antimicrobial Chemotherapy*, 39(6); 855–64.

Department of Clinical Epidemiology and Biostatistics (1981). Clinical epidemiology rounds: How to read a clinical journal. V: To distinguish useful from useful or even harmful therapy. *Can. Med. Assoc., J.*, 124; 1156–62.

Detsky, A. S. (1995). Evidence of effectiveness: evaluating its quality. In Sloan F. A. (ed) *Valuing health care*. Cambridge University Press, New York.

Doubilet, P., Weinstein, M. C., and McNeil, B. J. (1986). Use and misuse of the term cost-effective in medicine. *N. Eng. J. Med.*, 314, 253–6.

Drummond, M. F. and Stoddart, G. L. (1984). Economic analysis and clinical trials. *Controlled Clinical Trials*, 5, 115–28.

Drummond, M. F., Davies, L. M. (1991). Economic analysis alongside clinical trials: revisiting the methodological issues. *International Journal of Technology Assessment in Health Care*, 7(4), 561–573.

Fineberg, H. V. (1980). Decision trees: construction, uses, and limits. *Bull Cancer*, 67, 395–404.

Gerard, K., andMooney, G. H. (1993). QALY league tables: handle with care. *Health Economics*, 2(1), 59–64.

Gold, M. R., Siegel, J. E., Russell, L. B., and Weinstein, M. C. (ed.) (1996). *Cost-effectiveness in health and medicine*. Oxford University Press, New York.

Goldsmith, C. H., Gafni, A., Drummond, M. F., Torrance, G. W., and Stoddart, G. L. (1987). Sensitivity analysis and experimental design: the case for economic evaluation of health care programmes. In *Proceedings of the Third Canadian conference on health economics 1986*. (ed. J. M. Horn), pp. 129–48. Department of Social and Preventive Medicine, University of Manitoba, Winnipeg.

Grossman, M. (1972). *The demand for health: a theoretical and empirical investigation* NBER Occasional Paper 119. National Bureau of Economic Research, New York.

Guyatt, G. H., Feeny, D. H., and Patrick, D. L. (1993). Measuring health-related quality of life. *Annals of Internal Medicine* 118; 622–9.

Hillman, A. L. and Bloom. B. S. Economic effects of prophylactic use of misoprostol to prevent gastric ulcer in patients taking nonsteroidal anti-inflammatory drugs. *Archives of Internal Medicine*, **149**, 2061–65. (1989).

Hillner, B. E., Smith, T. J., and Desch, C. E. (1992). Efficacy and cost-effectiveness of autologous bone marrow transplantation in metastatic breast cancer. Estimates using decision analysis while awaiting clinical trial results. *J. A. M. A.*, **267**(15), 2055–61.

Hull, R. D., Hirsh, J., Sackett, D. L., and Stoddart, G. L. (1981). Cost-effectiveness of clinical diagnosis, venography and non-invasive testing in patients with symptomatic deep-vein thrombosis. *N. Engl. J. Med.* **304**, 1561–1567.

—, Hirsh, J., Sackett, D. L., and Stoddart, G. L. (1982). Cost-effectiveness of primary and secondary prevention of fatal pulmonary embolism in high-risk surgical patients. *Can. Med. Assoc. J.* **127**; 990–5.

Jefferson, T., Demicheli, V. (1994). Is vaccination against Hepatitis B efficient? A review of world literature. *Health Economics*, **3**(1), 25–37.

Karlsson, G. and Johannesson, M. (1996). The decision rules of cost-effectiveness analysis. *PharmacoEconomics*, **9**(2), 113–20.

Keeler, E. and Cretin, S. (1983). Discounting of life savings and other non-momentary effects. *Management Science*, **29**(3), 300–6.

Koopmanschap, M. A., Rutten F. F. H., van Ineveld, B. M., and van Roijen, L. (1995). The friction cost method for measuring indirect costs of disease. *J. Health Economics*, 14, 171–89.

Koomanschap, M. A., Rutten, F. F. H. (1996). Indirect costs: the consequence of production loss or increased costs of production. *Medical Care*, **34** (12), suppl., DS59–DS68.

L'Abbe, K. A., Detsky, A. S., O'Rourke, K. (1987). Meta-analysis in clinical research. *Annals of Internal Medicine*, **107**, 224–33.

Laupacis, A., Feeny, D., Detsky, A. S., and Tugwell, P. X. (1992). How attractive does a technology have to be to warrant adoption and utilization? Tentative guidelines for using clinical and economic evaluations. *Can Med Assoc J.*, **146**, 473–81.

Logan, A. G., Milne, B. J., Achber, C., Campbell, W. P., and Haynes, R. B. (1981). Cost-effectiveness of a worksite hypertension treatment programme. *Hypertension*, **3**(2), 211–18.

Magid, D., Schwartz, B., Craft, J., and Schwartz, J. S. (1992). Prevention of Lyme disease after tick bites. A cost-effectiveness analysis. *N. Engl. J. Med.*, **327**(8), 534–541.

Mark, D. B., Hlatky, M. A., Califf, R. M., Naylor, C. D., Lee, K. L., *et al.* (1995). Cost-effectiveness of thrombolytic therapy with tissue plasminogen activator as compared with streptokinase for acute myocardial infarction. *N. Engl. J. Med.*, **332**(21), 1418–24.

Mugford M. (1989). Reducing the incidence of infection after caesarian section: implications of prophylaxis with antibiotics for hospital resources. *British Medical Journal*, **299**, 10003–6.

O'Brien, B. (1994). Measurement of health-related quality of life in the economic evaluation of medicines. *Drug Information J.*, **28**, 45–53.

—, Goeree, R., Mohamed, A. H., and Hunt, R. (1995). Cost-effectiveness of Helicobacter pylori eradication for the long-term management of duodenal ulcer in Canada. *Archives of Internal Medicine*, **155**, 1958–64.

Olsen, J. A. (1994). Production gains: should they count in health care evaluations? *Scottish J. Political Economy*, **41**(1), 69–84.

Oster, G., and Epstein, A. M. (1987). Cost-effectiveness of antihyperlipidemic therapy in the prevention of coronary heart disease: the case of cholestyramine. *J. A. M. A.*, **258**, 2381–7.

Parsonage, M., and Neuburger, H. (1992). Discounting and health benefits. *Health Economics*, **1**, 71–6.

Posnett, J., Jan, S. (1996). Indirect cost in economic evaluation: the opportunity cost of unpaid inputs. *Health Economics*, **5**(1), 13–23.

van Roijen, L., Essink-Bot, M. L., Koopmanschap, M. A., Bonsel, G., Rutten, F. F. H. (1996). Labor and health status in economic evaluation of health care. *International Journal of Technology Assessment in Health Care*, **12**(3), 405–15.

Scandinavian Simvastatin Survival Study Group (1994). Randomised trial of cholesterol lowering in 4444 patients with coronary heart disease. *Lancet*, **344**, 1383–89.

Schulman, K. A., Kinosian, B., Jacobson, J. A., Glick, H., Willian, M. K., Koffer, H., et al. (1990). Reducing high blood cholesterol level with drugs. *J. A. M. A.*, **264**(23), 3025–33.

Sculpher, M. J., and Buxton, M. J. (1993). The episode-free day as a composite measure of effectiveness. *PharmacoEconomics*, **4**(5), 345–52.

—, Drummond, M. F., and Buxton, M. J. (1996). The iterative use of economic evaluation as part of the process of health technology assessment. *J. Health Services Research and Policy*, **1**(4).

Viscusi, W. K. (1995). Discounting health effects for medical decisions. In *Valuing health care: costs, benefits and effectiveness of pharmaceuticals and medical technologies*. Ed. F. A. Sloan, pp. 123–145. New York, Cambridge University Press.

Weinstein, M. C. (1990). Principles of cost-effective resource allocation in health care organizations. *Int J. Technology Assessment in Health Care*, **6**, 93–105.

— and Stason, W. B. (1977). Foundations of cost-effectiveness analysis for health and medical practices. *N. Engl. J. Medi.*, **296**, 716–21.

— and Fineberg, H. V. (1980). *Clinical decision analysis*. W. B. Saunders Company, Philadelphia.

6

Cost–utility analysis

6.1. SOME BASICS

Cost–utility analysis is a form of evaluation that focuses particular attention on the quality of the health outcome produced or averted by health programmes or treatments. It has many similarities to cost-effectiveness analysis, and thus all the points discussed in Chapter 4 on cost analysis and many of those discussed in Chapter 5 on cost-effectiveness analysis also apply here. The first section of this chapter reviews some of the general issues the analyst would need to consider when undertaking a cost–utility analysis. Later sections discuss particular issues in more detail.

6.1.1. How does cost–utility analysis differ from cost-effectiveness analysis?

In cost-effectiveness analysis (CEA), the incremental cost of a programme from a particular viewpoint is compared to the incremental health effects of the programme, where the health effects are measured in natural units related to the objective of the programme, e.g. average blood pressure improvement in mm Hg, cases found, cases of disease averted, patients significantly improved, lives saved, life-years gained. The results are usually expressed as a cost per unit of effect. In cost–utility analysis (CUA), the incremental cost of a programme from a particular viewpoint is compared to the incremental health improvement attributable to the programme, where the health improvement is measured in quality-adjusted life-years (QALYs) gained, or possibly some variant like healthy years equivalent (HYEs). The results are usually expressed as a cost per QALY gained. Thus, there are many similarities between CEA and CUA. For example, the questions of whether or not to include productivity changes (Section 5.1.4) and whether or not to discount future effects (Section 5.1.5) still apply.

CEA and CUA are similar, if not identical, on the cost side, but differ on the outcomes side. As described in Box 6.1, outcomes in CEA are single, programme-specific, and unvalued. In contrast, outcomes in CUA may be single or multiple, are general as opposed to programme-specific, and incorporate the notion of value.

Box 6.1. Why was cost–utility analysis developed?

In cost-effectiveness analysis the outcomes are measured in programme-specific units such as millimetres of blood pressure reduction, disability-days averted, cases cured, lives saved, and life-years gained. Typically the main outcome is designated as the primary effectiveness measure and used as the denominator in the cost/effectiveness ratio. There are three problems. First, because the measure of primary effectiveness may differ from programme to programme, cost-effectiveness analysis cannot be used to make comparisons across a broad set of interventions. Second, in any one programme there is often more than one outcome of interest. In fact, normally there is a large number of relevant outcomes; for example, outcomes of any specific intervention often include life extension, long-term quality of life changes, side effects both major and minor from the intervention, as well as the short-term quality-of-life effects of the intervention itself. Third, some outcomes are more important, or more valued, than others.

Cost–utility analysis was developed to address these problems. It enables a broad range of relevant outcomes to be included by providing a method through which the various disparate outcomes can be combined into a single composite summary outcome. This, in turn, allows broad comparisons across widely differing programs. And, finally, cost–utility analysis provides a method to attach values to the outcomes so the more important outcomes are weighted more heavily.

Both CEA and CUA require valid effectiveness data (from the literature, from your own study, or from expert judgement supplemented by sensitivity analysis), but in the case of CUA only final outcome effectiveness data will suffice (e.g. lives saved, disability-days averted). Intermediate output data (e.g., cases found, patients appropriately treated) are unsuitable, since they cannot be converted into an outcome measure like QALYs gained which is required for CUA. As an aside, intermediate outcomes may well be suitable for clinical decision analysis using a patient's utilities for the intermediate outcomes, but they are simply unsuitable for CUA where the outcomes must be expressed in an outcome measure like QALYs gained.

By converting the effectiveness data to a common unit of measure, like QALYs gained, CUA is able to incorporate simultaneously both the changes in the quantity of life (mortality) and the changes in the quality of life (morbidity). In the QALY approach, the quality adjustment is based on a set of values or weights called utilities, one for each possible health state, that reflect the relative desirability of the health state.

Because of the similarities between CUA and CEA some authors do not distinguish between the two, particularly in the United States. For example, Weinstein and Stason (1977) and Gold *et al.* (1996b) treat cost–utility analysis as a particular case of cost-effectiveness analysis. Thus, be aware in reading the literature that CUA may appear under other labels.

Although technically CUA can be seen as simply a specific type of CEA, we have continued to use the separate label because we believe it is useful for several reasons. First, it clearly distinguishes between those studies that use a generic measure of outcome and thus are potentially comparable across studies (CUA), and those that use a measure of outcome specific to the programme under study (CEA). Second, it highlights the crucial role of consumer preferences (utilities) in valuing the outcomes. Third, because of the need to incorporate consumer preferences, there is much that is special about CUA. And, finally, we have continued with the CUA label to maintain consistency with the first edition, and with much of the field of health economics which has now adopted the distinction. (See Box 6.2. for a brief history of cost–utility analysis.)

Box 6.2 History of cost–utility analysis

In the beginning the approach described in this chapter was not called cost–utility analysis. Because it relaxed the narrow restrictiveness of traditional cost-effective-ness analysis, it was first called generalized cost-effectiveness analysis (Torrance 1971). Later it was called utility maximization (Torrance *et al.* 1972) and the health status index model (Torrance 1976b). The health status index approach was also the initial label used for a similar development from the Bush group at San Diego (Fanshel and Bush 1970; Bush *et al.* 1972). The label 'cost–utility analysis' was first used by our group in 1981 (Sinclair *et al.* 1981) and by the Bush group in 1982 (Kaplan and Bush 1982). Since then the cost–utility label has stuck, except in the United States where many analysts still call it cost-effectiveness.

We adopted the CUA label to distinguish the approach from CEA. The distin-guishing features of CUA are that multiple outcomes can be incorporated and the outcomes are not just counted but are valued according to their desirability. In addition, a distinguishing feature of CUA, as we practise it, is that the relative desirability of outcomes is measured using von Neumann–Morgenstern utility theory. Hence, the origin of the name cost-UTILITY analysis. Although we believe the name is useful, it has caused its own confusion. On the one hand, there are those who correctly point out that, from a theoretical point of view, CUA as conventionally practised, even using von Neumann–Morgenstern utilities as the quality-adjustment weights, would maximize utility only under very restrictive assumptions (Weinstein and Fineberg 1980; Torrance and Feeny 1989; Mehrez and Gafni 1991; Garber and Phelps 1995) and so one might argue the label is misleading. On the other hand, there are many studies, including our own (Oldridge *et al.* 1993), that have used the CUA label regardless of how the quality-adjustment weights were determined (Kaplan and Bush 1982; Kaplan *et al.* 1988; Goel and Detsky 1989; Hall *et al.* 1992; Kennedy *et al.* 1995). Our view is that the CUA label is useful in describing a certain class of studies, and thus helps to communicate. However, use of the label does not guarantee that all studies have used a uniform methodology (Gerard 1992), and readers need to assess for themselves how the study has been conducted.

6.1.2 When should CUA be used?

The following are a number of situations where you might wish to use CUA:

(1) when health-related quality of life is *the* important outcome. For example, in comparing alternative programmes for the treatment of arthritis, no

programme is expected to have any impact on mortality, and the interest is focused on how well the different programmes improve the patient's physical function, social function, and psychological well-being;

(2) when health-related quality of life is *an* important outcome. For example, in evaluating neonatal intensive care for very-low-birth-weight infants, not only is survival an important outcome, but also the quality of that survival is critical;

(3) when the programme affects both morbidity and mortality and you wish to have a common unit of outcome that combines both effects. For example, treatments for many cancers improve longevity and improve long-term quality of life, but decrease quality of life during the treatment process itself.

(4) when the programmes being compared have a wide range of different kinds of outcomes and you wish to have a common unit of output for comparison. For example, if you are a health planner who must compare several disparate programmes applying for funding, such as an expansion of neonatal intensive care, a programme to locate and treat hypertensives, and a programme to expand the rehabilitative services provided to post-myocardial infarction patients;

(5) when you wish to compare a programme to others that have already been evaluated using cost–utility analysis.

6.1.3. When should it not be used?

The following are situations when CUA should not be used:

(1) when only intermediate outcome data can be obtained. For example, in a study to screen employees for hypertension and treat them for one year, Logan *et al.* (1981) used end points of mm Hg blood pressure reduction. Intermediate outcomes of this type cannot be readily converted into QALYs for use in CUA;

(2) when the effectiveness data show that the alternatives are equally effective in all respects of importance to consumers (eg. including side-effects). In this case cost-minimization analysis is sufficient; cost–utility analysis is not needed;

(3) when the effectiveness data show that the new programme is dominant; that is, the new programme is both more effective and less costly (win–win). In this case, no further analysis is needed;

(4) when the extra cost of obtaining and using utility values is judged to be in itself not cost effective. This is the case above in points 2 and 3. It would also be the case even when the new programme is more costly than the old, if effectiveness data show such an enormous superiority for the new programme that the incorporation of utility values could almost certainly not change the result. It might even be the case with a programme that is

more costly and only somewhat more effective, if it can be credibly argued that the incorporation of any reasonable utility values will show the programme to be overwhelmingly cost-effective. Note, however, that this does mean that the new programme could not be compared now or in the future to other programs competing for the same limited funding, because the complete CUA results for this programme would not be available. Moreover, one could argue that you must have performed a rough cost–utility analysis using judgemental utilities in order to reach these conclusions. Finally, with the advent of generic preference-weighted health state classification systems (see Section 6.4), the cost of obtaining and using utility values has been significantly reduced.

6.2. UTILITIES

The term 'utility' has been around for several centuries, has been used by a variety of disciplines, and has a number of related but different meanings (Cooper and Rappoport 1984; Miyamoto 1988; Sen 1991).Thus, it creates a significant potential for confusion and for people to talk past each other. In a broad way the term has always been synonymous with preference; the more preferable an outcome, the more utility associated with it. The differences in meaning arise when approaches are developed to define the concept more precisely and especially when attempts are made to measure it.

Measured preferences may be ordinal or cardinal. For ordinal preferences, outcomes simply need to be rank ordered, with ties allowed, from most preferred to least preferred. For cardinal preferences, a number must be attached to the outcome that in some sense represents the strength of preference for the outcome relative to the others. These numbers should be measured such that they fall on an interval scale, in two senses. First, in terms of measurement theory, the scale should be an interval scale as described later in Section 6.5.2; that is, a scale like temperature in degrees farenheit, that has no natural zero and is unique under a positive linear transformation. Second, in terms of the individual's preferences, the scale must have the equal interval property in the sense that the interval from 0.2 to 0.3 has the same meaning to the individual as the interval from 0.8 to 0.9 (Bossert 1991).

6.2.1. History of utility theories

This is an optional section that readers may skip, if they wish, without loss of continuity.

In 1944, a mathematician, John von Neumann, and an economist, Oscar Morgenstern, first published their theory of rational decision making under uncertainty, now called expected utility theory, or sometimes von Neumann–Morgenstern utility theory (von Neumann and Morgenstern 1944). Interestingly, they developed the theory, not for its own sake, but only because they needed it as a small part of a theory of games they were developing. History now remembers them only secondarily for their contributions to game theory, and primarily for their enormous contribution in developing a theory of decision making that has dominated the field for over half a century.

Box 6.3. Axioms of von Neumann–Morgenstern utility theory

The original axioms of von Neuman and Morgenstern have been refined and restated over the years by various authors. Bell and Farquhar (1986) present the axioms as follows.

Preference exist and are transitive. For any pair of risky prospects y and y' either y is preferred to y', y' is preferred to y or the individual is indifferent between y and y'. In addition, for any three risky prospects, y, y', and y'', if y is preferred to y', and y' is preferred to y'', then y is preferred to y''; similarly, if y is indifferent to y', and y' is indifferent to y'', then y is indifferent to y''.

Independence. An individual should be indifferent between a two-stage risky prospect and its probabilistically equivalent one-stage counterpart derived using the ordinary laws of probability. For example, consider two risky propects y and y', where y is made up of outcome x_1 with probability p_1 and outcome x_2 with probability $(1 - p_1)$, indicated symbolically as $y = \{p_1, x_1, x_2\}$, and $y' = \{p_2, x_1, x_2\}$. This axiom implies that an individual would be indifferent between the two-stage risky prospect $\{p, y, y'\}$, and its probabilistically equivalent one-stage counterpart $\{pp_1+(1 - p)p_2, x_1, x_2\}$.

Continuity of preferences. If there are three outcomes such that x_1 is preferred to x_2, which is preferred to x_3, there is some probability p at which the individual is indifferent between outcome x_2 with certainty or receiving the risky prospect made up of outcome x_1 with probability p and outcome x_3 with probability $1 - p$.

Von Neumann and Morgenstern developed a normative model; that is, they prescribed how a rational individual 'ought' to make decisions when faced with uncertain outcomes. To do this they defined, in a set of fundamental axioms, what they meant by rational behaviour under uncertainty (see Box 6.3). The axioms are compelling, have withstood vigorous debate, and have remained the dominant normative definition of rational behaviour under uncertainty for over half a century. The axioms are certainly not without controversy, and to this day they are constantly under attack with many variations and alternatives being proposed (Allais 1991; Schoemaker 1991; Currim and Sarin 1992; Schoemaker 1992; Tversky and Kahneman 1992; Kleindorfer *et al.* 1993; Wakker *et al.* 1994; Fishburn and Wakker 1995; Cohen 1996; Nease 1996). However, no alternative has dislodged them from their position as the dominant normative paradigm. The axioms of von Neumann and Morgenstern provide the foundation for modern decision theory, which has been widely applied in business, government, health care, and many other fields for several decades. Their work also represented a seminal contribution to the economic theory of behaviour under uncertainty.

It is doubly unfortunate, however, that von Neumann and Morgenstern called their new approach 'utility theory' and called the associated preference measures 'utilities'. First, in their usage, utility did not mean usefulness as it does in normal language. Second, in their usage utility meant neither what it had traditionally meant to economists and philosophers during the nineteenth century nor what it meant to modern economists. In developing consumer theory during the nineteenth century, economists assumed the existence of a cardinal utility function that represented the consumer's satisfaction for various bundles of commodities received with certainty. Nineteenth century philosophers used this concept of utility as the foundation for utilitarian ethics in which utilities among individuals were compared and aggregated to decide on the socially optimal policy. Ultimately, this approach, particularly the comparison and aggregation of these individual utilities, was rejected.

At the turn of the century, the Italian economist, Vilfredo Pareto, discovered that ordinal utilities were sufficient to support consumer theory. More recently, Arrow and Debreu (1954) further refined the theory based on the concept of consumers preference orderings, including risk. As a result, students of microeconomics have been taught that cardinal utility (under certainty) is unnecessary, probably unmeasurable, and may not even exist. For a discussion of this history see Russell and Wilkinson (1979) or Allais (1991). For a discussion of the relationship of von Neumann–Morgenstern utilities within microeconomics see Hey (1979).

The key point here is that cardinal utilities under uncertainty, as defined by von Neumann and Morgenstern, are quite different from both the ordinal utilities underlying contemporary microeconomics and the cardinal utilities (under certainty) of nineteenth-century economists. To avoid these potential confusions, it is frequently recommended that users of modern utility theory under uncertainty refer to their measures as 'von Neumann–Morgenstern (NM) utilities'. Unfortunately, very few writers take this precaution. From this point in the book, unless otherwise specified, we use utility to mean NM utility.

Following the initial work by von Neumann and Morgenstern, the field has expanded rapidly and there is now a vast literature. Some representative books include those by Luce and Raiffa (1957), Raiffa (1968), Holloway (1979), and Keeney and Raiffa (1976; 1993).

It is important to appreciate that the von Neumann–Morgenstern axioms and utility theory are not intended as descriptions of how individuals actually make decisions in the face of uncertainty, but as a prescriptive or normative model of how they 'ought' to make such decisions if they wish to act rationally as defined by the basic axioms. Although there is some evidence that individuals in some circumstances do follow the model (Fischer 1979; Currim and Sarin 1992; Nease 1996), there is much more evidence that they do not (Loomes 1991; Luce 1992).

We should not be surprised that individual behaviour does not necessarily follow a normative model; normative models are not behavioral models. Normative models are used to define approaches that individuals should take to be consistent with underlying theories; behavioral models are used to describe actual behavior as found in reality. As Howard points out, 'the whole idea of a normative model arises when we are not satisfied with our functioning ... [In] view of the many easily demonstrated lapses in human decision making that we can observe, who would want to rely on unaided judgement for a complex and important decision problem?' (1988).

6.2.2. Utility, value, and preference

Many people use the terms 'utility', 'value' and 'preference' interchangeably, but in fact there are differences. Preference is the umbrella term that describes the overall concept; utilities and values are different types of preferences. What you get depends on how you do the measurements (see Table 6.1). There are two key aspects of the measurement process. One is the way in which the question is framed, specifically whether the outcomes in the question are certain or uncertain. The other is the way in which the subject is asked to respond, specifically whether the subject is asked to perform a scaling task based on introspection or to make a choice.

Table 6.1. Methods of measuring preferences

Response method	Question framing	
	Certainty (values)	Uncertainty (utilities)
Scaling	1 Rating scale Category scaling Visual analogue scale Ratio scale	2
Choice	3 Time trade-off Paired comparison Equivalence Person trade-off	4 Standard gamble

Consider a subject being asked preference questions for health outcomes, where each outcome is a specific lifetime path for the subject. That is, each outcome describes a path from now to death consisting of one or more health states for specified time periods. This, in fact, is the most general case of measuring preferences for health outcomes, and all health state preference measurement uses, or should use, this format. Even measuring preferences for single temporary states, such as one week of hospitalization for an acute episode of some disease, cannot be done in isolation of what will follow. What will follow should always be described explicitly, else the subject will implicitly assume something and it will affect the measurement in unknown ways.

A question framed under certainty would ask the subject to compare two or more outcomes and to choose between them or to scale them. In thinking about each outcome, the subject is asked to assume that the outcome would occur with certainty. There are no unknowns and no probabilities in the way the various futures are described. A question framed under uncertainty would ask the subject to compare two alternatives, where at least one of the alternatives contained uncertainty; that is, it contained probabilities. The conventional standard gamble question, described in Section 6.3.2, is a common example. The difference between these two forms of questioning is that the certainty method does not capture the subject's risk attitude, while the uncertainty method does.

Risk attitude is a well-known concept in preference measurements and utility theory (Keeney and Raiffa 1976; Holloway 1979; Gafni and Torrance 1984). The intuitive notion is that if a person shies away from more risky alternatives in favour of less risky alternatives, they are risk averse. If they are indifferent, they are risk neutral, and if they prefer risky situations, they are risk-seeking. Mathematically, the concept can only be operationalized when measuring preferences over outcomes that are themselves defined on an interval scale. Then, the definition is that if the subject prefers the expected value of an uncertain alternative to the uncertain alternative itself, the subject is risk averse; indifference between the two represents risk neutrality; and a preference for the gamble indicates a risk-seeking attitude.

For example, a subject who prefers $100 for sure to a 50/50 gamble of receiving $0 or $200 would be said to be risk averse with respect to money. On the other hand, if the subject was indifferent between the two, he would be risk neutral; and if the gamble was preferred, he would be risk-seeking. Similarly, a subject who rated three health outcomes, A, B, and C, on a visual analogue scale as valued at 0.4, 0.6, and 0.8, who then preferred outcome B for sure to a 50/50 gamble of receiving outcome A or C, would be said to be risk averse with respect to value. As in the case for money, if the subject had been indifferent, he would have been classed as risk neutral; and if he had preferred the gamble, he would be called risk-seeking. Risk attitude with respect to values is sometimes called relative risk attitude (Dyer and Sarin 1979; Dyer and Sarin 1982; Torrance *et al.* 1995) to differentiate it from risk attitudes with respect to fundamental consequences like dollars or years of healthy life.

Note that the risk attitude really only pertains to a specific question. There is no requirement that a person have a consistent risk attitude over multiple questions. For example, it is often found empirically that people are risk averse for large gains, risk-seeking for small gains, and risk-seeking for losses (Holloway 1979; Fischer *et al.* 1986). However, the existence of a consistent risk attitude that can be modelled mathematically is often assumed for practical convenience. For example, the three generic types of relative risk attitude are shown in Fig 6.1. As the figure shows, a person whose relative risk attitude is consistently risk averse over the length of the scale will have utilities (preferences adjusted for risk) that exceed their values (riskless preferences). Empirically, this is the common finding.

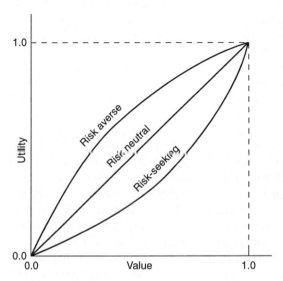

Figure 6.1. The three generic types of relative risk attitude.
Torrance *et al.*, PharmacoEconomics, 7(6), 1996, Fig. 1.

The second dimension of Table 6.1 refers to the response method. A subject can be asked to determine a strength of preference by introspection and to indicate the result on a numerical scale. Alternatively, a subject can be asked to choose between two alternatives, thus revealing the preference indirectly. The first approach is primarily rooted in psychology and psychometric scaling, although it is also described in the field of decision science as a measurable value function (Dyer and Sarin 1979; Dyer and Sarin 1982; Loomes 1995). The second method comes primarily from economics and decision sciences, and is a particular application of the revealed preference approach. (Revealed preference is a general approach in economics whereby the underlying preferences are revealed by the choices that individuals make.) The advantage of scaling is that it takes less respondent time. The advantage of the choice-based methods is that choosing, unlike scaling, is a natural human task at which we all have considerable experience, and furthermore it is observable and verifiable. Thus, many analysts, including ourselves, prefer the choice-based methods in designing studies.

Table 6.1 is divided into four cells. Cell 1 contains instruments that require the subject to think introspectively about outcomes presented with certainty and to provide a rating or a score. Rating scales (assign a number), category scales (assign a category), and visual analogue scales (mark a line) are all variations on the same theme. Ratio scaling, as used by Rosser and colleagues (1978), also belongs in this category. In ratio scaling, subjects were asked to indicate how many times worse one outcome was compared to the next best outcome. The outcomes were defined with certainty and the task was one of introspection. There are no instruments that fall in cell 2 to our knowledge, although presumably one could ask subjects to rate their preferences for gamble alternatives. Cell 3 contains the time trade-off approach (see Section 6.3.3), the paired comparison approach (Streiner and Norman 1989; Hadorn, *et al.* 1992; Hadorn and Uebersax 1995), and the old equivalence approach (Patrick *et al.* 1973; Patrick and Erickson 1993) now renamed the person trade-off approach (Nord *et al.* 1993; Nord 1995; 1996). Finally, cell 4 contains the well-known standard gamble in all its variations (Torrance 1986; Torrance and Feeny 1989; Furlong *et al.* 1990; O'Brien *et al.* 1994; Bennett and Torrance 1996).

To summarize, all of the methods in Table 6.1 measure preferences. Those in cells 1 and 3 measure values; those in cell 4 measure utilities. Because the task is different in each cell, one should not be surprised that the resulting preference scores will differ. Indeed, the common finding is that, for states preferred to death, standard gamble scores are greater than time trade-off scores, which in turn are greater than visual analogue scores (Torrance 1976a; Wolfson *et al.* 1982; Read *et al.* 1984; Churchill *et al.* 1987; Bass *et al.* 1994; Stiggelbout *et al.* 1994; O'Leary *et al.* 1995; Rutten-van Molken *et al.* 1995; Bennett and Torrance 1996). (However, one recent study produced the contrary finding of time trade-off scores exceeding standard gamble scores (Dolan *et al.* 1996a). The reason given for the differences between cells 3 and 4 is risk attitude, which is only captured in cell 4. The reason for the difference between cells 1 and 3 presumably lies in the difference between choosing and scaling.

Which method is best? As indicated earlier, other things being equal, we prefer choice-based methods over scaling methods. In practice, other things are not equal, notably the time required to use the different approaches, and we typically use a mixture of scaling and choice questions (see Section 6.4.4). In choosing between values and utilities we can get some help from the underlying theories. Von Neumann–Morgenstern utility theory indicates that utilities are appropriate for problems that involve uncertainty *or* certainty or both; note that outcomes with certainty can be included as a degenerate probability distribution (that is, a probability distribution with a single outcome that has a probability of 1.0). On the other hand, again based on the underlying theory, values are *only* appropriate for problems that involve certainty; thus, values are much more restricted in their applicability. Another way to think of it is that only utilities capture the individual's risk attitude and this is essential for problems that contain uncertainty. Hence we, and most researchers (Mehrez and Gafni 1991; Gold *et al*. 1996b), argue that because future health outcomes are clearly uncertain in the real world, the preferences measured under uncertainty (utilities) are the more appropriate. It should be noted, however, that these theoretical arguments are technically only valid at the individual level. Von Neumann–Morgenstern utility theory only covers individual decision-making, and once we aggregate the utilities across the respondents and use the results to inform societal decision making, the theory no longer directly applies. On the other hand, the theory would apply if we assume that society is a single individual with utilities equal to the mean utilities of the community. Finally, cells 3 and 4 are similar with respect to time and complexity of the methods. So, on balance, we recommend utilities rather than values.

As a final caveat, users of economic evaluation studies and preference-scored health status classification systems should be aware that all of these methods are in use. Users should check carefully to determine what method was used in studies or pre-scored instruments of interest to them, and to ensure that the method suits their purpose.

6.3. MEASURING PREFERENCES

The various methods for measuring preferences are summarized briefly in this section, and a simulated interview of the three main instruments is provided in Annex 6.1. Further descriptions of most of the methods are available in the literature. A detailed technical manual describing how to build and use standard gamble boards, time trade-off boards, and feeling thermometers (visual analogue scales) is available (Furlong *et al*. 1990). A video demonstrating an interview using these instruments can also be obtained (O'Brien *et al*. 1994). The book by Spilker (1996) contains descriptions of the standard gamble, the time trade-off, and visual analogue scales in Chapters 12 and 27. The book by Gold *et al*. (1996b) contains a brief summary of a variety of measurement approaches in Chapter 6. A journal article covering the three main techniques is also available (Torrance 1986).

The three most widely used techniques to measure directly the preferences of individuals for health outcomes are the rating scale and its variants, the standard gamble, and the time trade-off. These three are summarized below.

6.3.1. Rating scale, category scaling, visual analogue scale

The simplest approach to measuring preferences is to ask subjects first to rank health outcomes from most preferred to least preferred, and second, to place the outcomes on a scale such that the intervals or spacing between placements correspond to the differences in preference as perceived by the subject. That is, outcomes that are almost equally desirable would be placed close together while outcomes that are very different in desirability would be placed far apart. The subject should be instructed to concentrate on these intervals and comparisons of one interval to another, rather than on the scores themselves. The purpose is to encourage the subject to produce an interval scale of preferences. Note, because ratios of scale values are meaningless in an interval scale it is inappropriate for subjects to make comparisons like 'outcome A is twice as desirable as outcome B and so I will place it twice as high on the scale'. The correct comparisons are ones like, 'the difference in desirability between outcomes A and B is twice as great as the difference between C and D, hence I will make the interval between A and B twice as large'.

There are a number of variations on the rating scale approach. The scale can have numbers (eg. 0–100), categories (eg. 0–10), or just consist of a 10 cm line on a page. The different variations often have different names. Rating scale usually refers to a scale of numbers, often 0-100. Category rating or category scaling is the variation that consists of a small number of categories, often 10 or 11, that the subject is to assume to be equally spaced. Visual analogue scaling consists of a line on a page, often 10cm in length, with clearly defined endpoints and with or without other marks along the line. Sometimes several techniques are combined. For example, many of the studies from McMaster University use a 'feeling thermometer' which is a combination of visual analogue scale and rating scale (Furlong *et al.* 1990; Bennett and Torrance 1996; Feeny *et al.* 1996).

Preferences for chronic states can be measured on a rating scale. The chronic states are described to the subject as irreversible; that is, they are to be considered permanent from age of onset until death. The subject must be provided with the age of onset and the age of death, and these should be the same for all states that are measured together relative to each other in one batch. States with different ages of onset and/or ages of death can be handled by using multiple batches. Two additional chronic states are added to each batch as reference states for the scale – healthy (from age of onset to age of death) and death (at age of onset).

The subject is asked to select the best health state of the batch, which presumably would be 'normal healthy life' and the worst state, which may or may not be 'death at age of onset'. He or she is then asked to locate the other states on the rating scale relative to each other such that the distances between the locations are proportional to his or her preference differences. The rating scale is measured between 0 at one end and 1 at the other end. If death is judged to be the worst state and placed at the 0 end of the rating scale, the preference value for each of the other states is simply the scale value of its placement. If death is not judged to be the worst state but is placed at some intermediate point on the scale, say d, the preference values for the other states are given by the formula $(x - d)/(1 - d)$, where x is the scale placement of the health state.

Preferences for temporary health states can also be measured on a rating scale. Temporary states are described to the subject as lasting for a specified duration of time at the end of which the person returns to normal health. As with chronic states, temporary states of the same duration and same age of onset should be batched together for measurement. Each batch should have one additional state, 'healthy', added to it. The subject is then asked to place the best state (healthy) at one end of the scale and the worst temporary state at the other end. The remaining temporary states are located on the scale such that the distances between the locations are proportional to his or her preference differences.

If the programmes being evaluated involve only morbidity and not mortality and if there is no need to compare the findings to programmes that do involve mortality, the procedure described above for temporary health states is sufficient. However, if this is not the case, the interval preference values for the temporary states must be transformed onto the standard 0-1 health preference scale. This can be done by redefining the worst temporary health state as a chronic state of the same duration, and measuring its preference value by the technique described for chronic states. The values for the other temporary health states can then be transformed onto the standard 0–1 dead-healthy scale by a positive linear transformation (just like converting $^\circ$ F to $^\circ$ C).

Scores from a rating scale give the investigator a firm indication of the ordinal rankings of the health outcomes, and some information on the intensity of those preferences. However, rating scales are subject to measurement biases, and the empirical findings are that when compared to preferences measured by the standard gamble or the time trade-off; the rating scale scores are not an interval scale of preferences (Torrance 1976a; Torrance *et al.* 1982; Torrance *et al.* 1996b). Notable biases that seem to be at work are the end-of-scale bias in which subjects tend to shy away from using the ends of the scale, and the spacing out bias in which subjects tend to space out the outcomes over the scale regardless of the outcomes (Bleichrodt and Johannesson, 1997). Empirical findings indicate that rating scale scores can be converted to standard gamble or time trade-off scores by using a power curve conversion (Torrance 1976a; Torrance *et al.* 1982; Torrance *et al.* 1996b). Thus, one approach is to use the rating scale method, which is quick and efficient, and to convert the resulting scores to utilities by a suitable power curve conversion. A second approach, which is not mutually exclusive, is to use the rating scale task primarily as a warm up for subjects, to familiarize them with the descriptions of the outcomes, and to have them begin to think hard about their preferences prior to measuring the important preferences by some other technique.

6.3.2. Standard gamble

The standard gamble is the classical method of measuring cardinal preferences. It is based directly on the fundamental axioms of utility theory, first
presented by von Neumann and Morgenstern (1944) – see Box 6.3. In fact, the
standard gamble method is a direct application of the third axiom in Box 6.3.
The method has been used extensively in the field of decision analysis, and
good descriptions of the methods are available in books in this field; for
example, see Holloway (1979).

The method can be used to measure preferences for chronic states but
the method varies somewhat depending upon whether or not the chronic
state is preferred to death or considered worse than death. For chronic
states preferred to death the method is displayed in Fig. 6.2. The subject
is offered two alternatives. Alternative 1 is a treatment with two possible
outcomes: either the patient is returned to perfect health and lives for an
additional t years (probability p), or the patient dies immediately
(probability 1 – p). Alternative 2 has the certain outcome of chronic
state *i* for life (*t* years). Probability p is varied until the respondent is
indifferent between the two alternatives, at which point the required
preference score for state i for time t is simply p; that is, $h_i = p$.
Here, h_i is measured on a utility scale where perfect health for t years
is 1.0 and immediate death is 0.0.

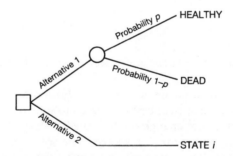

Figure 6.2.   Standard gamble for a chronic health state preferred to death.

Since most subjects cannot readily relate to probabilities, the standard
gamble is often supplemented with the use of visual aids, particularly a
probability wheel (Torrance 1976a; Furlong *et al.* 1990). This is an adjus-
table disk with two sectors, each of different colour, and constructed so that
the relative size of the two sectors can be readily changed. The alternatives are
displayed to the subject on cards, and the two outcomes of the gamble
alternative are colour-keyed to the two sectors of the probability wheel.
The subject is told that the chance of each outcome is proportional to the
similarly coloured area of the disk.

Preferences for temporary health states can be measured relative to each other using the standard gamble method as shown in Fig. 6.3. Here intermediate states i are measured relative to the best state (healthy) and the worst state (temporary state j). Note, that all states must last for the same duration, say t, followed by a common state, usually healthy. In this format the formula for the utility of state i for time t is $h_i = p + (1 - p)h_j$, where i is the state being measured and j is the worst state. Here h_i is measured on a utility scale where perfect health for duration t is 1.0. If death is not a consideration in the use of the utilities, h_j can be set equal to zero and the h_i values determined from the formula which then reduces to $h_i = p$. However, if it is desired to relate these values to the 0–1 dead-healthy scale, the worst of the temporary states (state j) must be redefined as a short duration chronic state for time t followed by death and measured on the 0-1 scale by the technique described above for chronic states. This gives the value for h_j for time t which can then, in turn, be used in above formula to find the value for h_i for time t.

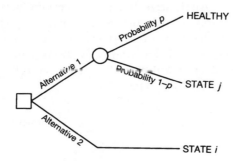

Figure 6.3.   Standard gamble for a temporary health state.

Variations on this method are also possible. For example, in Fig. 6.3 state j can be the state considered next best compared to state i, rather than being the worst state. This does not change the formula $h_i = p + (1 - p)h_j$ but it does mean that the h values for the states have to be solved in sequence, starting with the worst state. This variation is used in the simulated interview in Section 6.8 of this chapter.

6.3.3. Time trade-off

The time trade-off (TTO) method was developed specifically for use in health care by Torrance *et al.* (1972). It was originally developed as a simple, easy-to-administer instrument that gave comparable scores to the standard gamble (Torrance 1976a). Subsequently, its theoretical properties have been explored (Mehrez and Gafni 1990), and further empirical work indicates that TTO scores require adjustment before they can be used as von Neumann–Morgenstern utilities.

The application of the time trade-off technique to a chronic state considered better than death is shown in Fig. 6.4. The subject is offered two alternatives:

(1) state i for time t (life expectancy of an individual with the chronic condition) followed by death;
(2) healthy for time x < t followed by death.

Time x is varied until the respondent is indifferent between the two alternatives, at which point the required preference score for state i is given $h_i = x/t$.

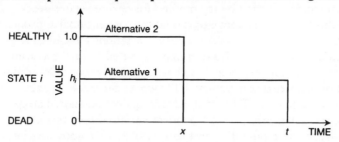

Figure 6.4.   Time trade-off for a chronic health state preferred to death.

Preferences for temporary health states can be measured relative to each other using the time trade-off method as shown in Fig. 6.5. As with the rating scale and the standard gamble, intermediate states i are measured relative to the best state (healthy) and the worst state (temporary state j). The subject is offered two alternatives:

(1) temporary state i for time t (the time duration specified for the temporary states), followed by healthy;
(2) temporary state j for x < t, followed by healthy.

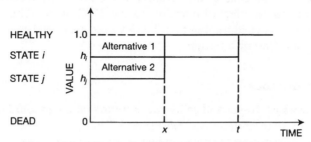

Figure 6.5.   Time trade-off for a temporary health state.

Time x is varied until the respondent is indifferent between the two alternatives, at which point the required preference score for state i is $h_i = 1-(1 - h_j)x/t$. If we set $h_j = 0$, this reduces to $h_i = 1 - x/t$. Figure 6.5 shows the basic format, but other variations are possible. State j need not be the worst state as long as it is any state worse than i. In using variations, however, care must be taken to ensure that all preference values can be calculated. In one systematic variation which has been used (Torrance *et al.* 1972; Torrancc 1976a; Sackett and Torrance 1978), state j is always the next worse state to state i. This variation is used in the simulated interview in this section. Although the formula is still the same, $h_i = 1 - (1 - h_j)x/t$, the states must now be solved in sequence from worst to best.

Finally, as with the rating scale and the standard gamble, if the preference scores for the temporary states are to be transformed to the 0–1 dead-healthy scale, the worst of the temporary states must be redefined as a short duration chronic state and measured by the method for chronic states described above.

The methods described above represent the conventional approach to TTO as developed by Torrance and colleagues. Variations have been suggested by others. Buckingham and colleagues experimented with three approaches to trading off time: conventional TTO where the respondent trades against unwanted premature death, annual TTO where the trade is against unwanted convalescence, and daily TTO with a trade against unwanted sleep. Based on ease of use and relationship to independent variables they recommended daily TTO. However, one potential problem with this recommendation is that if the TTO scores are used for calculating QALYs, they are in fact being used to represent trade-offs between living states and death, and it would seem that scores based on trades against death would be more appropriate for the task.

Cook and colleagues investigated the second stage of using TTO for temporary states (Cook *et al.* 1994). This is the stage where the worst temporary state is redefined as a short term chronic state followed by death and measured using the method for chronic states. They were concerned that the imminence of death in such a scenario would inappropriately distort the result. Accordingly, in an application where the short duration was 12 weeks, they chose to present the state at two longer durations, 12 months and 12 years, in part to determine if the duration would affect the results. To their surprise there was no effect of duration on the TTO score. Although this is only one study, it is encouraging that TTO scores measured at one duration also apply to a different duration.

6.3.4. Other methods

In the early work of Rosser and colleagues a 'ratio scaling' method was used to measure health state preferences (Rosser and Kind 1978). The method took advantage of the fact that the disability scale could be considered a ratio scale with perfect health representing a natural zero of no disability. Then each successively more undesirable disability was compared to the next better one, and the subject was asked how many times worse it was. The result was computed into a ratio scale of disability (x) and converted to an interval scale of preference (y) through the conversion $y = 1 - x$. This was the source of the scores for the original Rosser Index (Rosser and Kind 1978; Rosser and Watts

1978). Interestingly, the scores were very different from those obtained from the traditional instruments (Buxton and Ashby 1988). To our knowledge, the ratio scaling method has never been used since.

In the early work of the San Diego group that developed the Quality of Well-Being scale a preference measurement technique was used called 'equivalence' in which respondents were asked to state how many patients in the designated state of health should have their lives extended by one year in order to be equivalent to extending the lives of 100 healthy patients by one year (Patrick *et al.* 1973; Patrick and Erickson 1993) They reported that the technique gave similar values to their main technique, category scaling. Accordingly, there has been little further interest in the approach until recently. Now the approach has been revived under a new name, person trade-off (Nord *et al.* 1993; Nord 1995; Nord 1996). Nord reports that person trade-off (PTO) results do not match the results from traditional techniques like rating scale, standard gamble, and time trade-off and that the differences can be quite large. Moreover, Nord argues that the PTO scores are more appropriate for use in resource allocation, because they are based directly on the trade-offs that society considers appropriate. On the other hand, the traditional scores are based directly on the trade-offs that each person considers appropriate for themselves, while the PTO scores are based on trade-offs considered appropriate for others in general. The issue of which approach is best for resource allocation is currently unresolved, and may in the end be unresolvable other than by fiat. Further research and debate no doubt will enlighten the situation, but ultimately the choice between the two approaches hinges less on analytical correctness than it does on normative values.

6.4. MULTI-ATTRIBUTE HEALTH STATUS CLASSIFICATION SYSTEMS WITH PREFERENCE SCORES

Measuring preferences for health outcomes, as described in the previous section, is a very time consuming and complex task. A recent alternative that is very attractive and being widely used is to bypass the measurement task by using one of the pre-scored multi-attribute health status classification systems that exist. Currently there are three main systems available: Quality of Well-Being (QWB), Health Utilities Index (HUI), and EuroQol (EQ-5D), although others may well be developed.

In this section we first describe the applicable theory, multi-attribute utility theory, and then the three main systems.

6.4.1. Multi-attribute utility theory

Traditional von Neumann–Morgenstern utility theory was extended to cover multi-attribute outcomes by Keeney and Raiffa (1976). To accommodate the extension they had to add one additional assumption to the three axioms of utility theory. This assumption is that the utility independence among the attributes can be represented by at least first-order utility independence, and perhaps by stronger utility independence (mutual utility independence, additive independence). This is best explained by example. Consider the Health Utilities Index Mark 2 (HUI2) which is a multi-attribute health status classification system consisting of the following six core attributes: sensation, mobility, emotion, cognition, self-care, pain. Each attribute in turn consists of four or five levels of specified impairment from no impairment to full impairment. See Section 6.4.4 for a full description of the system.

First-order utility independence implies that there is no interaction (synergism or antagonism) between preferences among levels on any one attribute and the fixed levels for the other attributes. An example would be the case where level 3 mobility has a utility of 0.6 on the mobility subscale, regardless of the health status levels on the other attributes. The mobility subscale is the single attribute utility function for mobility, scaled such that the best level of mobility is 1.0 and the worst level of mobility is zero. Note that the overall weight for mobility could change on the basis of health status on the other attributes, and thus the overall effect of changes in mobility could change without violating first-order utility independence. For example, a change from level 1 mobility to level 3 mobility could reduce overall utility by 0.2 if that were the only health status deficit, but by less than 0.2 if the individual already had other major health status deficits. All that is required for first-order utility independence is that the relative scaling *within* the mobility subscale stays constant.

Mutual utility independence is a stronger assumption. It requires that there be no interaction between preferences for levels on *some* attributes and the fixed levels for other attributes. This characteristic must hold for all possible subsets of attributes. An example of mutual utility independence would be the case where level 2 on sensation coupled with level 3 on mobility has a utility of 0.7 on the sensation–mobility subscale, regardless of the health status levels on the other attributes. The sensation–mobility subscale is the subscale for these two attributes combined, such that the worst level on sensation coupled with the worst level of mobility is zero and the best level on sensation coupled with the best level on mobility is 1. Note that the weight of this subscale for sensation and mobility could change given different health status on other attributes, so that the overall impact of changes within sensation and mobility could differ without violating mutual utility independence. For example, a change from level 1 on sensation and level 1 on mobility to level 2 on sensation and level 3 on mobility could reduce overall utility by 0.25 if those were the only deficits, but by less than 0.25 if the individual already had other major deficits. What is required for mutual utility independence is that the relative scaling *within* the sensation–mobility subscale stays constant.

Additive utility independence implies that there is no interaction for preferences among attributes at all. That is, the overall preference depends only on the individual levels of the attributes and not on the manner in which the levels of the different attributes are combined. An example of additive independence would be the case where a change from level 1 mobility to level 3 mobility would reduce the overall utility by 0.2 regardless of the levels on the other attributes.

The three independence assumptions lead to three different multi-attribute functions. The simplest assumption, first order utility independence, leads to the most complex mathematical function, the multi-linear function. The second possible assumption, mutual utility independence, leads to the multiplicative function. The strongest assumption (most difficult to fulfil), additive independence, leads to the simplest function, the additive function. See Box 6.4 for the three multi-attribute utility functions.

Box 6.4. Types of multi-attribute utility functions

Additive:

$$u\ (x) = \sum_{j=1}^{n} k_j\ u_j\ (x_j)$$

where $\sum_{j=1}^{n} k_j = 1$

Multiplicative:

$$u\ (x) = (1/k)\ [\prod_{j=1}^{n}\ (1+k\ k_j\ u_j\ (x_j)) - 1]$$

where $(1+k) = \prod_{j=1}^{n}\ (1+k\ k_j)$

Multilinear:
$$u\ (x) = k_1\ u_1(x_1) + k_2\ u_2(x_2) + \ldots$$
$$+ k_{12}\ u_1(x_1)\ u_2(x_2) + k_{13}\ u_1(x_1)\ u_3(x_3) + \ldots$$
$$+ k_{123}\ u_1(x_1)\ u_2(x_2)\ u_3(x_3) + \ldots$$
$$+ \ldots$$
where the sum of all *K*'s equals 1.

Hybrid:
Various hybrid models are possible, based on hierarchically nested subsets of attributes.

Notation: $u_j(x_j)$ is the single attribute utility function for attribute j.
  $u(x)$ is the utility for health state x, represented by an n-element vector.
  k and k_j are model parameters.
  Σ is the summation sign.
  Π is the multiplication sign.

The multiplicative model contains the additive model as a special case. In fitting the multiplicative model, if the measured k_j sum to 1, then k=0 and the additive model holds.

6.4.2. Quality of Well-Being (QWB)

The QWB scale (Kaplan and Anderson 1988; Kaplan and Anderson 1996) classifies patients according to four attributes: mobility, physical activity, social activity, and symptom-problem complex. If the patient has multiple symptoms or problems, the one the patient finds to be most undesirable is used. The scoring function is based on category scaling measurements on a random sample of the general public. Thus the scores are values, not utilities. Respondents were asked to rate a single day in the various states on a scale anchored by death and perfect health. The resulting scoring function is on the 0.0 (death) to 1.0 (full health) preference scale. The original QWB was time consuming to use, taking about 15 minutes for a patient to be classified, but a shorter version is being developed.

The full system and scoring function is shown below in Tables 6.2 and 6.3.

6.4.3. EuroQol (EQ-5D)

The EuroQol Group, a consortium of investigators in Western Europe, initially developed a system with six attributes: mobility, self-care, main activity, social relationships, pain, and mood (EuroQol Group 1990). Subsequently it was revised to include five attributes: mobility, self-care, usual activity, pain/discomfort, anxiety/depression (Essink-bot *et al.* 1993; Brooks 1996; Kind 1996). Each attribute has three levels: no problem, some problems, major problems, thus defining 243 possible health states, to which has been added 'unconscious' and 'dead' for a total of 245 in all. Preferences for the scoring function were measured with the time trade-off technique on a random sample of approximately 3000 members of the adult population of the United Kingdom (Dolan *et al.* 1995; Dolan *et al.* 1996b). The scores fall on the 0.0 (dead) to 1.0 (perfect health) value scale.

The full system and scoring function is shown below in Tables 6.4 and 6.5.

6.4.4. Health Utilities Index (HUI)

There are three HUI systems: HUI1, HUI2, and HUI3. Each system consists of a health status classification system and one or more scoring formulae. In all cases the scores are preference-based, interval-scaled, and on the 0.0 (dead) to 1.0 (perfect health) scale. Scores are derived from preferences of members of the general public. The systems were developed over time, each building in part on the previous one.

HUI1 was based in part on the QWB system and contains four attributes: physical function including mobility and physical activity, role function including self-care and role activity, social–emotional function including emotional well-being and social activity, and health problem. Preference scores were measured using the time trade-off technique on a random sample of

Table 6.2. Quality of Well-Being classification system

PART 1. Quality of Well-Being/general health policy model: function scales with step definitions and calculating weights.

Step no.	Step definition	Weight
	Mobility Scale (MOB)	
5	No limitations for health reasons	–.000
4	Did not drive a car, health related; did not ride in a car as usual for age (younger than 15 yr), health related, and/or did not use public transportation, health related; or had or would have used more help than usual for age to use public transportation, health related	–.062
2	In hospital, health related	–.090
	Physical Activity (PAC)	
4	No limitations for health reasons	–.000
3	In wheelchair, moved or controlled movement of wheelchair without help from someone else; or had trouble or did not try to lift, stoop, bend over, or use stairs or inclines, health related; and/or limped, used a cane, crutches, or walker, health related; and/or had any other physical limitation in walking, or did not try to walk as far or as fast as other the same age are able, health related.	–.060
1	In wheelchair, did not move or control the movement of wheelchair without help from someone else, or in bed, chair, or couch for most or all of the day, health related	–.077
	Social Activity Scale (SAC)	
5	No limitations for health reasons	–.000
4	Limited in other (e.g., recreational) role activity, health related	–.061
3	Limited in major (primary) role activity, health related	–.061
2	Performed no major role activity, health related, but did perform selfcare activities	–.061
1	Performed no major role activity, health related, and did not perform or had more help than usual in performance of one or more selfcare activities, health related	–.106

PART 2. Quality of Well-Being/general health policy model: symptom/problem complexes (CPX) with calculating weights

CPX no.	CPX definition	Weights
1	Death (not on respondent's card)	–.727
2	Loss of consciousness such as seizure (fits), fainting, or coma (out cold or knocked out)	–.407
3	Burn over large areas of face, body, arms, or legs	–.387
4	Pain, bleeding, itching, or discharge (drainage) from sexual organs – does not include normal menstrual (monthly) bleeding	–.349
5	Trouble learning, remembering, or thinking clearly	–.340
6	Any combination of one or more hands, feet, arms, or legs either missing, deformed (crooked), paralyzed (unable to move), or broken – includes wearing artificial limbs or braces	–.333
7	Pain, stiffness, weakness, numbness or other discomfort in chest, stomach (including hernia or rupture), side, neck, back, hips, or any joints or hands, feet, arms, or legs	–.299
8	Pain, burning, bleeding, itching, or other difficulty with rectum, bowel movements, or urination (passing water)	–.292
9	Sick or upset stomach, vomiting or loose bowel movement, with or without chills, or aching all over	–.290
10	General tiredness, weakness, or weight loss	–.259
11	Cough, wheezing, or shortness of breath, with or without fever, chills, or aching all over	–.257
12	Spells of feeling, upset, being depressed, or of crying	–.257
13	Headache, or dizziness, or ringing in ears, or spells of feeling hot, nervous, or shaky	–.244
14	Burning or itching rash on large areas of face, body, arms, or legs	–.240
15	Trouble talking, such as lisp, stuttering, hoarseness, or being unable to speak	–.237
16	Pain or discomfort in one or both eyes (such as burnign or itching) or any trouble seeing after correction	–.230
17	Overweight for age and height or skin defect of face, body, arms, or legs, such as scars, pimples, warts, bruises, or changes in colour	–.188
18	Pain in ear, tooth, jaw, throat, lips, tongue, several missing or crooked permanent teeth – includes wearing bridges or false teeth, stuffy, runny nose; or any trouble hearing – includes wearing a hearing aid	–.170
19	Taking medication or staying on a prescribed diet for health reasons	–.144
20	Wore eyeglasses or contact lenses	–.101
21	Breathing smog or unpleasant air	–,101
22	No symptoms or problem (not on respondent's card)	–.000
23	Standard symptom/problem	–.257
X24	Trouble sleeping	–.257
X25	Intoxication	–.257
X26	Problems with sexual interest or performance	–.257
X27	Excessive worry or anxiety	–.257

Note: x indicates that a standardized weight is used.

Adapted from Kaplan and Anderson 1996, Tables 1 and 2.

Table 6.3.   Quality of Well-Being scoring formula

	Calculating formulas	

Formula 1. Point-in-time well-being score for an individual (W):

$$W = 1 + (CPXwt) + (MOBwt) + (PACwt) + (SACwt)$$

where *wt* is the preference-weighted measure for each factor
and CPX is symptom/problem complex. For example, the
W score for a person with the following description
profile may be calculated for one day as:

CPX-11	Cough, wheezing, or shortness of breath, with or without fever, chills, or aching all over	–.257
MOB-5	No limitations	–.000
PAC-1	In bed, chair, or couch for most or all of the day, health related	–.077
SAC-2	Performed no major role activity health related, but did perform self-car	–.061

$$W = 1 + (-.257) + (-.000) + (-.077) + (-.061) = .605$$

Formula 2. Well-years (WY) as an output measure:

$$WP = [\text{No. of persons} \times (CPXwt + MOBwt + PACwt + SACwt) \times \text{Time}]$$

Adapted from Kaplan and Anderson 1996, Table 1.

parents living in the City of Hamilton and obtained from the Hamilton Board
of Education. States worse than death were measured as a negative score. The
value scoring formula is a multiplicative multi-attribute preference function,
on the 0.0 (dead) to 1.0 (perfect health) scale, with some states taking on
negative scores (see first edition of this book for the HUI1 system and scoring
formula). The system was originally developed for the evaluation of outcomes, including long-term outcomes, of neonatal intensive care (Torrance *et
al.* 1982; Boyle *et al.* 1983), but was later used more broadly (Gold *et al.*
1996*a*).

The HUI system was further extended, initially for paediatric applications, by
Cadman and colleagues (Cadman *et al.* 1986). As part of their study, 84 parent
and child pairs rated attributes for importance and the results identified six
attributes that constitute the core of health-related quality of life: sensory and
communications ability (comprising vision, hearing, and speech); happiness;
self-care ability; pain or discomfort; learning and school ability; and physical
activity ability. These six attributes formed the core of the HUI2 system. The
initial application of the HUI2 system was in childhood cancer, and accordingly,
the levels on the attributes were described appropriately for children and an
additional attribute, fertility, was added that was specific to the disease and its
treatment (Feeny *et al.* 1992; Feeny *et al.* 1995; Torrance *et al.* 1995; Torrance *et
al.* 1996*b*). Subsequently, the HUI2 system has been modified for adult
applications. In addition, the fertility attribute can be easily dropped from
both the classification system and from the scoring formula, if not needed.

Table 6.4 EuroQol classification system

Mobility
1. No problems walking
2. Some problem walking about
3. Confined to bed

Self-care
1. No problems with self-care
2. Some problems washing or dressing self
3. Unable to wash or dress self

Usual activities
1. No problems with performing usual activities (e.g. work, study, housework, family or leisure activities)
2. Some problems with performing usual activities
3. Unable to perform usual activities

Pain/discomfort
1. No pain or discomfort
2. Moderate pain or discomfort
3. Extreme pain or discomfort

Anxiety/depression
1. Not anxious or depressed
2. Moderately anxious or depressed
3. Extremely anxious or depressed

Note: For convenience each composite health state has a five digit code number relating to the relevant level of each dimension, with the dimensions, always listed in the order given above. Thus 11223 means:
1 No problems walking about
1 No problems with self-care
2 Some problems with performing usual activities
2 Moderate pain or discomfort
3 Extremely anxious or depressed

Dolan, Gudex, Kind and Williams 1995, Figure 1.

Preferences for the HUI2 scoring function were measured on a random sample of parents of schoolchildren in the City of Hamilton and surrounding district using both a visual analogue technique and a standard gamble instrument. Thus, both value and utility functions are available, although the utility function is the one recommended for most applications. States worse than death were identified, but were scored as equal to death. The scoring formula is a multiplicative multi-attribute utility function, with scores that fall on the 0.0 (dead) to 1.0 (perfect health) scale.

The HUI3 classification system was based closely on that of the HUI2. The application-specific attribute, fertility, was dropped. The sensory attribute of

Cost-utility analysis

Table 6.5.   EuroQol scoring formula

Coefficients for TTO tariffs

DIMENSION	COEFFICIENT
Constant	0.081
Mobility	
level 2	0.069
level 3	0.314
Self-care	
level 2	0.104
level 3	0.214
Usual activity	
level 2	0.036
level 3	0.094
Pain/discomfort	
level 2	0.123
level 3	0.386
Anxiety/depression	
level 2	0.071
level 3	0.236
N3	0.269

Dolan, Gudex, Kind and Williams (1995), Table 1.

EuroQol TTO scores are calculated by subtracting the relevant coefficients from 1.000. The constant term is used if there is any dysfunction at all. The N3 term is used if any dimension is at level 3. The term for each dimension is selected based on the level of that dimension. The algorithm for computing the tariff is quite straightforward. For example, consider the state 11223:

Full health	= 1.000
Constant term (for any dysfunctional state)	− 0.081
Mobilty (level 1)	− 0
Self-care (level 1)	− 0
Usual activities (level 2)	− 0.036
Pain or discomfort (level 2)	− 0.123
Anxiety or depression (level 3)	− 0.236
N3 (level 3 occurs within at least one dimension)	− 0.269
Therefore, the estimated value for 11223	= 0.255

HUI2 was expanded in HUI3 into the three attributes: vision, hearing and speech. The remaining changes were made to increase the structural independence (orthogonality) of the attributes. An attribute is structurally independent of other attributes if it is conceivable for an individual to function at any level on that attribute, regardless of the levels on the other attributes. If all attributes are structurally independent of each other, all combinations of levels in the system are possible. This goal has been achieved in the HUI3. Structural independence is not only useful for the descriptive classification system, but it greatly simplifies the estimation of the scoring function.

Preferences for the HUI3 were measured on a random sample of general population adults living in the City of Hamilton using both a visual analogue technique and a standard gamble instrument. States worse than death were measured as negative scores on the 0.0 (dead) to 1.0 (perfect health) scale. Both a multiplicative model and a multi-linear model are being estimated.

Shown below are the HUI2 system (Table 6.6), the HUI2 scoring formula (Table 6.7) and the HUI3 system (Table 6.8). The HUI3 scoring formula is still under development. An exercise on calculating HUI scores is provided in Box 6.5.

To use the system, researchers must describe the health states of subjects according to an HUI classification system, and then use the corresponding scoring formula. For clinical studies or population studies, questionnaires have been developed for self administration or interviewer administration to collect sufficient data to classify the patient or subject into both the HUI2 and the HUI3. The questionnaire takes under 10 minutes for self administration and only two to three minutes for interviewer administration, and are available in an increasing number of languages.

6.5. QUALITY-ADJUSTED LIFE-YEARS (QALY)

One of the key features of conventional CUA is its use of the QALY concept; results are reported in terms of cost per QALY gained.

6.5.1. What is the QALY concept?

The concept of the QALY was first introduced in 1968 by Herbert Klarman and colleagues in a study on chronic renal failure (Klarman *et al.* 1968). They noted that the quality of life with a kidney transplant was better than that with dialysis, and estimated that it was 25% better. The cost per life-year gained by the different treatment options was calculated with and without this quality adjustment. Although they did not use the term 'quality-adjusted life-year', the concept was identical.

As was first mentioned in Chapter 2, the advantage of the QALY as a measure of health outcome is that it can simultaneously capture gains from reduced morbidity (quality gains) and reduced mortality (quantity gains), and combine these into a single measure. Moreover, the combination is based on

Table 6.6 Health Utilities Index mark 2 classification system

Attribute	Level	Level description
Sensation	1	Ability to see, hear, and speak normally for age
	2	Requires equipment to see or hear or speak
	3	Sees, hears, or speaks with limitations even with equipment
	4	Blind, deaf, or mute
Mobility	1	Able to walk, bend, lift, jump, and run normally for age
	2	Walks, bends, lifts, jumps, or runs with some limitations but does not require help
	3	Requires mechanical equipment (such as canes, crutches, braces, or wheelchair) to walk or get around independently
	4	Requires the help of another person to walk or get around and requires mechanical equipment as well
	5	Unable to control or use arms and legs
Emotion	1	Generally happy and free from worry
	2	Occasionally fretful, angry, irritable, anxious, depressed, or suffering "night terrors"
	3	Often fretful, angry, irritable, anxious, depressed, or suffering "night terrors"
	4	Almost always fretful, angry, irritable, anxious, depressed
	5	Extremely fretful, angry, irritable, anxious, or depressed usually requiring hospitalization or psychiatric institutional care
Cognition	1	Learns and remembers schoolwork normally for age
	2	Learns and remembers schoolwork more slowly than classmates as judged by parents and/or teachers
	3	Learns and remembers very slowly and usually requires special educational assistance
	4	Unable to learn and remember
Self-care	1	Eats, bathes, dresses, and uses the toilet normally for age
	2	Eats, bathes, dresses, or uses the toilet independently with difficulty
	3	Requires mechanical equipment to eat, bathe, dress, or use the toilet independently
	4	Requires the help of another person to eat, bathe, dress, or use the toilet
Pain	1	Free of pain and discomfort
	2	Occasional pain. Discomfort relieved by non-prescription drugs or self-control activity without disruption of normal activties
	3	Frequent pain. Discomfort relieved by oral medicines with occasional disruption of normal activities
	4	Frequent pain, frequent disruption of normal activities. Discomfort requires prescription narcotics for relief
	5	Severe pain. Pain not relieved by drugs and constantly disrupts normal activities
Fertility[1]	1	Able to have children with a fertile spouse
	2	Difficulty in having children with a fertile spouse
	3	Unable to have children with a fertile spouse

[1]Fertility attribute can be deleted if not required. Contact developers for details.
Torrance *et al.* 1996, *Medical Care*, **34**, Table 1.

Table 6.7. Health Utilities Index mark 2 scoring formula

Sensation		Mobility		Emotion		Cognition		Self-care		Pain		Fertility	
x_1	b_1	x_2	b_2	x_3	b_3	x_4	b_4	x_5	b_5	x_6	b_6	x_7	b_7
1	1.00	1	1.00	1	1.00	1	1.00	1	1.00	1	1.00	1	1.00
2	0.95	2	0.97	2	0.93	2	0.95	2	0.97	2	0.97	2	0.97
3	0.86	3	0.84	3	0.81	3	0.88	3	0.91	3	0.85	3	0.88
4	0.61	4	0.73	4	0.70	4	0.65	4	0.80	4	0.64		
		5	0.58	5	0.53					5	0.38		

Formula:
$u^* = 1.06(b_1 \times b_2 \times b_3 \times b_4 \times b_5 \times b_6 \times b_7) - 0.06$
where u^* is the utility of the health state on a utility scale where dead has a utility of 0.00 and healthy has a utility of 1.00. Because the worst possible health state was judged by respondents as worse than death, it has a negative utility of -0.03. The standard error of u^* is 0.015 for measurement error and sampling error, and 0.06 if model error is also included.
x_i is attribute level code for attribute i; b_i is level score for attribute i.
Torrance *et al.*, (1996), *Medical Care*, 34, Table 8.

the relative desirability of the different outcomes. A simple example is displayed in Fig 6.6. Without the intervention the individual's health-related quality of life would deteriorate according to the lower path and the person would die at time Death 1. With the intervention the person would deteriorate more slowly, would live longer, and would die at time Death 2. The area between the two curves is the QALY gained by the intervention. For instructional purposes the area can be divided into two parts, A and B, as shown. Part A is the amount of QALY gained due to quality improvement (the gain in health-related quality of life during the time that the person would have otherwise been alive anyhow) and part B is the amount of QALY gained due to quantity improvement (the amount of life extension but factored by the quality of that life extension).

Much more complicated cases can be handled. The paths may cross each other. For example, many cancer treatments cause a QALY loss in the short term in order to achieve a QALY gain in the longer term. The paths may be identical for a long time after the intervention and only diverge in the distant future. An example of this pattern could be a hypertension drug that is well tolerated and has no side-effects but eventually averts serious cardiovascular events. The paths may be probabilistic. Often the paths are not precisely known; rather the probabilities are known for the various adverse and beneficial events. In this case the QALY gained can be calculated using the probabilities to determine one or more of the following: the mean, variance, and probability distribution for the QALY gained.

6.5.2. What are the quality weights?

To operationalize the QALY concept, as described above, one needs quality weights that represent the health-related quality of life of the health states under consideration. These quality weights are the scale for the vertical axis in Fig 6.6. The instruments that we have just discussed in Sections 6.3 and 6.4 are used to obtain the required weights.

Table 6.8. Health Utilities Index mark 3 classification system

Attribute	Level	Level description
Vision	1	Able to see well enough to read ordinary newsprint and recognize a friend on the other side of the street, without glasses or contact lenses.
	2	Able to see well enough to read ordinary newsprint and recognize a friend on the other side of the street, but with glasses
	3	Able to read ordinary newsprint with or without glasses but unable to recognize a friend on the other side of the street, even with glasses
	4	Able to recognize a friend on the other side of the street with or without glasses but unable to read ordinary newsprint, even with glasses
	5	Unable to read ordinary newsprint and unable to recognize a friend on the other side of the street, even with glasses
	6	Unable to see at all
Hearing	1	Able to hear what is said in a group conversation with at least three other people, without a hearing aid
	2	Able to hear what is said in a conversation with one other person in a quiet room without a hearing aid, but requires a hearing aid to hear what is said in a group conversation with at least three other people
	3	Able to hear what is said in a conversation with one other person in a quiet room with a hearing aid, and able to hear what is said in a group conversation with at least three other people with a hearing aid
	4	Able to hear what is said in a conversation with one other person in a quiet room without a hearing aid, but unable to hear what is said in a group conversation with at least three other people even with a hearing aid
	5	Able to hear what is said in a conversation with one other person in a quiet room with a hearing aid, but unable to hear what is said in a group conversation with at least three other people even with a hearing aid
	6	Unable to hear at all
Speech	1	Able to be understood completely when speaking with strangers or friends
	2	Able to be understood partially when speaking with strangers but able to be understood completely when speaking with people who know me well
	3	Able to be understood partially when speaking with strangers or people who know me well
	4	Unable to be understood when speaking with strangers but able to be understood partially by people who know me well
	5	Unable to be understood when speaking to other people (or unable to speak at all)

Table 6.8. *contd*

Attribute	Level	Level description
Ambulation	1	Able to walk around the neighborhood without difficulty, and without walking equipment
	2	Able to walk around the neighborhood with difficulty; but does not require walking equipment or the help of another person
	3	Able to walk around the neighborhood with walking equipment, but without the help of another person
	4	Able to walk only short distances with walking equipment, and requires a wheelchair to get around the neighborhood
	5	Unable to walk alone, even with walking equipment. Able to walk short distances with the help of another person, and requires a wheelchair to get around the neighborhood
	6	Cannot walk at all
Dexterity	1	Full use of two hands and ten fingers
	2	Limitations in the use of hands or fingers, but does not require special tools or help of another person
	3	Limitations in the use of hands or fingers, is independent with use of special tools (does not require the help of another person)
	4	Limitations in the use of hands or fingers, requires the help of another person for some tasks (not independent even with use of special tools)
	5	Limitations in use of hands or fingers, requires the help of another person for most tasks (not independent even with use of special tools)
	6	Limitations in use of hands or fingers, requires the help of another person for all tasks (not independent even with use of special tools)
Emotion	1	Happy and interested in life
	2	Somewhat happy
	3	Somewhat unhappy
	4	Very unhappy
	5	So unhappy that life is not worthwhile
Cognition	1	Able to remember most things, think clearly and solve day to day problems
	2	Able to remember most things, but have a little difficulty when trying to think and solve day to day problems
	3	Somewhat forgetful, but able to think clearly and solve day to day problems
	4	Somewhat forgetful, and have a little difficulty when trying to think or solve day to day problems
	5	Very forgetful, and have great difficulty when trying to think or solve day to day problems
	6	Unable to remember anything at all, and unable to think or solve day to day problems
Pain	1	Free of pain and discomfort
	2	Mild to moderate pain that prevents no activities
	3	Moderate pain that prevents a few activities
	4	Moderate to severe pain that prevents some activities
	5	Severe pain that prevents most activities

Box 6.5 Exercise: Health Utilities Index

In the HUI2 system (Table 6.6), the health state of an individual is described as a six or seven element vector with each element denoting the level on an attribute. For example, 1321221 would be an individual who was at level 1 sensation, level 3 mobility, level 2 emotion, level 1 cognition, level 2 self-care, level 2 pain, and level 1 fertility. Because the fertility attribute is optional in the system, if only six elements are specified they refer to the first six attributes.

The utility score for a health state is determined using the formula from Table 6.7. If only six elements are specified, b_7 is omitted from the formula (or equivalently, b_7 is set equal to 1).

1. Determine the HUI2 utility score for the following health states:
(a) 1321221
(b) 2132113
(c) 111111
(d) 112114
(e) 332325

Answers: 0.72, 0.62, 1.00, 0.57, 0.17.

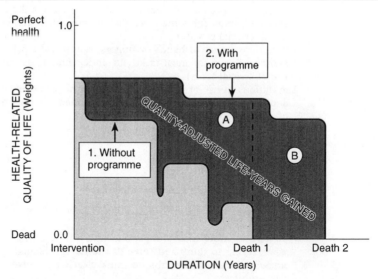

Figure 6.6. Quality-adjusted life years gained from an intervention.
Torrance, Chap. 114 in Spilker, 1996, Fig. 1.
Also, Chap. 4 in Gold et al., 1996, Fig. 4.2.

To satisfy the QALY concept, as described in the previous section, the quality weights must be (a) based on preferences, (b) anchored on perfect health and death, and (c) measured on an interval scale.

The QALY weights for health states should be based on preferences for the health states. This way the more desirable (more preferred) health states receive greater weight and will be favoured in the analysis. Other potential approaches to assigning QALY weights, such as the impact of the health state on earnings, the impact of the health state on health care utilization, the prevalence of the health state in the population, or psychometric scaling techniques are not appropriate for identifying those outcomes that are better or more desirable and differentiating from those that are worse or less desirable.

The scale of QALY weights may contain many points, but two points that must be on the scale are perfect health and death. These two are required because they will both occur in programmes being evaluated with the QALY model, and weights will be required for them. Because these two must always be on the scale, and because they are well specified and understood, they have been selected to be the two anchor points (actually, a better term would be reference points) for the interval scale of QALY weights. This is akin to selecting the freezing point and the boiling point of water to be the anchor points for the interval scale of temperature. To define an interval scale of QALY weights, death and perfect health can be given any two arbitrary values as long as the value for death is smaller than the value for perfect health. The pair of values could be (32, 212), (0, 100), (-5.9, 2.3), (0, 1) or whatever, and the resulting scale would be an interval scale of QALY weights. However, one pair of scores stands out as particularly convenient (death = 0 and perfect health = 1), and this has become the conventional scale for QALY weights. Note, this still allows states worse than death, which would have scores less than zero, and indeed states better than perfect health, if they exist, which would have scores greater than one.

There are a number of reasons why zero and one are particularly convenient scores to assign to death and perfect health respectively. First, take death. Because death is a permanent state, if any score other than zero were used for death, it would mean that in all analyses the (non-zero) death score would be assigned to the state of death for each year off into the future for as long as the death lasted (ie. forever). Thus, the analyses would have streams of numeric outcomes going to infinite – not a pretty picture. Accordingly, zero is the only practical score that can be used for death. Now, take perfect health. The advantage of using one for perfect health is that the resulting QALY is then measured in units of 'perfect health years' (ie. one year in perfect health = 1 QALY, half a year in perfect health = 0.5 QALY, one year in a health state with a QALY weight of 0.5 = 0.5 QALY, and so on). Indeed, at least one agency uses Years of Healthy Life (YHL) as the term for the concept being described here (see Box 6.6).

Scales of measurement can be nominal (eg. colours: red, blue, green), ordinal (eg. size: small, medium, large, extra large, extra extra large), or cardinal (eg. length: in metres; or temperature: in ° C). Cardinal scales can be interval (eg. temperature) or ratio (eg. length). The difference between these two is that the ratio scale has an unambiguous zero point that indicates there is absolutely none of the phenomenon being measured. For example, if something has a length of zero, it has no length. However, if something has a temperature of zero, it still has a temperature. A convenient memory aid that lists the types of scales in increasing order of their mathematical properties is the French word for black, NOIR, standing for Nominal, Ordinal, Interval, Ratio.

Box 6.6. QALY and aliases

In the beginning the composite summary outcome measure was not called quality-adjusted life years (QALY). The concept first appeared in 1970 under the term *function years* (Fanshel and Bush 1970). Two years later, in an application to tuberculin testing, the same group mentioned, as an aside, that function years gained are equivalent to 'additional quality-adjusted years of life' (Bush *et al.* 1972). In our early work it was originally called the *index day* (Torrance 1971) and then the *health day* (Torrance *et al.* 1972), and the health status unit day and health status unit year (Torrance 1976b). The term *quality-adjusted life year* with its well-known acronym *QALY* was first popularized by a landmark 1977 paper from Harvard University, published in the *New England Journal of Medicine* (Weinstein and Stason 1977).

Note that all QALYs are not the same. Weights may be based on standard gamble utility measurements, time trade-off value measurements, visual analogue scale value measurements, estimates by physicians or researchers, or preference weighted systems like the Health Utilities Index, the Quality of Well-Being, or the EuroQol-5D. When weights are based on measured preferences, the preferences may be measured on patients, on the general public, or on some other group. The QALY can be constructed in the conventional way by adding up its parts, or can be determined in a holistic way by measuring utilities for paths of health states.

QALYs also go by other names. The United States National Centre for Health Statistics use the term Years of Healthy Life (YHL) (Erickson *et al.* 1995), while Statistics Canada uses Health-Adjusted Person Years (HAPY) and Health-Adjusted Life Expectancy (HALE) (Berthelot *et al.* 1996).

Because it has an absolute zero, a ratio scale is unique under a positive multiplicative transformation. This means that any ratio scale can be multiplied by any positive constant and the result is still a ratio scale of the same phenomenon, just in different units. This property is used, for example, to convert feet to yards, or metres to miles. Because it has no natural zero, an interval scale is unique under a positive linear transformation. This means that any interval scale x can be transformed to a scale y using a function $y = a + bx$, where a can be any constant and b can be any positive constant. The result will still be an interval scale of the same phenomenon, but in different units and with a different zero. This property is used to convert degrees F to degrees C.

An interval scale has the property that ratios of intervals have meaning, but ratios of scale quantities do not. In a ratio scale both types of ratios have meaning. For example, with temperature, the interval scale property means that it is correct to state that the gain in temperature in going from 40° F to

80° F is twice as much as the gain in going from 40° F to 60° F, but it is incorrect to state that 80° F is twice as hot as 40° F. The former statement holds true whether the temperature is measured in ° F or ° C, while the latter does not. Conversely, in length, it is both correct to state that the gain in length from 40 metres to 80 metres is twice as much as the gain from 40 metres to 60 metres, and that 80 metres is twice as long as 40 metres. Both statements remain true whether the lengths are measured in metres, inches, miles, fathoms, light-years, or any other unit of length.

At first glance it may seem that a scale of health-related quality of life does have a natural zero at death. After all, death represents no health-related quality of life. The problem here is that there can be states worse than death (Torrance *et al.* 1982; Torrance 1984; Patrick *et al.* 1994), and these states require a score for their health-related quality of life. Thus, death is not the bottom of the scale. In fact, there is no well defined bottom of the scale. Conventionally, as discussed above, death is assigned a zero score and states worse than death take on negative scores. This is akin to the temperature at which water freezes being assigned 0° C and temperatures colder than that are then negative.

Alternatively, it may seem that if you reverse the scale so that perfect health has a score of zero and death has a score of one, there would be a natural zero at perfect health. Such a scale would represent health-related reductions in quality of life, and numerically would be obtained by taking one minus the scale of health-related quality of life. For example, a state with a score of 0.8 on the conventional scale would have a score of 0.2 on the reductions scale. A state worse than death with a score of -0.1 on the conventional scale would have a score of 1.1 on the reductions scale. If perfect health can be considered to be a natural zero for the reductions scale, the reductions scale would qualify as a ratio scale as opposed to an interval scale. This assumption was invoked in the original scaling work of Rosser and colleagues (Rosser and Kind 1978; Rosser and Watts 1978) who used a ratio scaling technique to measure reductions in health-related quality of life. Subjects ranked states in order of severity, and then went down the list comparing each state to the next less severe one. Specifically, for each pair they asked 'how many times more ill is a person described as being in state 2 as compared with state 1?' (Rosser and Kind 1978). Finally, the subject was asked to place death on the scale.

Many students of this field have been confused by the seemingly contradictory statements by Rosser and colleagues that the measurements are on a ratio scale and by others like ourselves that the scale is not a ratio scale and the measurements are on an interval scale. The fact is that there are two different scales. The scale of health-related quality of life is an interval scale, and is not a ratio scale. The scale of reductions in health-related quality would be a ratio scale if perfect health is a natural endpoint of the scale at the upper end, and this assumption was invoked in the ratio scaling method of Rosser and colleagues.

Finally, it is useful to note that for economic evaluation an interval scale is required for the QALY weights, but an interval scale is all that is required. First, an interval scale is required because it is important that intervals of equal length on the scale have equal interpretation, and this is the fundamental nature of an interval scale. That is, it is important that a gain from 0.2 to 0.4 on the scale represents the same increase in desirability as a gain from 0.6 to 0.8. This is required because in the QALY calculations those two types of gains will appear equal.

Second, an interval scale is all that is required; there is no need to have a ratio scale. There are two reasons. First, because an interval scale is a type of cardinal scale, all parametric statistical calculations are allowed; e.g. mean, standard deviation, t-test, analysis of variance, etc. Second, because all economic evaluations are comparative, the analysis is always dealing with differences between the programme and the comparator, and all mathematical manipulations on differences (intervals) are valid with an interval scale. That is, it is valid to take ratios of differences (the incremental QALYs gained in programme A are twice those of programme B), and to use the differences in other ratios (the incremental cost per incremental QALY for programme A is one-third of that for programme B), as well as to perform the statistical tests (the incremental QALYs gained in programme A are not statistically significantly different from those gained in programme B at the 5% level).

6.5.3. How are QALYs calculated?

Conceptually, the QALY calculation is very straightforward. Referring to Fig 6.6, the incremental QALYs gained is simply the area under path 2 less the area under path 1. The area under a path can be thought of as the sum of the areas under each component health state on the path, where the area under a health state is the duration of the health state in years, or fraction of a year, multiplied by the quality weight for the health state. This is the QALYs gained without discounting.

Because individuals, and society, generally prefer gains of all types, including health gains, to occur earlier rather than later, future amounts are multiplied by a discount factor to account for this time preference. Recent guidelines have recommended various discount rates, for example 5% (Canadian Coordinating Office for Health Technology Assessment 1994; Haddix *et al.* 1996; Torrance *et al.* 1996a) and 3% (Gold *et al.* 1996b). The technique of discounting, as applied to costs, is described in detail in Chapter 4. The method is the same when applied to QALYs. Essentially the method consists of taking the amounts that will occur in future years and moving them year by year back to the present, reducing the amount each year by r% of the remaining amount, where r% is the annual discount rate.

Examples of QALY calculations with and without discounting are shown in Boxes 6.7 and 6.8.

Box 6.7. Exercise: simple QALY calculations

The following exercise will give you practice in calculating QALYs in simple cases. Once you have mastered these examples you will be able to handle much more complicated cases by simply following the same principles. In solving these problems you should always begin by sketching a QALY diagram to clarify the calculations required. A QALY diagram is a sketch like Fig 6.6 that shows the health-related quality of life path taken by the patient with the programme and the path without the programme. The solutions are given in Box 6.8, but try not to look ahead until you have either solved the problems or given up in total frustration.

Questions 1–4 are taken from the first edition of the book. They are still good exercises although the clinical content and the utility scores may be somewhat dated. The only change we made to these questions is to change the discount rate to 5%, which is more consistent with contemporary standards. Questions 5–7 are new in this edition.

In order to calculate QALYs you need two pieces of data: (1) the path of health states and the duration of each health state over the time span for which QALYs are to be calculated, and (2) the preference weights for the health states for the same durations (see Section 6.5.2). The preference weights for questions 1–4 are shown below and came from TTO measurements on a random sample of the general public (Sackett and Torrance 1978). The preference weights for questions 5–7 are shown in Table 6.7.

Part (b) of some questions involves discounting. For discounting methods see Chapter 4. For discounting purposes assume that all health gains or losses that occur throughout a year take place at the beginning of the year.

Preference Weights for Questions 1–4

Duration	Health state	Weight
3 months	Hospital dialysis	0.62
3 months	Home confinement for tuberculosis	0.68
8 years	Home dialysis	0.65
8 years	Mastectomy for breast cancer	0.48

1. Sketch the QALY diagram and determine how many QALYs are gained if a person achieves an eight-year life extension on home dialysis,
   (a) assuming no discounting
   (b) assuming discounting at a rate of 5 per cent per annum.

2. Sketch the QALY diagram and determine how many QALYs are gained if a person achieves a three-month life extension on hospital dialysis,
   (a) assuming no discounting
   (b) assuming discounting at 5 per cent per annum.

3. Sketch the QALY diagram and determine how many QALYs are gained by preventing a case of tuberculosis which would have been treated at home for three months,
   (a) assuming no discounting
   (b) assuming discounting at 5 per cent.

4. Assume a breast-cancer patient will become symptomatic, have a mastectomy, and live an additional six years. By screening, you can detect the breast cancer one year earlier, perform the mastectomy one year earlier, and add two years to the patient's life (that is, she now lives nine years from the mastectomy instead of

six). Sketch the QALY diagram and determine how many QALYs are gained by screening,
(a) assuming no discounting
(b) assuming discounting at 5 per cent.

5. Sketch the QALY diagram and determine how many QALYs are achieved during the year by a patient in a one year clinical trial who has a baseline HUI2 health state of 133114, a six month HUI2 health state of 122112, and a one-year HUI2 health state of 112111. Assume that health status changes between measurements are smooth and gradual over time so that changes in utility scores can be approximated by a straight line.

6. Suppose the patient in question 5 was the typical patient in the treatment group, and the typical patient in the control group has a baseline HUI2 health state of 133114, a six month HUI2 health state of 132113 and a one year HUI2 health state of 132113. Sketch the QALY diagram for the two patients and determine the QALYs gained over the year for the treatment patient compared to the control patient.

7. In actually implementing the HUI in a clinical trial the patient is asked to think of her health-related quality of life over a defined recall period and to answer the HUI questions accordingly. Redo questions 5 and 6 assuming the interviews were done precisely at months 0, 6 and 12, the recall period was 4 weeks, and thus the HUI2 score from each interview represents the average health-related quality of life during the recall period.

6.5.4. Alternatives to QALYs

The QALY concept is not without controversy. For a sample of the current debate, see the following references (Carr-Hill 1991; Carr-Hill and Morris 1991; Spiegelhalter *et al.* 1992; Broome 1993; Nord 1993; Williams 1995) plus the material in this section. The critics range from those who argue that the QALY approach is needlessly complex and should be replaced by simpler disaggregated measures (Cox *et al.* 1992) to those who claim that the QALY approach is overly simplistic and should be replaced by more complex methods (Mehrez and Gafni 1989, 1991, 1992). Several alternatives to QALYs have been suggested, and the following two are described briefly below: healthy-years equivalents and saved-young-life equivalents.

Healthy-year equivalents (HYE) have been proposed as a theoretically superior alternative to QALYs, but one that is more challenging to execute (Mehrez and Gafni 1989, 1991, 1992). An example of HYE measurement is given in Box 6.9. Essentially, the HYE approach, as proposed by Mehrez and Gafni, differs from the conventional approach to QALYs in two respects. First, it measures the preferences over the entire path (also called profile) of health states through which the individual would pass, rather than for each state alone. Second, it measures the preferences using a two-stage standard gamble measurement procedure that first measures the conventional utility for the path and then measures the number of healthy years that would give the same utility (see Box 6.9).

Box 6.8. Solutions: Simple QALY Calculations

These are the solutions for the exercises in Box 6.7.

1.

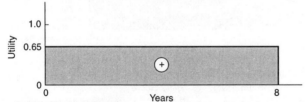

(a) 0.65 x 8 = 5.2 QALYs
(b) 0.65 x (5.7864 + 1.0000) = 4.4 QALYs

2.

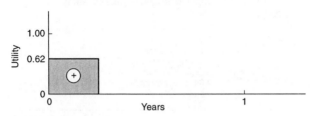

(a) 0.62 x 0.25 = 0.16 QALY
(b) 0.62 x 0.25 = 0.16 QALY

3.

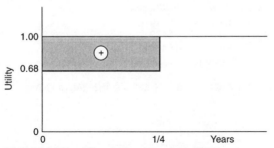

(a) (1.00-0.68) x 1/4 = 0.32 x 1/4 = 0.08 QALY
(b) (1.00-0.68) x 1/4 = 0.32 x 1/4 = 0.08 QALY

4.

(a) 0.48 x 2 − (1 − 0.48) x 1 = 0.96 − 0.52 = 0.44 QALY
(b) 0.48 x 0.7107 + 0.48 x 0.6768 − 0.52 x 1.00 = 0.67 − 0.52 = 0.15 QALY

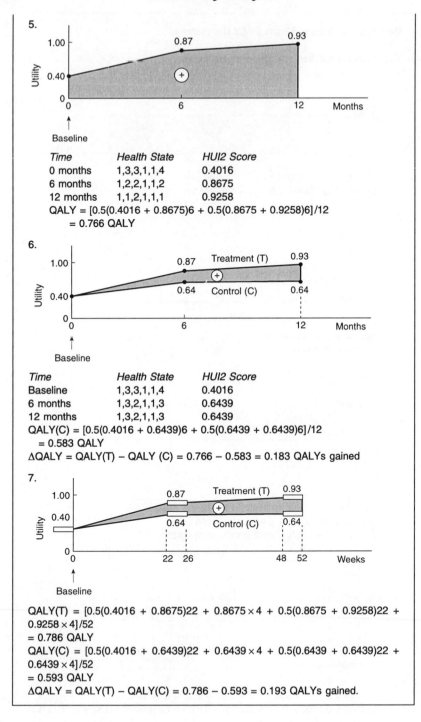

5.

Time	Health State	HUI2 Score
0 months	1,3,3,1,1,4	0.4016
6 months	1,2,2,1,1,2	0.8675
12 months	1,1,2,1,1,1	0.9258

QALY = [0.5(0.4016 + 0.8675)6 + 0.5(0.8675 + 0.9258)6]/12
   = 0.766 QALY

6.

Time	Health State	HUI2 Score
Baseline	1,3,3,1,1,4	0.4016
6 months	1,3,2,1,1,3	0.6439
12 months	1,3,2,1,1,3	0.6439

QALY(C) = [0.5(0.4016 + 0.6439)6 + 0.5(0.6439 + 0.6439)6]/12
   = 0.583 QALY
ΔQALY = QALY(T) – QALY (C) = 0.766 – 0.583 = 0.183 QALYs gained

7.

QALY(T) = [0.5(0.4016 + 0.8675)22 + 0.8675 × 4 + 0.5(0.8675 + 0.9258)22 + 0.9258 × 4]/52
= 0.786 QALY
QALY(C) = [0.5(0.4016 + 0.6439)22 + 0.6439 × 4 + 0.5(0.6439 + 0.6439)22 + 0.6439 × 4]/52
= 0.593 QALY
ΔQALY = QALY(T) – QALY(C) = 0.786 – 0.593 = 0.193 QALYs gained.

Box 6.9. Healthy years equivalents (HYE) measurement

This simple example illustrates the measurements process for the HYE (Mehrez and Gafni 1989; 1991; 1992). Consider a health path (also called a health profile) over time as shown below.

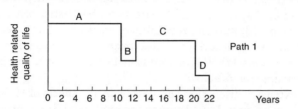

The path, of course, can have any length and any pattern. This particular path (Path 1) consists of four different health states for different periods of time totalling 22 years, followed by death.

Step 1. Determine utility of path 1
The utility for path 1 is determined using a conventional standard gamble question anchored on perfect health for 22 years and immediate death as shown below. As in any conventional standard gamble, the probability p is varied systematically to find the indifference probability p*. The result p* is the von Neumann–Morgenstern utility for path 1 on a utility scale where immediate death has a utility of zero and perfect health for 22 years has a utility of 1.

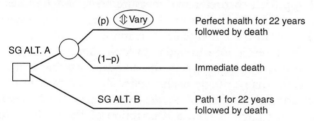

Step 2. Determine HYE for utility of path 1
Step 2 consists of a second standard gamble shown below that determines the number of healthy years followed by death that would yield the same utility as path 1.

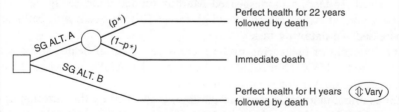

In this standard gamble, H is varied systematically to find the value H* where the respondent is different between the two alternatives in the standard gamble. Thus, H* is the number of healthy years followed by death that has a utility of p*, the same utility as path 1. Thus, H* is the HYE of path 1.

Variations on the HYE measurement procedure described above are also possible. A simpler variation occurs when the health path consists of only one chronic health state until death (Mehrez and Gafni 1989). Then the result of the two stage measurement procedure is the HYE for the chronic health state for the duration specified. A more complex variation occurs when the health path is a decision tree; that is, the health path is probabilistic, consisting of multiple branches each with its own probability of occurance. In this case, the HYE for the probabilistic health path has been called 'extended HYE' (Wakker 1996) and '*ex ante* HYE' (Johannesson 1995a; 1995b), and is more complicated to measure (see 6 below).

There has been extensive discussion and debate on all aspects of HYEs, and the debate may not yet be over. In addition to the references listed throughout this section, other articles on the HYE debate include the following (Culyer and Wagstaff 1993; Fryback 1993; Gafni and Birch 1993; Mehrez and Gafni 1993; Bleichrodt 1995; Culyer and Wagstaff 1995). In this book we are not able to go into all the intricacies of the entire debate; interested readers can go to the original sources for that. However, a few of the key points are summarized below.

1. Measuring preferences over a path of health states is theoretically attractive but more difficult in practice. It is theoretically attractive because it is a more general approach to preference measurement, and imposes fewer restrictive assumptions. Thus, it is more likely to capture more accurately the true preferences of the individuals. It is more difficult in practice for two reasons. First, each measurement task is more difficult for the respondent; the certain alternative in the standard gamble is a path of health states rather than a single health state. Because each health state often requires considerable detail to describe appropriately (examples include up to a half page of text, a description of the health status on eight attributes, or even videos to describe a single health state), one may quickly run into cognitive overload with many subjects. Second, in many practical problems there may be a large number of health paths to be assessed. Indeed, a modest-sized Markov model could easily have eight states and 20 cycles, which would give over 10^{18} unique health paths to be assessed – a daunting task.

2. The concept of measuring preferences over a path of health states is not restricted to HYEs, but could also be used with QALYs, if desired. In such a case, the QALY for a path would be the utility of the path, as measured for example in a single standard gamble, multiplied by the duration of the path. Note that the standard gamble referred to here is identical to step 1 of the HYE procedure (see Box 6.9). Note also, that this path-based QALY procedure is just a simple (in concept) variation of the regular QALY procedure. It is just the regular QALY procedure as it would normally be applied to a single chronic state, but with the chronic state replaced in the

preference measurement task by the path. Note, finally, that such a path-based QALY is also a utility (see Section 6.6.1), because it is calculated by multiplying a utility by a positive constant.

3. All researchers who have independently evaluated the HYE have concluded that the two-stage standard gamble measurement procedure originally proposed for the HYE is theoretically equivalent to a one-stage time trade-off procedure (Buckingham 1993; Johannesson *et al.* 1993; Loomes 1995; Williams 1995; Wakker 1996; Weinstein and Pliskin 1996). This conclusion does not imply that the two measurement procedures will give identical results, but it does imply that if the two procedures differ empirically, there is no theoretical grounds for choosing one over the other. Presumably one would choose the procedure with the least potential for measurement error, which would seem to be the time trade-off method (Wakker 1996; Weinstein and Pliskin 1996). Note, also, that neither the HYE nor the TTO captures the individual's risk attitude, so neither captures fully the individual's preferences under risk.

4. The HYE is not a utility and is not intended an an alternative to utility theory (Gafni 1996; Wakker 1996). Under von Neumann–Morgenstern utility theory, the appropriate approach for an individual is to solve his decision problem using conventional utility theory. This would involve measuring utilities for each health path (the first standard gamble in the HYE approach), taking expected utilities, and selecting the alternative with the largest expected utility.

5. The HYE may be a useful communication tool for those not trained in decision theory or utility theory. For example, in the case given above, the result could usefully be explained to the decision maker by converting the expected utility for each alternative into its HYE. This could be done by using a standard gamble like the second one in the HYE approach, except the probability in the gamble alternative of the standard gamble would be based on the expected utility of each decision alternative in the problem, not on the utility of each health path in the problem.

6. As pointed out above in points 3 and 4 the original HYE does not capture an individual's risk attitude and is not a replacement for utility theory. However, an extension to the HYE approach called 'extended HYEs' by Wakker (1996) and 'the certainty–equivalent number of HYEs' or '*ex ante* HYE' by Johannesson '(Johannesson 1995a; 1995b) does indeed rank risky health paths according to the individual's preferences. Extended HYEs are defined as the number of healthy years that has the same utility as the gamble rather than the sure thing. More precisely, it is the number of healthy years that has the same utility as the gamble defined over all possible health paths for the alternative under consideration. For example, a patient facing three treament options, A, B, and C, would be presented with the full decision tree flowing from option A. This decision tree would take the place of the path in step 1 of the HYE measurement procedure (see

Box 6.9). The HYE obtained in step 2 would be the HYE for option A. Similarly, the HYE for each of the other two options would be determined. Then, these HYEs would indeed rank the three options according to the patient's preferences. However, the problem with this approach is that as an analytic model it provides no advantage over descriptive empirical reality because it simply replicates the full preference order of the individual. That is, you might just as well have asked the patient to select his or her preferred option from among A, B, and C, and dispensed with all the measurements. In addition, except in simple problems, the cognitive demands of this approach to measurement would be extremely severe.

An approach using person trade-offs (PTO) to determine saved-young-life equivalents (SAVE) has been suggested as an alternative to the conventional QALY (Nord *et al.* 1993; Nord 1995; 1996). The basic argument is that the weights for conventional QALYs, and thus the QALYs themselves, reflect an individualistic perspective and not a societal perspective, and thus the conventional QALY does not measure social value. Specifically, it is noted that the weights for conventional QALYs represent an aggregation of preferences and trade-offs that individuals hold for their own health. That is, they represent the trade-offs among various living states and between living states and death that the individuals would want for themselves. In aggregating, all persons preferences are considered equal, although other weighting schemes are possible (Williams 1988), and so the resulting QALY is equity neutral. Researchers have found that when members of the general public are asked specific PTO questions, like how many patients of type A should be cured to be equivalent in social value to curing 10 patients of type B, the results do not match conventional QALYs. The reasons often seem to relate to equity considerations; help the sicker people first, treat all equally regardless of capacity to benefit, and perhaps to the 'rule of rescue' (Hadorn 1991) in which life-saving is always given the highest priority. The SAVE is the common metric that can be used with the PTO approach. All programmes are converted through PTO measurements to their SAVE value, and programmes are compared on the basis of costs and SAVEs.

Conventional QALYs and SAVEs take different approachs to the definition and measurement of preferences from a societal perspective. In the QALY approach, each member of society is asked what kinds of trade-offs they would like *for themselves*, and the societal decision making is made consistent with these trade-offs. In the SAVE approach each member of society is asked what kinds of trade-offs they would like *for others*, and this forms the basis for the societal decision making. It is not clear on theoretical or ethical grounds that one is better than the other. There would be no problem if the two approaches gave similar results, but it appears they do not. The SAVE approach appears to give more emphasis to quantity of life, and less to quality of life. That is, compared to the QALY approach the SAVE approach is less willing to take mortality risks to improve quality of life. This may represent the human tendency, also seen in other fields, of being more conservative when giving advice than when taking it.

The SAVE approach is new and the measurement techniques are still under development (Ubel *et al.* 1996). So, what should an analyst do? Currently, the default method is still the QALY, and generally this should be the primary approach taken by analysts. However, in some studies, or for some decision makers, analysts may wish also to explore the impact of using a SAVE approach. If the two approaches give dramatically different answers to the resource allocation question, a discussion of the reasons could be quite enlightening for the decision makers.

6.6. ADVANCED TOPICS

6.6.1. Is a QALY a utility?

QALYs are used as the denominator in cost–utility analysis, so it is natural to think that a QALY is somehow also a utility. In general, it is not.

A utility, in our context here, is a von Neumann–Morgenstern utility. So all QALYs that are formed from preferences measured in any way other than with a standard gamble, by definition, can not be utilities. But what about QALYs formed from preferences for health states measured with a standard gamble? Can they not be utilities? It turns out they can be, but only under quite restrictive assumptions (Weinstein and Fineberg 1980; Torrance and Feeny 1989). The two attributes of quality and quantity must be mutually utility-independent (preferences for gambles on the one attribute are independent of the amount of the other attribute); the trade-off of quantity for quality must exhibit the constant proportional trade-off property (the proportion of remaining life that one would trade off for a specified quality improvement is independent of the amount of remaining life), and the single attribute utility function for additional healthy life-years must be linear with time (for a fixed quality level ones utilities are directly proportional to longevity, a property also referred to as risk neutrality with respect to time). These conditions, particularly the latter one, are uncommon in practice, and thus even a utility-weighted QALY is generally not in itself a utility.

However, could a utility-weighted QALY turn out to be a good approximation of a utility? Garber and Phelps (1995) argue that it could, and describe a set of assumptions under which decisions based on cost/QALY would be entirely consistent with welfare economic theory (see also Garber *et al.* 1996). Empirically, it may turn out that QALYs are an adequate approximation of utilities, at least under most situations. So far, there are few data. One study has found that the approximation is not adequate at the individual level, but at the group level it looks promising to use a regression approach to predict path utilities from the utilities of the component states (Kuppermann *et al.* 1997).

Similarly, a yet unpublished McMaster University study on preferences for knee disability states found that the QALY is a good approximation of the path utility at the group level. More research is clearly needed to determine the situations where a QALY is a good approximation of a utility and where it is not.

Finally, does it really matter whether or not a QALY is a utility? Some think not (Culyer 1989). The view is that the QALY is a good basic definition of what we are trying to achieve in health care, and maximizing QALYs is quite an appropriate goal. Because this view is not based on economic welfare theory it has been called the 'extra welfarist' foundation for cost–utility analysis.

6.6.2. Is it double-discounting to discount QALYs?

It is sometimes argued that it is double discounting to discount QALYs if the preference instrument used to measure the QALY weight already incorporated the respondents time preference (Krahn and Gafni 1993). For example, the time trade-off method is often said to capture the subjects time preference because it asks time-based questions. So, it would not make sense to discount again, or would it?

To explore this issue we need to look at exactly how a subject's time preference affects the QALY. Time preference in health is normally modelled as a constant discount rate (r) over time (Lipscomb *et al.* 1996). Consider a subject who initially has no time preference (r = 0) and rates a state as 0.5 on the TTO. Now, assume the subject suddenly takes on positive time preference (r > 0), the normal kind of time preference where we prefer good things to happen earlier and bad things to happen later. The t option in the TTO would now diminish in utility proportionately more than the shorter x option, and to maintain utility indifference the subject would reduce x, thus reducing the TTO score. So, TTO scores would be negatively related to the subjects degree of time preference, but not in direct proportion. For example, if the subjects time preference was 10% per year (r = 0.1), this does not mean that the TTO score would reduce by 10%. Large TTO scores would reduce by only a small amount, while small TTO scores would be affected proportionally much more.

Johannesson and colleagues (1994) point out that, at the individual level, depending upon the shape of the individual's utility function, discounted QALYs can lead to programme rankings that violate the individual's preferences. In the special case where the shape of the individual's utility function matches the discounting model with a rate r, and the quality weights are being derived using a TTO method, the problem can be avoided by calculating the TTO score by dividing the discounted (at rate r) years in full health by the discounted (at rate r) years in the index health state. The difficulty, however, for programme evaluation, is that this method only applies at the individual level. Even there it would be complex to implement, probably only applies to a subset of individuals, and would lead to a different discount rate for each individual. In programme evaluation the discount rate reflects the time preference of the decision maker, not necessarily that of the patients, the discount rate must apply to all patients regardless of their individual rates, and in many applications it applies to outcomes achieved by both current and future patients, thus capturing the intergenerational time preference as well.

Now consider the standard gamble. It incorporates the subject's risk preference, but not time preference. Even though the alternatives of the gamble have time in them, the time is the same in each alternative and if the subjects time preference changes (r changes), it affects each alternative proportionally the same, so the utility indifference is not disturbed. Thus, different time preferences do not lead to different scores from the standard gamble. Finally, visual analogue scale (VAS) scores also are not affected by time preference for the same reasons.

So, to summarize, preference scores measured by SG or VAS are not affected by time preference so there is no issue. Preference scores measured by TTO are indeed affected by the subjects time preference, but not in any uniform or proportionate way. Moreover, the subject's time preference may be much different from the modest-sized social rate of discount of 3–5 per cent recommended by most guidelines for economic evaluation (Canadian Coordinating Office for Health Technology Assessment 1994; Gold *et al.* 1996b; Torrance *et al.* 1996a). Individual time preferences for health have been found to be highly variable, even within subject, and to include both positive and negative rates of discount (Fuchs 1982; Dolan and Gudex 1995). Thus, even with the TTO it is not a simple case that the recommended social rate of discount has been incorporated by the subjects who rated the outcomes. Although a method has been suggested for adjusting TTO scores to account for an individual's time preference (Johannesson *et al.* 1994), it is not clear how this can be used in programme evaluations. It appears to us that more thought and research is needed to clarify this fully, but at the moment our advice would be to continue to discount at the recommended social rate of discount regardless of how the preference weights were obtained.

6.7. CRITICAL APPRAISAL OF A PUBLISHED ARTICLE

Reference: Boyle, M. H., Torrance, G. W., Sinclair, J. C., and Horwood, S. P. (1983). Economic evaluation of neonatal intensive care of very-low-birth-weight infants. *N. Engl. J. Med.*, **308**, 1330–7.

This article, although somewhat dated, has been retained in the second edition as it is still considered one of the better example of a comprehensive cost–utility analysis (Gerard 1992). Note, however, that the article preceeded the introduction of willingness to pay into the cost–benefit methodology in health. Note, also, that the technology under evaluation is now dated. Despite these shortcomings we believe the article still makes a useful teaching example.

The paper is assessed below using the 10 questions set out in Box 3.1. It is suggested that you locate the article and attempt the exercise before reading the assessment.

1. Was a well-defined question posed in answerable form?

    __X__ YES   _____ NO   _____ CAN'T TELL

The study examines both the costs and health outcomes of management of very-low-birth-weight babies either by a regional programme with a specialized neonatal intensive care unit or by previously existing facilities within the region.

The viewpoint for the analysis is clearly that of society since, as the authors explain, '...we measured all the costs and benefits of providing neonatal intensive care, *regardless of who pays or who benefits*' (p.1330 of the paper).

2. Was a comprehensive description of the competing alternatives given?

    __X__ YES   _____ NO   _____ CAN'T TELL

The intervention under study is the neonatal intensive care component of the McMaster regional perinatal programme. This intervention, therefore, consists of both specific clinical services (the neonatal intensive care unit itself and the specialized procedures performed therein) and the programmatic aspects of the management of very-low-birth-weight babies within the region (consultation, referral, transport, etc.). A general description of the setting, population served, levels of care provided, frequency of neonatal intensive care, and hospitals involved is provided on pp. 1330–1. For more detailed description, readers are provided with references to recommendations for the regional development of perinatal health services (p. 1331, col. 1) to which this programme conformed, and with a reference to an earlier article by the same authors [(1981) Evaluation of neonatal intensive care programs. *N Eng. J. Med.*, **305**, 489–94] which identified several specific clinical manoeuvres typically included in a neonatal intensive care programme (Table 1, p. 490). The neonatal intensive care 'programme' is compared to the 'no programme' situation in which care was previously delivered in individual hospitals within the region in the absence of a specialized neonatal intensive care unit at McMaster and an organized referral network.

3. Was there evidence that the programmes' effectiveness had been established?

    __X__ YES   _____ NO   _____ CAN'T TELL

This assessment might be questioned; however, in their previous article, cited above, the authors reviewed the evidence on efficacy and effectiveness of several practices involving the respiratory, nutritional, and environmental management of sickness in infants. They found experimental evidence supporting the efficacy of many of the specific manoeuvres typically included in a neonatal intensive care programme. Yet, they also emphasized that methodological difficulties clouded conclusions on whether regional neonatal intensive care programmes were effective (p. 490).

In their economic evaluation of the neonatal intensive care (NIC) component of the McMaster regional perinatal programme, the effectiveness of the intervention is evaluated simultaneously with its efficiency through a 'before–after' research design. The health outcomes of all live-born infants weighing 500–1499 g, born to residents of Hamilton-Wentworth County, were compared for two groups: infants born from 1964–1969 (before the NIC programme) and infants born from 1973–1977 (after the introduction of NIC). Rate of survival to hospital discharge, life-years per live birth, and quality-adjusted life-years per live birth, all increased with NIC, thereby indicating programme effectiveness.

The before–after design is, of course, a less powerful research design than the randomized controlled trial. There was no concurrent control group and a major concern is whether the comparability of the two groups on factors other than NIC may have influenced infant outcomes. For example, there may have been differences between the groups in neonatal mortality risk. The authors were clearly aware of the limitations of the research design that they were forced to use. They performed such analyses as were possible in order to minimize potential bias, and identified potential confounding variables. For example, as noted on p. 1334, col. 2, they carried out birth-weight specific comparisons to minimize confounding from factors such as maternal age, parity and socioeconomic status known to affect the birth-weight distribution of live births. They also ascertained that other factors capable of influencing birth-weight specific mortality risk at the time of birth (e.g. mode of delivery), did not represent an important difference between the groups.

4. Were all the important and relevant costs and consequences for each alternative identified?

___X___ YES _____ NO _____ CAN'T TELL

With respect to the costs of organizing and operating NIC, the authors identified hospital costs (including both capital and labour costs generated in the NIC unit and various wards, support services such as housekeeping and overhead services such as administration), physician services, convalescent care in community hospitals outside Hamilton, and ambulance transport (p. 1331, col. 2). They also identified as 'follow-up' costs the costs of caring for infants post discharge, including both items such as hospital and physician services/dental services/drugs and items such as special institutional care applied and the extra cost of special education (p. 1331, col. 2). (Note that although the authors label these follow-up items as 'costs' of the programmes, the items could have been treated as 'consequences' of the programmes. As consequences, they would have counted as 'changes in future resource use' and any savings here would have appeared as a direct benefit in later calculations. Although some intermediate calculations would have shown different absolute figures, any calculation of net economic benefit would not have changed and the conclusions would, of course, be unaffected by this alternative formulation.)

The authors also identified important intangible and emotional costs and consequences of the programme (p. 1335, col. 1), although these items were not measurable. While they did not include direct or indirect costs incurred by families up to the point of discharge, they did identify and impute a value to the provision of care to handicapped children by parents in their homes.

The consequences of the alternatives included both their health outcomes and the ensuing quality of life for survivors. In addition, the impact on the ability of the survivors to eventually perform productive economic roles was included. Thus a comprehensive range of costs and consequences was identified, consistent with the adoption of a societal viewpoint.

5. Were costs and consequences measured accurately in appropriate physical units?

___X__ YES   _____ NO   _____ CAN'T TELL

In order to measure hospital services consumed, the authors first identified, in specific measurement units, the different types of service which might be utilized during an episode of care (e.g. patient days for nursing and 'hotel' services, work units for radiology, operations for surgical services, etc.) and then recorded through chart review the actual utilization of services by infants in the study. Actual utilization of physician services, convalescent care, and ambulance services was also obtained from appropriate records (p. 1331, col. 2). Types and quantities of health care and other services utilized by surviving children were obtained in a home interview with a random sample of families (p. 1331, col. 2). As the authors noted on p.1334, col. 2, the direction of bias resulting from parental recall is uncertain.

Programme effects were measured initially by lives saved, obtained from hospital discharge data. However, effectiveness was also measured by life-years gained, both to age 15 and to death. In addition, what the authors term the 'social value', also called the 'utility' of the programme consequences, was measured by quality-adjusted life-years gained, again both to age 15 and to death.

An important element in the physical measurement of both costs and effects was the estimation of both lifetime health outcomes and utilization of services for surviving children. The authors employed their own data (based on a sophisticated, multi-attribute, classification system for health states employed in the home interview) to make the estimates up to age 15 where necessary. They employed forecasts made independently by two developmental paediatricians using the available health history for each child to make the projections past age 15 (p. 1131). In order to reflect uncertainty about the future, probability distributions of outcomes rather than point estimates were made by the paediatricians, and the authors later conducted sensitivity analyses on life expectancies.

6. Were costs and consequences valued credibly?

___X__ YES   _____ NO   _____ CAN'T TELL

Costs and benefits were valued in 1978 Canadian dollars. State-of-the-art methods were employed in two instances – the valuation of hospital neonatal care services and the establishment of utility values for the complex array of possible health states for surviving children.

In order to cost NIC, the authors established a 'fully allocated unit price' (cost) for each of the services previously identified as potentially contributing to an episode of hospital care. This involved the use of a mathematical model which employed hospital budget data and cost allocation criteria to apportion an appropriate share of the expense of all relevant hospital departments to services used in NIC. Reference is provided to a separate publication containing the exact data and detailed methods employed (p. 1331). (A key feature of this methodology is that it not only provides a method for sorting out situations of joint use of resources by more than one ward or unit, but it also sorts out situations in which two hospital departments simultaneously provide services to each other.) The cost of an NIC episode was then calculated by summing the quantities of each service used, multiplied by its unit price.

The costs of other services used were established from actual records of charges or operating expenses, the sources of which are noted by the authors. In the case of costs for the future care of handicapped children at home or in institutions, estimates were based on previous studies or obtained from the responsible paying agencies (p. 1332, col. 1). Future health care cost estimates were based on age and sex-specific normal utilization patterns adjusted for children in this study by health states. The value of their economic productivity was based on official census data on normal age and sex-specific earnings patterns, adjusted by forecasts of their productive ability as a percentage of normal ability (pp. 1331–2.)

The valuation of life-years gained by surviving children in terms of their quality was accomplished by multiplying time spent or forecasted to be spent in any specific health state by the utility value of that health state. The utility values were based upon the preferences of a local random sample of parents with schoolchildren (p. 1331). Note that these utility values were based on actual measurement of preferences rather than an arbitrary assignment of values, and included parents with and without normal children (which is consistent with a societal viewpoint). The authors refer readers interested in more details of the specific multi-attribute utility theory approach (employed to deal with the complex range of health outcomes) to a separate publication (p. 1331, col. 2, note 12).

As a result of these identification, measurement, and valuation procedures, the authors were in a position to conduct any one or all of the cost-effectiveness, cost–benefit, or cost–utility analyses.

7. Were costs and consequences adjusted for differential timing?

     X YES   NO   CAN'T TELL

A discount rate of 5 per cent per annum was applied to costs, earnings, and effects occurring in the future in order to convert the future values to their equivalent present value. Although no rationale was provided for the choice of a 5 per cent discount rate, the authors considered values from 0–10 per cent in the sensitivity analysis – a range which is likely to encompass the rates typically employed in economic evaluations (and recommended by most governments).

It is interesting to note the impact that discounting has on the results of this study. Tables 3 and 4 differ only in that, in the latter, all future costs and effects have been discounted to their present value. The first line of both tables is identical since all costs and effects measured to the point of hospital discharge occur within year one. However, as the analysis is extended to age 15 of the survivors and to death, the effects of discounting become apparent. As the authors explain, 'Since neonatal intensive care has high initial costs in order to achieve later gains in numbers of life-years, numbers of quality-adjusted life-years, and productivity, discounting affects the later gains more than the initial costs and adversely affects the measures of economic evaluation' (p. 1333).

8. Was an incremental analysis of costs and consequences of alternatives performed?

     X YES   NO   CAN'T TELL

Although the costs and outcomes of the two alternative programmes are calculated separately, the results of the study are presented in incremental form, that is, as the *additional* cost of the NIC programme per *additional* effect (e.g. life saved, life-year gained, QALY gained) it achieves. Details of how the incremental data were calculated are provided in the appendix. As well, the appendix demonstrates that all of the data used to derive the efficiency estimates were introduced into the calculations in their incremental form.

9. Was allowance made for uncertainty in the estimation of costs and consequences?

    __X__ YES   _____ NO   _____ CAN'T TELL

Four factors were chosen for testing in the sensitivity analysis: the discount rate, life expectancy, condition of those lost to follow-up and utility values. Of these four, varying the discount rate appears to have the greatest impact on the results (see Fig. 2, p. 1325). In fact, the sensitivity analysis demonstrates that the choice of discount rate can be pivotal for at least one of the indicators of efficiency in one birth-weight group. The net economic benefit per live birth for the 1000–1499 g birth-weight group was positive at discount rates lower than approximately 3.5 per cent but negative at higher discount rates.

This study demonstrates that sensitivity analyses can also be used to increase confidence in the original results. For example, the authors emphasize that, 'A major finding of this study – that by every economic measure neonatal intensive care for infants weighing 1000–1499 g is superior to neonatal intensive care for infants weighing 500–999 g – is robust with respect to all sensitivity analyses investigated' (p. 1335).

10. Did the presentation and discussion of study results include all issues of concern to users?

    __X__ YES   _____ NO   _____ CAN'T TELL

The authors did not rely upon a single index on which to base their conclusions but rather calculated their results using three different economic evaluation techniques (CEA, CBA, and CUA), each of which incorporates different value judgements. It is left to the reader to decide which index is most appropriate for evaluating NIC programmes. As well, the results are calculated for two distinct weight groups and three time horizons, again allowing the reader to judge the programme according to the criteria he feels are most important and relevant.

The authors explicitly acknowledge that many of the intangible factors that affect the value of NIC programmes have been excluded from the analysis (p. 1335, col. 1). It is unrealistic to expect, though, that these factors could be sufficiently quantified so as to permit inclusion. The authors' discussion of this point is a good demonstration of the principle that although certain costs and consequences may be immeasurable (for practical purposes), nonetheless they may be included in the analysis in a qualitative manner.

A great deal of discussion is devoted to the generalizability of the study results. A strong case is presented to support the assumption that the findings about health outcomes can be generalized to NIC programmes in similar urban settings during the period studied. With respect to the economic outcomes, costs and earnings appear to be generalizable over time and financing mechanisms, but perhaps not across settings where service intensities may vary.

Finally, the authors caution against comparing their results with the results of other studies (evaluating different interventions) in an attempt to assess the relative efficiency (or merit!) of NIC programmes. Differences in the viewpoint for the analysis, methodological approach or assumptions used to derive estimates of costs and outcomes may have dramatic effects on the results (as we saw earlier with the case of the discount rate). The authors are reluctant therefore to interpret their results normatively, and instead emphasize that, 'A judgement concerning the relative economic value of neonatal intensive care of very-low-birth-weight infants will require the economic evaluation of other health programmes by similar methods.' (p. 1336).

REFERENCES

Allais, M. (1991). Cardinal utility history, empirical findings, and applications: an overview. *Theory and Decision*, **31**, 99–140.

Arrow, K.J., and Debreu, G. (1954). Existence of equilibrium for a competitive economy. *Econometrica*, **22**, 265–90.

Bass, E. B., Steinberg, E., Pitt, H., Griffiths, R., Lillemoe, K., Saba, G., *et al.* (1994). Comparison of the rating scale and the standard gamble in measuring patient preferences for outcomes of gallstone disease. *Medical Decision Making*, **14** (4) Oct–Dec, 307–14.

Bell, D. and Farquhar, P. (1986). Perspectives on utility theory. *Oper. Rsch.*, **34**(1) Jan–Feb, 179–83.

Bennett, K.J. and Torrance, G.W. (1996). Measuring health state preferences and utilities: rating scale, time trade-off and standard gamble techniques. In *Quality of life and pharmacoeconomics in clinical trials* (2nd edn) (ed. B. Spilker), pp. 253–65. Lippincott–Raven, Philadelphia.

Berthelot, J., Roberge, R., and Wolfson, M. (1993). The calculation of health-adjusted life expectancy for a Canadian province using a multi–attribute utility function: a first attempt. In *Calculation of health expectancies: harmonization, consensus and future perspectives*, (ed. J. M. Robine, C.D. Mathers, M.R. Bone, and I. Romieu), Vol. 226, pp. 161–72. John Libbey Eurotext Ltd.

Bleichrodt, H. (1995). QALYs and HYEs: Under what conditions are they equivalent? *J. Health Economics*, **14**, 17–37.

—, and Johannesson, M. (1997). An experimental test of the theoretical foundation for rating-scale valuations. *Medical Decision Making*, **17**(2), Apr–Jun, 208–16.

Bossert, W. (1991). On intra– and interpersonal utility comparisons. *Social Choice and Welfare*, **8**, 207–19.

Boyle, M.H., Torrance, G.W., Sinclair, J.C., and Horwood, S.P. (1983). Economic evaluation of neonatal intensive care of very–low–birth–weight infants. *N. Eng. J. Med.*, **308**, 1330–7.

Brooks, R. with the EuroQol Group. (1996). EuroQol: the current state of play. *Health Policy*, **37**, 53–72.

Broome, J. (1993). QALYS. *J. Public Economics*, 50, 149–67.

Buckingham, K. (1993). A note on HYE (healthy years equivalent). *J. Health Economics*, 11, 301–9.

Bush, J., Fanshel, S., and Chen, M. (1972). Analysis of a tuberculin testing program using a health status index. *Socio–Econ. Plan. Sci.*, 6, 49–68.

Buxton, M. and Ashby, J. (1988). The time trade-off approach to health state valuation. In: *Measuring health: a practical approach* (ed. G. Teeling Smith), pp. 69–87. John Wiley & Sons Ltd, Chichester.

Cadman, D., Goldsmith, C., Torrance, G.W., Boyle, M., and Furlong, W. (1986). Development of a health status index for Ontario children. Final report to Ontario Ministry of Health for research grant DM648 (00633). McMaster University, Centre for Health Economics and Policy Analysis, Hamilton, Ontario.

Canadian Coordinating Office for Health Technology Assessment. (1994) Guidelines for Economic Evaluation of Pharmaceuticals: Canada (1st end).

Carr-Hill, R. (1991). Allocating resources to health care: is the QALY (quality-adjusted life year) a technical solution to a political problem? *Int. J. Health Serv. Res.*, 21, 351–63.

—, and Morris, J. (1991). Current practice in obtaining the 'Q' in QALYs: a cautionary note. *Brit. Med. J.*, 303, 699–701.

Churchill, D., Torrance, G., Taylor, D., Barnes, C., Ludwin, D., Shimizu, A., *et al.* (1987). Measurement of quality of life in end-stage renal disease: The time trade-off approach. *Clinical and Investigative Medicine*, 10(1), 14–20.

Cohen, B.J. (1996). Is expected utility theory normative for medical decision-making? *Medical Decision Making*, 16, 1–14.

Cook, J., Richardson, J., and Street, A. (1994). A cost–utility analysis of treatment options for gallstone disease: metholological issues and results. *Health Economics*, 3, 157–68.

Cooper, R., and Rappoport, P. (1984). Were the ordinalists wrong about welfare economics? *J. Economic Literature*, 22, 507–30.

Cox, D., Fitzpatrick, R., Fletcher, A., Gore, S., Spiegelhalter, D., and Jones, D. (1992). Quality-of-life assessment: can we keep it simple? *J. R. Statist. Soc. A.*, 155, Part 3, 353–93.

Culyer, A. (1989). The normative economics of health care finance and provision. *Oxford Review of Economic Policy*, 5(1), 34–58.

—, and Wagstaff, A. (1993). QALYs versus HYEs. *J. Health Economics*, 11, 311–23.

—, (1995). QALYs versus HYEs: A reply to Gafni, Birch and Mehrez. *J. Health Economics*, 14, 39–45.

Currim, I. and Sarin, R. (1992). Robustness of expected utility model in predicting individual choices. *Organizational Behavior and Human Decision Processes*, 52, 544–68.

Dolan, P., and Gudex, C. (1995). Time preference, duration and health state valuations. *Health Economics*, 4, 289–99.

—, Gudex, C., Kind, P., and Williams, A. (1995). A social tariff for EuroQol: Results from a UK general population survey. Discussion Paper No. 138, Centre for Health Economics, University of York, York.

—, —, —, —, (1996a). Valuing health states: a comparison of methods. *J. Health Economics*, 15, 209–31.

—, —, —, —, (1996b). The time trade-off method: results from a general population study. *Health Economics*, 5, 141–54.

Dyer, J. and Sarin, R. (1979). Measurable multi-attribute value functions. *Operations Research*, 27, 810–22.

—, —, (1982). Relative risk aversion. *Management Science*, **28**(8), 875–86.

Erickson, P., Wilson, R., and Shannon, I. (1995). *Years of healthy life*. Statistical Notes, Number 7, April 1995. National Center for Health Statistics, Hyattsville, Maryland.

Essink-bot, M., Stouthard, M., and Bonsel, G. (1993). Generalizability of valuations on health states collected with the EuroQol – questionnaire. *Health Economics*, **2**, 237–46.

EuroQol Group. (1990). EuroQol – a new facility for the measurement of health-related quality of life. *Health Policy*, **16**, 199–208.

Fanshel, S. and Bush, J. (1970). A health status index and its application to health services outcomes. *Operations Research*, **18**(6) Nov.–Dec. 1021–66.

Feeny, D., Furlong, W., Torrance, G., Rosenbaum, P., and Weitzman, S. (1992). A comprehensive multi-attribute system for classifying the health status of survivors of childhood cancer. *Journal of Clinical Oncology*, **10**(6), 923–28.

—, Furlong, W., Boyle, M., and Torrance, G. (1995). Multi-attribute health status classification systems: Health utilities index. *PharmacoEconomics*, **7**, 490–502.

—, Torrance, G.W., and Labelle, R. (1996). Integrating economic evaluations and quality of life assessments. In *Quality of life and pharmacoeconomics in clinical trials* (2nd edn) (ed. B. Spilker), pp. 85–95. Lippincott–Raven, Philadelphia.

Fischer, G.W. (1979). Utility models for multiple objective decisions: Do they accurately represent human preferences. *Decision Sciences*, **10**, 451–79.

Fischer, G., Kamlet, M., Fienberg, S., and Schkade, D. (1986). Risk preferences for gains and losses in multiple objective decision making. *Management Science*, **32**(9), 1065–86.

Fishburn, P. and Wakker, P. (1995). The invention of the independence condition for preferences. *Management Science*, **41**, 1130–44.

Fryback, D. (1993). QALYs, HYEs, and the loss of innocence [editorial]. *Medical Decision-Making*, 13 Oct.–Dec., 271–2.

Fuchs, V.R. (1982). Time preference and health: an exploratory study. In *Economic aspects of health* (ed. V. R. Fuchs), (pp. 93–120. The University of Chicago Press, Chicago.

Furlong, W., Feeny, D., Torrance, G., Barr, R., and Horsman, J. (1990). *Guide to design and development of health-state utility instrumentation*. Working Paper No. 90–9. McMaster University, Centre for Health Economics and Policy Analysis, Hamilton, Ontario.

Gafni, A., (1996). HYEs: Do we need them and can they fulfil the promise? *Medical Decision Making*, **16**, 215–16.

—, and Torrance, G. (1984). Risk attitude and time preference in health. *Management Science*, **30**(4), 440–51.

—, and Birch, S. (1993). Economics, health and health economics: HYEs versus QALYs. *J. Health Economics*, **11**, 325–39.

Garber, A.M. and Phelps, C.E. (1995). *Economic foundations of cost-effectiveness analysis*. National Bureau of Economic Research, Stanford, California.

—, Weinstein, M.C., Torrance, G.W., and Kamlet, M.S. (1996). Theoretical foundations of cost-effectiveness analysis. In *Cost-effectiveness in health and medicine*. (ed. M.R. Gold, J.E. Siegel, L.B. Russell, and M.C. Weinstein), pp. 25–53. Oxford University Press, New York.

Gerard, K. (1992). Cost–utility in practice: A policy maker's guide to the state of the art. *Health Policy*, **21**, 249–79.

Goel, V, and Detsky, A. (1989). A cost–utility analysis of preoperative total parenteral nutrition. *Int. J. Technology Assessment in Health Care*, **5**, 183–94.

Gold, M., Franks, P., and Erickson, P. (1996a). Assessing the health of the nation: The predictive validity of a preference–based measure and self–related health. *Medical Care*, 34(2), 163–77.

Gold, M.R., Siegel, J.E., Russell, L.B., and Weinstein, M.C. (1996b). *Cost-effectiveness in health and medicine.* Oxford University Press, New York.

Haddix, A., Teutsch, S., Shaffer, P., and Dunet, D. (1996). *Prevention effectiveness: A guide to decision analysis and economic evaluation.* Oxford University Press, Oxford.

Hadorn, D. (1991). Setting health care priorities in Oregon: cost-effectiveness meets the rule of rescue. *J.A.M.A.*, 265(17), 2218–25.

Hadorn, D.C., Hays, R.D., and Hauber, T. (1992). Improving task comprehension in the measurement of health state preferences. *J. Clin. Epid.*, 45, 233–43.

— and Uebersax, J. (1995). Large scale outcome evaluation: how should quality of life be measured? I. Calibration of a brief questionnaire and a search for preference subgroups. *J. Clin. Epid.*, 48, 607–18.

Hall, J., Gerard, K., Salkeld, G., and Richardson, J. (1992). A cost–utility analysis of mammography screening in Australia. *Soc. Sci. Med.* 34(9), 993–1004.

Hey, J. (1979). *Uncertainty in microeconomics.* New York University Press, New York.

Holloway, C. (1979). Decision making under uncertainty: Models and choices. *Prentice–Hall, Englewood Cliffs, NJ.*

Howard, R. (1988). Decision analysis: Practice and promise. *Management Science*, 34(6), 679–95.

Johannesson, M., (1995a). Quality-adjusted life years versus healthy-years equivalents – A comment. *J. Health Economics*, 14, 9–16.

—, (1995b). The ranking properties of healthy-years equivalents and quality-adjusted life-years under certainty and uncertainty. *Int. J. Technology Assessment in Health Care*, 11, 40–8.

—, Pliskin, J., and Weinstein, M. (1993). Are healthy-years equivalents an improvement over quality-adjusted life-years? *Medical Decision-Making*, 13(4) Oct.–Dec. 281–6.

—, —, — (1994). A note on QALYs, time trade-off and discounting. *Medical Decision Making*, 14(2) Apr–June, 188–93.

Kaplan, R.M. and Anderson, J.P. (1996). The general health policy model: an integrated approach. In *Quality of life and pharmacoeconomics in clinical trials* (2nd edn), (ed. B. Spilker), pp. 309–22. Lippincott–Raven, Philadelphia.

— and Bush, J. (1982). Health-related quality of life measurement for evaluation research and policy analysis. *Health Psychology*, 1, 61–80.

— and Anderson, J. (1988). A general health policy model: Update and applications. *Health Services Research*, 23(2) June, 203–35.

—, Atkins, C.J., and Wilson, D.K. (1988). The cost–utility of diet and exercise interventions in non–insulin–dependent diabetes mellitus. *Health Promotion*, 2, 331–40.

Keeney, R. and Raiffa, H. (1976). *Decisions with multiple objectives: preferences and value tradeoffs.* Wiley, New York.

— and Raiffa, H. (1993). *Decisions with multiple objectives: preferences and value tradeoffs.* (2nd edn). Cambridge University Press, Cambridge.

Kennedy, W., Reinharz, D., Tessier, G., Contandriopoulos, A.P., Trabut, I., Champagne, F., *et al.* (1995). Cost-utility of chemotherapy and best supportive care in non–small cell lung cancer. *PharmacoEconomics*, 8, 316–23.

Kind, P. (1996). The EuroQol instrument: an index of health-related quality of life. In *Quality of life and pharmacoeconomics in clinical trials.* (2nd edn) (ed. B. Spilker), pp. 191–201. Lippincott–Raven, Philadelphia.

Klarman, H., Francis, J., and Rosenthal, G. (1968). Cost-effectiveness analysis applied to the treatment of chronic renal disease. *Medical Care*, 6(1), 48–54.

Kleindorfer, P., Kunreuther, H., and Schoemaker, P. (1993). *Decision sciences – an integrative perspective*. Cambridge University Press, New York.

Krahn, M., and Gafni, A. (1993). Discounting in the economic evaluation of health care interventions. *Medical Care*, 31, 403–18.

Kuppermann, M., Shiboski, S., Feeny, D., Elkin, E.P., and Washington, A.E. (1997). Can preference scores for discrete states be used to derive preference scores for an entire path of events? An application to prenatal diagnosis. *Medical Decision-Making*, 17(1), Jan–Mar, 42–55.

Lipscomb, J., Weinstein, M.C., and Torrance, G.W. (1996). Time preference. In *Cost-effectiveness in health and medicine* (ed. M.R. Gold, J.E. Siegel, L.B. Russell, and M.C. Weinstein), pp. 214–46. Oxford University Press, New York.

Logan, A., Milne, B., Achber, C., Campbell, W., and Haynes, R. (1981). Cost-effectiveness of a worksite hypertension program. *Hypertension*, 3(2) Mar–Apr, 211–18.

Loomes, G. (1991). Evidence of a new violation of the independence axiom. *J. Risk and Uncertainty*, 4(1), 91–108.

— (1995). The myth of the HYE. *J. Health Economics*, 14, 1–7.

Luce, R. (1992). Where does subjective expected utility fail descriptively? *J. Risk and Uncertainty*, 5, 5–27.

— and Raiffa, H. (1957). *Games and decisions*. Wiley, New York.

Mehrez, A. and Gafni, A. (1989). Quality-adjusted life years, utility theory, and healthy-years equivalents. *Medical Decision-Making*, 9(2) Apr–June, 142–9.

—, — (1990). Evaluating health-related quality of life: An indifference curve interpretation for the time trade-off technique. *Social Science in Medicine*, 31(11), 1281–3.

—, — (1991). The healthy-years equivalents: how to measure them using the standard gamble approach. *Medical Decision-Making*, 11(2), Apr–June, 140–6.

—, — (1992). Preference based outcome measures for economic evaluation of drug interventions: quality adjusted life years (QALYs) versus healthy years equivalents (HYEs). *PharmacoEconomics*, 1(5), 338–45.

—, — (1993). Healthy-years equivalents versus quality-adjusted life years: In pursuit of progress. *Medical Decision-Making*, 13(4) Oct.–Dec. 287–92.

Miyamoto, J.M. (1988). Generic utility theory: measurement foundations and applications in multiattribute utility theory. *J. Mathematical Psychology*, 32, 357–404.

Nease, R.F. (1996). Do violations of the axioms of expected utility theory threaten decision analysis? *Medical Decision-Making*, 16(4), Oct–Dec, 399–403.

Nord, E. (1993). Toward quality assurance in QALY calculations. *Int. J. Technology Assessment in Health Care*, 9(1), 37–45.

— (1995). The person-trade-off approach to valuing health care programs. *Medical Decision-Making*, 15(3), Jul–Sep, 201–8.

— (1996). Health status index models for use in resource allocation decisions: A critical review in the light of observed preferences for social choice. *Int. J. Technology Assessment in Health Care*, 12(1), 31–44.

—, Richardson, J., and Macarounas-Kirchmann, K. (1993). Social evaluation of health care versus personal evaluation of health states. *Int. J. Technology Assessment in Health Care*, 9(4), 463–78.

O'Brien, B.J., Torrance, G.W., and Moran, L.A. (1994). *A practical guide to health state preference measurement: a video introduction*. Working Paper No. 95–2, Centre for Health Economics and Policy Analysis, McMaster University, Hamilton, Ontario.

O'Leary, J.F., Fairclough, D.L., Jankowski, M.K., and Weeks, J.C. (1995). Comparison of time trade-off utilities and rating scale values of cancer patients and their relatives: evidence for a possible plateau relationship. *Medical Decision Making*, 15(2), Apr–June, 132–7.

Oldridge, N., Furlong, W., Feeny, D., Torrance, G., Guyatt, G., Crowe, J., *et al.* (1993). Economic evaluation of cardiac rehabilitation soon after acute myocardial infarction. *Amer. J. Cardiol.*, 72, 154–61.

Patrick, D., Bush, J., and Chen, M. (1973). Methods for measuring levels of well-being for a health status index. *Health Services Research*, 8(3) Fall, 228–45.

— and Erickson, P. (1993). *Health status and health policy: quality of life in health care evaluation and resource allocation.* Oxford University Press, Inc., New York.

—, Starks, H., Cain, K., Uhlmann, R., and Pearlman, R. (1994). Measuring preferences for health states worse than death. *Medical Decision-Making*, 14(1), Jan–Mar, 9–18.

Raiffa, H. (1968). *Decision analysis: introductory lectures on choices under uncertainty.* Addison–Wesley, Reading, MA.

Read, J., Quinn, R., Berwick, D., Fineberg, H., and Weinstein, M. (1984). Preferences for health outcomes – Comparisons of assessment methods. *Medical Decision-Making*, 4(3), 315–29.

Rosser, R. and Kind, P. (1978). A scale of valuations of states of illness: Is there a social consensus. *Int. J. Epid.*, 7(4), 347–58.

— and Watts, V. (1978). The measurement of illness. *J. Operational Research Society*, 29(6), 529–40.

Russell, R. and Wilkinson, M. (1979). *Microeconomics: a synthesis of modern and neoclassical theory.* Wiley, New York.

Rutten-van Molken, M.P.M.H., Bakker, C.H., van Doorslaer, E.K.A., and van der Linden, S. (1995). Methodological issues of patient utility measurement: experience from two clinical trials. *Medical Care*, 33, 922–37.

Sackett, D. and Torrance, G. (1978). The utility of different health states as perceived by the general public. *J. Chron. Dis.*, 31(11), 697–704.

Schoemaker, P. (1991). Choices involving uncertain probabilities – tests of generalized utility models. *J. Economic Behavior and Organization*, 16, 295–317.

— (1992). Subjective expected utility theory revisited: a *reductio ad absurdum* paradox. *Theory and Decision*, 33, 1–21.

Sen, A. (1991). Utility: ideas and terminology. *Economics and Philosophy*, 7, 277–83.

Sinclair, J., Torrance, G., Boyle, M., Horwood, S., Saigal, S., and Sackett, D. (1981). Evaluation of neonatal intensive care programs. *New Eng. J. Med.*, 305(9), Aug.27, 489–94.

Spiegelhalter, D., Gore, S., Fitzpatrick, R., Fletcher, A., Jones, D., and Cox, D. (1992). Quality-of-life measures in health care. III: Resource allocation. *Brit. Med. J.*, 305, 1205–9.

Spilker, B. (1996). *Quality of life and pharmacoeconomics in clinical trials* (2nd edn). Lippincott-Raven, Philadelphia.

Stiggelbout, A., Kiebert, G., Kievit, J., Leer, J., Stoter, G., and de Haes, J. (1994). Utility assessment in cancer patients: adjustment of time tradeoff scores for the utility of life years and comparison with standard gamble scores. *Medical Decision-Making*, 14(1) Jan–Mar, 82–90.

Streiner, D.L and Norman, G.R. (1989). *Health measurement scales: a practical guide to their development and use.* Oxford University Press, Oxford.

Torrance, G.W. (1971). *A generalized cost-effectiveness model for the evaluation of health programs* [doctoral dissertation]. State University of New York at Buffalo, Buffalo.

— (1976a). Social preferences for health states: An empirical evaluation of three measurement techniques. *Socio–Economic Planning Sciences*, 10(3), 129–36.

— (1976b). Health status index models: A unified mathematical view. *Management Science*, 22(9) May, 990–1001.

— (1984). Health states worse than death. In *Proceedings of Third International Conference on Systems Science in Health Care.* (ed. W.V. Eimeren, R. Engelbrecht, and C.D. Flagle), pp. 1085–9. Springer–Verlag, Berlin.

— (1986). Measurement of health-state utilities for economic appraisal: A review. *J. Health Economics*, 5, 1–30.

—, Thomas, W., and Sackett, D. (1972). A utility maximization model for evaluation of health care programs. *Health Services Research*, 7(2) Summer, 118–33.

—, Boyle, M.H., and Horwood, S.P. (1982). Application of multi-attribute utility theory to measure social preferences for health states. *Operations Research*, 30, 1043–9.

— and Feeny, D. (1989). Utilities and quality-adjusted life years. *Int. J. Technology Assessment in Health Care*, 5, 559–75.

—, Furlong, W.J., Feeny, D.H., and Boyle, M. (1995). Multi-attribute preference functions: health utilities index. *PharmacoEconomics*, 7, 503–20.

—, Blaker, D., Detsky, A., Kennedy, W., Schubert, F., Menon, D., et al.. (1996a). Canadian guidelines for economic evaluation of pharmaceuticals. *PharmacoEconomics*, 9, 535–59.

—, Feeny, D.H., Furlong, W.J., Barr, R.D., Zhang, Y., and Wang, Q. (1996b). Multi-attribute utility function for a comprehensive health status classification system: health utilities index mark 2. *Medical Care*, 34, 702–22.

Tversky, A. and Kahneman, D. (1992). Advances in prospect theory: cumulative representation of uncertainty. *J. Risk and Uncertainty*, 5(4), 297–323.

Ubel, P.A., Loewenstein, G., Scanlon, D., and Kamlet, M. (1996). Individual utilities are inconsistent with rationing choices: a partial explanation of why Oregon's cost-effectiveness list failed. *Medical Decision-Making*, 16(2) Apr–June, 108–16.

von Neumann, J. and Morgenstern, O. (1944). *Theory of games and economic behaviour*. Princeton University Press, Princeton, NJ.

Wakker, P. (1996). A criticism of healthy years equivalents. *Medical Decision-Making*, 16, 207–14.

Wakker, P., Erev, I, and Weber, E. (1994). Comonotonic independence: the critical test between classical and rank-dependent utility theories. *J. Risk and Uncertainty*, 9, 195–230.

Weinstein, M. and Stason, W. (1977). Foundations of cost-effectiveness analysis for health and medical practices. *New Eng. J. Med.*, 296(13) Mar.31, 716–21.

— and Fineberg, H.C. (1980). *Clinical decision analysis*. W.B. Saunders Co, Philadelphia.

— and Pliskin, J. (1996). Perspectives on healthy years Equivalents (HYEs): What are the Issues? *Medical Decision-Making*, 16, 205–6.

Williams, A. (1988). Ethics and efficiency in the provision of health care. In *Philosophy and Medical Welfare* (ed. M. Bell and S. Mendux), pp. 111–26. Cambridge University Press, Cambridge.

— (1995). Economics, QALYs and medical ethics – A health economist's perspective. *Health Care Analysis: J. Health Philosophy and Policy*, 3(3), 221–6.

Wolfson, A.D., Sinclair, A.J., Bombardier, C., and McGeer, A. (1982). Preference measurements for functional status in stroke patients: inter-rater and inter-technique comparisons. In *Values and Long Term Care* (ed. R. Kane and R. Kane), pp. 191–214. D.C. Heath, Lexington.
Wolfson, M.C. (1996). Health-adjusted life expectancy. *Health Reports*, **8**, 41–6.

ANNEX 6.1. SIMULATED INTERVIEW

The following example and exercise is provided to give some feeling for how the main preference measurement instruments described in sections 6.3.1, 6.3.2 and 6.3.3 are actually used in practice. This example is unchanged from the first edition of the book. The example is still valid, but note that now it is considered better technique to use a converging ping-pong strategy for changing the probabilities offered in the standard gamble, or the times offered in the time trade-off (Furlong *et al.* 1990). In addition, we now recommend that if a visual analogue scale (feeling thermometer) instrument is used, it should precede the standard gamble or time trade-off.

Consider the following simulated interview between an interviewer (I) and a subject (S) to measure the preference scores for three chronic health states (A,B,C) and three temporary states (D,E,F). The preference scale is the conventional one anchored by dead = 0 and healthy = 1. In this example each state is measured three times, by three different techniques: standard gamble, time trade-off, and category scaling. The task is to determine the 18 preference scores (six states, three techniques). (Answers in Table 6.9.)

Hint: In the standard gamble and the time trade-off methods you must determine the subject's 'indifference point'. This is the point at which the subject is indifferent between (cannot decide between) choice 1 and choice 2. If the subject switches his choice on two adjacent questions, the indifference point is taken to be halfway between. If the subject expresses indifference on a particular question, that is taken as the indifference point.

Notation: I = Interviewer
         S = Subject
         A > B means A is preferred to B

1. Chronic health states

I: Thank you for agreeing to participate. On each of these three sheets is a description of a chronic condition. Each sheet is labelled A, B, or C. [*Note to reader*: The conditions can be quite disparate, like kidney dialysis, blind, mental retardation.] Please imagine that you will have to spend the rest of your life in one of these conditions. Rank the conditions in order of preference, and relative to 'healthy' and 'dead'. That is, if any of the conditions are better than being healthy or worse than being dead, please indicate.

S: Alright, healthy > A > B > C > dead.

I: Good. Now I have a device here called a probability wheel. [References: Torrance 1976, p. 131; Torrance 1982, p. 41.] The wheel is divided into two sectors; a blue sector and a yellow sector. First let us adjust the wheel so it is half blue and half yellow. Now consider the following choices; which do you prefer, choice 1 or choice 2? In choice 1 you get chronic condition C for the rest of your life. In choice 2 you get either 2a or 2b described below depending on the outcome of the spin of this pointer on the wheel. That is, if you choose 2, I am going to spin this pointer on the wheel and if it stops on blue you get 2a but if it stops on yellow you get 2b. 2a is healthy for the rest of your life. 2b is immediate death. Now which do you choose, 1 or 2?

S: Well C is pretty bad, I think I'd take my chances and select choice 2.

I: Alright. Now I am going to adjust the wheel so it is only 40 per cent blue and 60 per cent yellow. Now the pointer has a greater chance of stopping on yellow in which case you get 2b, immediate death. Would you still select choice 2?

S: Yes.

I: OK, now I'll adjust the wheel again so it is 30 per cent blue, 70 percent yellow. Would you still select choice 2?

S: No, I don't think so. That's too risky now, I'd take choice 1.

I: OK, that's the end of that one, thank you. Now, imagine a new situation. Here you again have two choices, and I want to know which you prefer. choice 1 is condition B for the rest of your life. choice 2 is the same as before. Let's reset the wheel to 50 per cent blue and 50 per cent yellow. Now, which choice do you prefer?

S: I think I'd take choice 1.

I: OK, now I'll adjust the wheel to 60 per cent blue, 40 per cent yellow. Now, how do you feel about the choices?

S: Oh, that makes choice 2 more attractive. I think I'll switch to it.

I: Fine, thank you. Now we have another new situation. This time choice 1 is condition A for the rest of your life. choice 2 is the same as before. Let's reset the wheel to 50/50, now which do you prefer?

S: Choice 1 definitely.

I: OK, now I'll adjust the wheel to 60 per cent blue, 40 per cent yellow. Now what do you think?

S: Still choice 1.

I: OK, let's move the wheel to 70 per cent blue, and 30 per cent yellow.

S: Still choice 1.

I: OK, let's move the wheel to 80 per cent blue, 20 per cent yellow.

S: Now, that makes it difficult to decide. I think choice 1 and choice 2 now seem about the same to me. I really don't much care which I get.

I: OK, fine thank you. Now I have a new type of question for you. Given your age, your remaining life expectancy is another 40 years. I am going to give you some choices and ask you which you prefer. Choice 1 is to live your remaining 40 years in condition C. Choice 2 is to live a shorter time, but healthy. For example, let's say in choice 2 you get to live only 20 more years, but healthy. Which would you take, choice 1 or choice 2?

S: I'd say choice 2, because C is really pretty bad.

I: OK, what if choice 2 was only 15 years, but still healthy.

S: Oh, that's getting pretty tough, but I think I'd still take choice 2.

I: OK, what if choice 2 is only 14 years?

S: That's about my limit. Any less than 14 years I'll switch to choice 1. Fourteen years is right on the knife edge, I could go either way.

I: OK, fine thank you. Now a new situation. Choice 1 is condition B for your remaining 40 years. In choice 2 you will have only 20 years to live, but they will be healthy years.

S: Well that's pretty hard to choose. I think those two choices are about the same.

I: Fine. Now for the last situation concerning these chronic states. Choice 1 is condition A for your remaining 40 years. In choice 2 your will have only 20 years to live but they will be healthy years.

S: Well, I think this time I would take choice 1.

I: OK, let's make choice 2, 25 years, all healthy.

S: I'd still take choice 1.

I: OK, let's make choice 2, 30 years, all healthy.

S: I'd still take choice 1.

I: OK, let's make choice 2, 35 years, all healthy.

S: OK, this time I would take choice 2.

I: Fine, thank you. Now for the last type of question relating to these health states, I have here a device we call a 'feeling thermometer'. [*See* Torrance 1982; p. 40.] As you can see it is a thermometer-shaped 0-100 scale on a felt board, with 0 labelled 'least desirable' and 100 labelled 'most desirable'. I also have these five narrow foam sticks pointed at each end labelled respectively healthy, dead, A,B, and C. I want you to select the foam stick that represents the most desirable way to spend the rest of your life and place it on the felt board beside the thermometer at 100. Similarly, please select the least desirable and place it at 0. Now place the other sticks somewhere between the top and the bottom of the thermometer depending on how you feel about spending the rest of your life in each condition. If you feel the same about two sticks just put them on top of each other. The distance between the sticks should all be relative to each other. For example, if you feel that the difference in desirability between healthy and A is twice as great as the difference between A and B, the spacing between the sticks healthy and A should be adjusted to be twice that between A and B.

S: OK, I think that's it.

I: Thinking it over, are there any changes you would like to make?

S: No, I think not.

I: Fine, now please read out the sticks and the thermometer values they are beside.

S: OK, Healthy 100, A 80, B 52, C 35, Dead 0.

I: Fine, thank you very much, that completes this phase of the interview.

2. Temporary health states

I: Here are three different sheets. Each sheet describes a temporary dysfunctional health condition which you would have for three months. At the end of the three months you will be completely recovered. Each sheet is labelled D,E or F [*Note to reader*: The conditions can be quite disparate like mononucleosis for three months, hospital confinement with kidney dialysis for three months for the treatment of temporary kidney failure, clinical depression for three months.] Imagine that you will have to spend the next three months in one of these conditions. Please rank them in order of preference.

S: OK, I'd say D > E > F.

I: Good, now I'm going to get out the probability wheel and give you some choices again. For this first situation imagine that, unfortunately, you have only 3 months to live. Choice 1 is to spend these 3 months in condition F. In choice 2 you get either 2a or 2b depending on the spin of the pointer on the wheel; blue gives you 2a, yellow 2b: 2a is healthy for the 3 months, 2b is immediate death. With the wheel at 50 per cent blue, 50 per cent yellow which would you choose?

S: F is pretty bad, I'll take choice 2.

I: OK, 40 per cent blue, 60 per cent yellow.

S: That's about my indifference point. Any less blue and I'll switch for sure.

I: Fine, now here's a completely new situation, that fortunately does not involve dying. This time you will always completely recover at the end of the three months. Choice 1 is condition E for the three months. Choice 2 is either 2a (if blue) or 2b (if yellow) depending on the outcome of the spin. 2a is immediate cure; 2b condition F for three months. With the wheel at 50 per cent blue, 50 per cent yellow which would you choose?

S: Choice 1.

I: OK, 60 per cent blue, 40 per cent yellow.

S: Choice 2.

I: Good, thanks. Now for a similar question. Choice 1 is condition D for three months followed by cure. Choice 2, is a spin leading to: 2a (blue), immediate cure; 2b (yellow), condition E for three months followed by cure. With the wheel at 50/50 which would you choose?

S: Choice 2.

I: OK, 40 per cent blue, 60 per cent yellow?

S: Still choice 2.

I: OK, 30 per cent blue, 70 per cent yellow?

S: OK, now I'll switch to choice 1.

I: Good, thanks. That completes the probability wheel questions. Now, here's a new question. Unfortunately, in this question we must again assume you have only three months to live. Choice 1 is to spend this last 12 weeks in condition F. In choice 2 you live for a shorter period of time, but healthy. Let's say six weeks.

S: I'd take Choice 2.

I: OK, what if it was only five weeks?

S: That's about my indifference point.

I: Good, now we'll change the situation so you no longer die. Now, you will be completely cured at the end of the temporary condition. Which would you prefer: choice 1, 12 weeks of E; choice 2, 6 weeks of F?

S: Choice 1.

I: OK, what if choice 2 is only five weeks?

S: OK, now I'd take choice 2.

I: Good, now for the last situation. Again the choices are followed by complete cure. Choice 1, 12 weeks of D; choice 2, 6 weeks of E.

S: Choice 2.

I: OK, what if choice 2 is 7 weeks?

S: I'd still take it.

I: What if it is 8 weeks?

S: Now I can't tell. That's my indifference point. Any longer than that and I'd switch to choice 1.

I: Good, that completes these questions. Now we just have the feeling thermometer to do again and then we're finished. This time the five sticks are labelled healthy, dead D, E, and F. Furthermore, this time we must assume that you have only three months to live. Please place the five sticks on the feeling thermometer following the same instructions as the last time. When you're ready please read them out to me.

S: OK, here they come. Healthy 100, D 81, E 75, F 41, Dead 0.

I: OK, terrific. That completes the interview. Thank you very much. You have been very helpful.

Table 6.9 Calculation of health state preference scores from the simulated interview

	Standard gamble	Time trade-off	Rating Scale (thermometer)
Cronic states			
lifetime			
Healthy	1.00	1.00	1.00
A	0.80	0.81	0.80
B	0.55	0.50	0.52
C	0.35	0.35	0.35
Dead	0.00	0.00	0.00
Temporary states			
3 months			
Healthy	1.00	1.00	1.00
D	0.82	0.82	0.81
E	0.73	0.73	0.75
F	0.40	0.42	0.41
Dead	0.00	0.00	0.00

Calculations

$C = 14/40 = 0.35$
$B = 20/40 = 0.50$
$A = 32.5/40 = 0.81$

$F = 0.40$
$E = 0.55 \times 1.00 + 0.45 \times 0.40 = 0.73$
$D = 0.35 \times 1.00 + 0.65 \times 0.73 = 0.82$

$F = 5/12 = 0.42$
$E = 1 - (1 - 0.42)(5.5/12) = 0.73$
$D = 1 - (1 - 0.73)(8/12) = 0.82$

7

Cost-benefit analysis

7.1. SOME BASICS

The feature that distinguishes among techniques of economic evaluation is the way in which the consequences of health care programmes are valued. Cost–benefit analysis (CBA) requires programme consequences to be valued in monetary units, thus enabling the analyst to make a direct comparison of the programmes incremental cost with its incremental consequences in commensurate units of measurement, be they dollars, pounds or yen. In this chapter we briefly examine the theoretical underpinnings of CBA and clarify the ways in which CBA differs from CEA and CUA. Recent texts giving more detailed exposition of the theory and practice of CBA in health care include Johansson (1995) and Johannesson (1996). Perhaps not surprisingly, the major portion of this chapter is given over to measurement issues concerning how consequences of health care programmes can be valued in terms of money. We trace a brief history of money valuation for health outcomes and lay out the advantages and disadvantages, conceptual and practical, of different approaches.

7.1.1 CBA: an approach or an analysis?

In casual conversation it might be reasonable to refer to all the evaluation techniques in this book as being 'cost–benefit analysis'. Indeed, in an influential early article, Williams (1974) used the phrase the 'cost–benefit approach' as a generic description of the way of thinking that economics brings to health care evaluation, where the problem is framed in terms of a production relationship between resource inputs and health outputs. But in defining cost–benefit analysis (CBA) as a specific technique of evaluation we need to be much more precise with the use of language. As shown in Box 7.1, CBA compares the discounted future streams of incremental programme benefits with incremental programme costs; the difference between these two streams being the net social benefit of the programme. In simple terms, the goal of analysis is to identify whether a programme's benefits exceed its costs, a positive net social benefit indicating that a programme is worthwhile. Although, as we will discuss below, the precise decision rule for CBA will depend upon the context of the evaluation and specifically if one is allocating resources within a fixed budget or not. (Pauly 1995). An alternative formulation considers whether the ratio of benefit to cost is greater than unity, although this formulation is generally regarded as problematic because the location of items in numerator or denominator can easily change the ratio (see Birch and Donaldson 1987 and Box 2.4 in Chapter 2).

Box 7.1.   Cost–Benefit Analysis: A formulation in search of data

Given i = 1, . . . I possible investments:

$$NSB_i = \sum_{t=1}^{n} \frac{b_i(t) - c_i(t)}{(1 + r)^{t-1}}$$

NSB_i	= net social benefit of project i (discounted)
$b_i(t)$	= benefits (in money terms) derived in year t
$c_i(t)$	= costs (in money terms) in year t
$1/(1 + r)$	= discount factor at annual interest rate r
n	= lifetime of project

The primary goal of CBA is to identify projects where NSB > 0. It will also be useful, for allocation within a fixed budget, to rank projects according to their NSB. The major issue for health care CBA is the valuation of health outcomes in money $b_i(t)$.

CBA is a full economic evaluation because programme outputs must be measured and valued. However, there is significant mislabeling of studies in the health care literature with studies that compare only programme costs (i.e., partial evaluation) using the term 'cost–benefit analysis'. In a recent literature review, Zarnke *et al.* (1997) found that 60 per cent of studies claiming to be CBA were actually cost comparisons where no attempt had been made to value benefits in monetary terms. As illustrated in Box 7.2, such restricted cost comparison formulations of cost–benefit analysis can be misleading for resource allocation because only programmes that generate cost savings would be seen as worthwhile.

7.1.2. The CBA question: Is the programme worthwhile?

As we have seen in previous chapters CEA and CUA are well suited to the task of allocating a fixed budget to competing programmes so as to maximize the selected effectiveness measure (e.g., life years saved, QALYs gained, HYEs gained). However, to do so requires both complete and comparable data on all alternatives and requires a formal periodic budget allocation process during which all programmes are assessed simultaneously – both of these requirements seldom exist in health care. More commonly, programmes are discussed one at a time, or a few at a time, and decisions are required without the

---

Box 7.2. Cost comparisons labelled as CBA: pertussis vaccination

In this study by Koplan *et al*, (1979), of pertussis vaccination, costs were measured as the resource cost of the vaccine, the treatment of complications resulting from the vaccine, and the treatment of cases of pertussis that resulted despite being vaccinated. These were called the costs with the programme. Benefits were defined as the savings in medical care costs by preventing pertussis and its sequelae. These were called the costs without the programme. The authors computed the following ratio:

$$\frac{\text{costs without programme}}{\text{cost with programme}} = \frac{\$1\,866\,153}{\$\,720\,862} = 2.6:1$$

This means that the benefits outweighed the costs incurred by 2.6 times. But this formulation does not meet a contemporary definition of CBA because no attempt was made to value, in money terms, the health consequences of the vaccination programme. Benefits have only been defined as cost savings. Consider what would happen if the above ratio had been less than 1, i.e. the programme is cost increasing but it provided health benefits. Using this type of partial evaluation we would only implement programmes that were cost saving.

---

luxury of complete data on all alternatives. Arguably, in this one-at-a-time decision-making, CBA has an advantage over CEA/CUA.

Given the difficulties in attaching money values to health outcomes, which we describe below, it is useful to outline some of the key differences between CBA and the techniques of cost-effectiveness and cost–utility analysis. As we have seen, in non-dominance circumstances where the new programme produces better outcomes at additional costs, both CEA and CUA tell us the price of achieving a particular goal whether it is the incremental cost of a life-year gained, case of disease detected, or a QALY gained. What CEA/CUA cannot tell us, is whether such a goal is *worth* achieving given the opportunity costs of the resources consumed. Hence, to *make decisions* using CEA/CUA we must invoke some external criterion of value, either through the use of implied values from cost per QALY league tables or published threshold values which are often arbitrary (see Chapter 9). Ultimately, although both CEA/CUA avoid money valuation of health outcomes *as part of the analysis*, to make any resource allocation decision using CEA/CUA data a decision-maker (implicitly or explicitly) must place a money value on the health outcomes and any other programme benefits.

The fact that both CEA/CUA and CBA ultimately require money valuation of health outcomes has led some authors (Phelps and Mushlin 1991) to argue that the techniques are nearly equivalent. However, there is a fundamental philosophical difference. Following Sugden and Williams (1979), CEA/CUA is based on a 'decision-making' philosophy where elected or appointed decision makers review results and decide on the relative values assigned to competing programmes and goals. In contrast, the philosophical foundation of CBA is in principles of welfare economics where the relevant source of values is believed to be individual consumers. A basic tenet of CBA therefore is that individual consumers are deemed to be the relevant source of money values for programme outcomes. This issue is explored further in Chapter 9.

7.1.3. CBA has broader scope than CEA/CUA

In many respects CBA is broader in scope than CEA/CUA. Because CBA converts all costs and benefits to money it is not restricted to comparing programmes within health care but can be used (although not without problems) to inform resource allocation decisions both within and between sectors of the economy (Drummond and Stoddart 1995). Some analysts have attempted to use WTP to compare health and non-health for programmes (Olsen and Donaldson 1997a). Indeed, in public sector economic evaluation in areas such as transport and environment, the application of CBA has a long history (Sugden and Williams 1979) and is the most widely used form of economic evaluation. In contrast CEA/CUA is necessarily restricted to the comparison of health care programmes that produce similar units of outcome such as QALYs. CEA/CUA address mainly questions of *production efficiency* with outcomes restricted to health benefits. In contrast, CBA is broader in scope and able to inform questions of *allocative efficiency*, because it assigns relative values to health and non-health related goals to determine which goals are worth achieving, given the alternative uses of resources, and thereby determining which programmes are worthwhile.

Some researchers have attempted to quantify some of the non-health benefits that consumers derive from health care programmes such as 'reassurance value' arising from knowledge of a test or procedure. This source of value has been called 'process utility' (as distinct from the utility of health outcomes) by Donaldson and Shackley (1997) and an application to quantify the monetary value of reassurance and information can be found in Donaldson *et al.* (1995) and Donaldson *et al.* (1997b). The analysis of WTP by pregnant women for additional (non-diagnostic) ultrasound could also be framed in this way (Berwick and Weinstein 1985). Another perspective on this point, however, is that if a person exhibits anxiety because they are not reassured in the process of care, then such anxiety could be measured as impairment of their psychological well-being and hence be a measurable component of quality-of-life or utility.

Another contrasting feature of CEA/CUA and CBA is that the former techniques are typically more narrowly client-focused. For example, in a clinical evaluation the focus of a CEA would typically be the expected health outcome for the patients treated. As argued by Labelle and Hurley (1992), the standard CEA/CUA framework does not capture effects that spill over to other persons – which can be positive or negative – known as externalities in economics. (In theory, it is possible to capture such effects in CEA/CUA, but in practice, this has not yet been done.) In contrast, as will be discussed later, using techniques of willingness-to-pay the CBA framework can quantify these effects. For example, the total societal willingness to pay for a new AIDS drug is the sum of the value accruing directly to the patients but also the value that others (current non-patients) attach to the new treatments.

7.2. ASSIGNING MONEY VALUES TO HEALTH OUTCOMES

There are three general approaches to the monetary valuation of health outcomes: (1) human capital; (2) revealed preferences; (3) stated preferences of willingness-to-pay (contingent valuation). We discuss each of these approaches and review both theoretical and practical strengths and weaknesses. As illustrated by the quotations in Box 7.3, the whole topic of attempting to assign money values to health outcomes explicitly as part of CBA has been, and remains, controversial. What is often overlooked, however, is that such valuations occur – often implicitly – everyday when decisions are made by both individuals and societies that trade-off health objectives against other benefits.

Box 7.3. The rhetoric of assigning money values to health

'The major disadvantage of the benefit–cost framework is the requirement that human lives and quality of life be valued in monetary units. Many decision makers find this difficult or unethical or do not trust analyses that depend upon such valuations.' (Weinstein and Fineberg 1980, p.240)

'To be trained in medicine, nursing or one of the other 'sharp end' disciplines and then be faced with some hard-nosed, cold-blooded economist placing money values on human life and suffering is anathema to many.' (Mooney 1992)

7.2.1. The human capital approach

The utilization of a health care programme can be viewed as an investment in a person's human capital. In measuring the pay-back on this investment the value of the healthy time produced can be quantified in terms of the person's renewed or increased production in the market-place. Hence the human capital method places monetary weights on healthy time using market wage rates and the value of the programme is assessed in terms of the present value of future earnings. This human capital method of valuing health status has been used for many years (for an early application see Mushkin *et al.* 1978). We can distinguish between two uses of the human capital concept: (1) as the *sole* basis for valuing all aspects of health improvements, and (2) as a method of valuing *part* of the benefits of health care interventions, using earnings data as a means of valuing productivity changes only. For an illustration of the human capital approach to health care CBA, consider the rubella vaccination example in Box 7.4.

Box 7.4.   CBA using human capital method: rubella vaccination

This study examined the costs and consequences of providing rubella vaccination. The consequences were conceptualized as those costs that would be avoided with the vaccination programme. Consequences included not only the averted medical costs associated with acute rubella and congenital rubella syndrome, but also the reduced economic productivity that results from a disability or premature death. In order to place a monetary value on reduced productivity, the authors computed average lifetime earnings and estimated the amount of earnings that would be lost if no rubella vaccination programme were in effect. They found that the costs of the programme totalled $28 937 400 and the value of lost productivity totalled $9 521 200 for both medical conditions (Schoenbaum *et al.* 1976).

There are a number of measurement difficulties with the human capital approach. First, although in theory wage rates reflect the marginal productivity of a worker there are often imperfections in labour markets and wage rates may reflect, *inter alia*, inequities such as discrimination by race or gender. Second, if the study is from a societal perspective the analyst would need to consider the value of healthy time gained that is not sold for a wage. This raises a general class of problems of how economists place shadow prices on non-marketed resources. For example, suppose a homemaker receives some treatment and is now able to return to his or her duties looking after the children, whereas previously he or she could not. There are two methods for attaching a shadow price to this time: (1) An *opportunity cost of time* argument would be that the value of this production in the home must be *at least* as great as what could be earned in the labour market, otherwise the homemaker would choose to enter the labour market. Hence, the time would be valued according to the wage rate forgone; (2) a *replacement cost* approach would attempt to quantify how much it would cost to replace the homemaker in the home with services from the market (e.g. cleaning, child minding, etc.). Both of these approaches have been used to value homemakers' time in studies; see Klarman (1967) for the opportunity cost and Weisbrod (1968) for the replacement cost approaches.

7.2.2. Human capital and welfare economics

In addition to some of the practical measurement problems of using the human capital approach, it came under attack in the 1970s by economists who argued that this production-based method for valuing health improvements was not consistent with the theoretical foundation of cost–benefit analysis from welfare economics. The most notable contribution to this debate was by Mishan (1971).

Although this book is intended for a practical audience of persons who wish to use economic evaluation, it is useful to spend a few sentences explaining some of the welfare economic underpinnings of CBA (for a more detailed conceptual approach see Johansson, 1995). First, welfare economics is a branch of economics that can address *normative* questions because it embodies certain value judgements. In contrast, most of economics is *positive* because it makes predictions without value judgements (e.g. raising the price of a product *will* reduce its demand). What do we mean by a value judgement in this context? Examine Box 7.5 for the two key value judgements of welfare economics. The proposition (and judgement) is that social welfare *should* comprise individuals welfare and that individuals *should* be considered the best source of information on their own welfare. Further, it is assumed that resource allocation is proceeding by the forces of a competitive market which is in equilibrium and that current (i.e. pre-programme) income distribution is appropriate. These propositions form the foundation for the Pareto principles in Box 7.5 which are central to cost–benefit analysis. Specifically, it is the contemporary reinterpretation of the Pareto principles by British economists Nicholas Kaldor (1939) and Sir John Hicks (1939, 1941) that forms the basis for CBA to be operationalized, with programme benefits being valued using a compensation test and the principles of willingness to pay.

Box 7.5. Pareto principles in brief

Vilfredo Pareto was a nineteenth century sociologist who is best known for his thoughts on the general principles of economic policy evaluation. He worked in the efficiency tradition of utilitarianism, with its focus on the 'greatest good of the greatest number', with less attention to distributional or equity issues. The general question he sought to answer was: How would we judge whether society as a whole was better off from a policy or programme?

Key assumptions
1. Social welfare is made up from the welfare (or utilities) of each individual member of society.
2. Individuals are the best judges of their own welfare (consumer sovereignty).

Principles
1. *Actual Pareto Improvement.* A policy that makes one or more persons better off and makes no person any worse off.
2. *Potential Pareto Improvement.* (Kaldor–Hicks criterion): A policy that creates gainers and losers in welfare, but if the gainers *could* compensate the losers and remain better off themselves after the change then society as a whole has benefited. Because compensation does not actually have to be paid, this principle raises some equity issues about who gains and who loses.

Returning to the critique of the human capital approach, Mishan (1971) pointed out that the valuation method was not consistent with the principles of welfare economics (see Box 7.5) because it offers a narrow view of the utility consequences of a project restricted to impacts on labour productivity. The more fundamental and relevant notion of value embedded in welfare economics is what consumers who gain from the programme are willing to *sacrifice* to have the programme in question. It is this collective willingness to pay (i.e. willingness to sacrifice other goods and services) which is the focus of CBA, recognizing that not all consumers will benefit and some may lose and require compensation. Mishan's contribution was to shift the focus of the debate and practical measurement toward contemplating what monetary compensation individuals required for reduced health, or how much they would be willing to pay for improved health.

Advocates of this Pareto school of compensation test were also quick to point out that study should focus on an individual's health–money decisions *under uncertainty* rather than certainty (Jones-Lee, 1976). Under a certainty scenario a person might (quite reasonably) request infinite compensation for, say, loss of life which would make CBA intractable. Rather, the argument was that valuations should be made on money versus health risk trade-offs. Based on this notion of valuing a so-called statistical life rather than an actual life, two types of enquiry emerged. The first was revealed preference studies looking at wage-risk trade-offs. The second was stated preference studies examining hypothetical scenarios and willingness to pay. This second type of survey method has become known as contingent valuation.

7.2.3. Revealed preference studies

A number of wage–risk studies have been published, in which the goal is to examine the relationship between particular health risks associated with a hazardous job and wage rates that individuals require to accept the job (Marin and Psacharopoulos 1982). This approach is consistent with the welfare economics framework just discussed, because it is based on individual preferences regarding the value of increased (decreased) health risk, such as injury at work, as a trade-off against increased (decreased) income, which represents all other goods and services the person might consume. An example of the wage–risk approach is given in Box 7.6.

Box 7.6. Value of a statistical life

Wage–risk example
'Suppose jobs A and B are identical except that workers in job A have higher annual fatal injury risks such that, on average, there is one more job-related death per year for every 10 000 workers in job A than in job B, and workers in job A earn $500 more per year than those in job B. The implied value of statistical life is then $5 million for workers in job B who are each willing to forgo $500 per year for a 1-in-10 000 lower annual risk' (Fisher *et al.* 1989).

The strength of the wage–risk approach is that it is based on actual consumer choices involving health versus money, rather than hypothetical scenarios and preference statements. However, a weakness of the approach is that estimated values have varied widely and estimation seems to be very context and job-specific. Using observed data there is always the problem of disentangling the many factors that will confound the relationship between wage and health risk. Furthermore, for use in a specific CBA of a treatment programme it is necessary to observe an occupational choice where the relevant health outcome is the focus of compensation or payment. A more fundamental concern is that the observed risk–money trade-offs may not reflect the kind of rational choice revealing preferences that economists believe because of the many imperfections intervening in labour markets and limitations in how individuals perceive occupational risks. It is not possible to review comprehensively the volume of work that has been done in this area but the interested reader should consult Viscusi (1992) for a good review.

It is worth noting at this point that there is another valuation principle that might also be referred to as revealed preference but is not based on individual consumers. This approach is a review of past decisions, such as court awards for injury compensation, to elicit the minimum value that society (or its elected representatives) places on health outcomes (Mooney 1977). In practice, how-ever, many such legal awards are actually based on human capital calculation of discounted earnings streams. Shifting the focus slightly, one might also be tempted to review previous government health care funding decisions as a source of revealed preference to determine dollar values assigned to health outcomes. But the danger here is one of circularity because we would use previous decisions in future analyses in the belief that some rational process had truthfully revealed societal values for health outcomes in the prior decision.

7.2.4. Contingent valuation studies

As the name suggests, contingent valuation studies use survey methods to present respondents with hypothetical scenarios about the programme or problem under evaluation. Respondents are required to think about the *con-tingency* of an actual market existing for a programme or health benefit and to reveal the maximum they would be willing to pay for such a programme or benefit. Why are we interested in the *maximum* willingness-to-pay? Consider a simple consumer decision to buy a chocolate bar. A measure of how much she values the chocolate bar is the maximum that she would be willing to pay. The difference between this value and the price she has to pay in the market is known as consumer surplus. Of course, for products like chocolate bars one does not need to hire high-priced economists to do a formal CBA; each consumer does this calculation in his own head. However, the logic carries over to contingent valuation studies for non-marketed goods such as a health care programme where we are trying to estimate value in relation to cost for purposes of collective funding. Hence in contingent valuation studies consumers are asked to consider what they would be willing to pay, and thereby sacrifice in terms of other commodities, for the programme benefits if they were in the market-place .

Here we take health programme benefits to be broadly defined; some may be improvements in health status while others may be attributes such as the value of information or the value associated with the process of care (Donaldson and Shackley 1997). It is the aggregation of this consumer surplus – which can be large, small, positive or negative – across individuals which forms the basis of the cost–benefit calculus. In many ways, therefore, CBA studies based on contingent valuation and statements of willingness-to-pay can be thought of as attempts to replace missing markets, albeit hypothetically, in an attempt to measure underlying consumer demand and valuation for non-marketed social goods such as health care programmes.

Before reviewing the use of contingent valuation methods in health care it is important to recognize that the need to value health gains and losses for inclusion in CBA has arisen in other public sectors such as transport and environment. Indeed, much of the pioneering for contingent valuation methods was undertaken in transport CBA by economists such as Jones-Lee (1976). An example of a contingent valuation question to estimate a money value for loss of life in the context of road safety is given in Box 7.7. As can be seen, an important advantage of this example is its realism, because it involves an easily understood choice that many people have faced – albeit with a little less precision on the risk of death! Hence in this example the contingency is not difficult to imagine because actual markets for cars do exist where price is related to safety features (e.g. inclusion/exclusion of air bags). Indeed, with this example one can even compare stated preferences with revealed preferences from actual market data.

Box 7.7. Value of a statistical life: road safety contingent valuation example

'Suppose that you are buying a particular make of car. You can, if you want, choose to have a new kind of safety feature fitted to the car at an extra cost. The next few questions will ask about how much extra you would be prepared to pay for some different types of safety feature. You must bear in mind how much you personally can afford.

As we said earlier, the risk of a car driver being killed in an accident is 10 in 100 000. You could choose to have a safety feature fitted to your car which would halve the risk of the car driver being killed, down to 5 in 100 000. Taking into account how much you can personally afford, what is the most that you would be prepared to pay to have this safety feature fitted to the car?' (Jones-Lee *et al.* 1985).

Hypothetical example

Current risk of death without safety feature	= 10 in 100 000
New risk with safety feature	= 5 in 100 000
Reduction in risk (dR)	= 5 in 100 000
Maximum (e.g.) premium willing to pay (dV)	= £50
Implied value of life	= dV/dR
	= £50/5 x 10^{-5}
	= £1m

Box 7.8. Use of willingness-to-pay and willingness-to-accept questions in the contexts of compensating variation and equivalent variation. Source: (O'Brien and Gafni, 1996)

Temporal perspective and programme status:		Does this consumer gain or lose in utility from before–after change?	Compensating variation (CV)	Equivalent variation (EV)
Before	After		$+/- required *after* the change to make utility same as before the change	$+/- required *before* the change to make utility the same as after the change
Project A		Gain	**A₁** Willingness-to-pay (WTP): Maximum amount that must be taken from gainer to maintain at current (before) level of utility	**A₃** Willingness-to-accept (WTA): Minimum amount that must be paid to *potential* gainers to forgo the gain and make utility equal to what it would have been after the change
No programme	Programme	Loss	**A₂** Willingness-to-accept (WTA): Minimum amount that must be paid to loser to maintain at current (before) level of utility	**A₄** Willingness-to-pay (WTP): Maximum amount that must be taken from *potential* loser to forgo the loss and make utility level equal to what it would have been after the change
Project B		Loss	**B₁** Willingness-to-accept (WTA): Minimum amount that must be paid to loser to maintain at current (before) level of utility	**B₃** Willingness-to-pay (WTP): Maximum amount that must be taken from *potential* loser to forgo the loss and make utility level equal to what it would have been after the change
Programme	No programme	Gain	**B₂** Willingness-to-pay (WTP): Maximum amount that must be taken from gainer to maintain at current (before) level of utility	**B₄** Willingness-to-accept (WTA): Minimum amount that must be paid to *potential* gainers to forgo the gain and make utility equal to what it would have been after the change

Another set of conceptual distinctions are shown in Box 7.8. Studies can use either the utility concept of compensating or equivalent variation and can ask questions of willingness to pay (WTP) or willingness to accept (WTA) depending upon whether a programme is being introduced or removed. For example, in Box 7.8 under the concept of compensating variation and for the introduction of a programme for an individual who gains from this programme, we would wish to find out the maximum amount that must be taken from the gainer to maintain them at the current (before programme) level of utility. This would be the maximum they would be willing to pay for the project to go ahead. In contrast, equivalent variation for the same individual would be the minimum amount that must be paid to this *potential* gainer to *forgo* the gain and to make his utility equal to what it would have been after the change. Hence the equivalent variation is the minimum the individual would be willing to accept in compensation to forgo the project. A more rigorous derivation and discussion of these concepts can be found in Johansson (1995), and this text also gives a discussion of the circumstances under which these concepts yield the same money values. Reviews of studies conducting money valuations of health programme benefits indicate that the majority of studies use WTP in the context of programme introduction and compensating variation (Diener *et al.* 1997).

Box 7.9. Health care contingent valuation studies
Here are some examples of published contingent valuation studies in health care.
Most of them are feasibility or pilot studies of WTP and not full CBA studies.

Thompson (1986)	– new arthritis drug
Appel *et al.* (1990)	– non-ionic contrast media
Donaldson (1990)	– care of the elderly
Berwick and Weinstein (1985)	– ultrasound with pregnancy
Johannesson and Jönsson (1991)	– hypertension/cholesterol lowering
Neumann and Johannesson (1994)	– *in vitro* fertilization
O'Brien and Viramontes (1994)	– chronic obstructive pulmonary disease
O'Brien *et al.* (1995)	– new antidepressant drug
Ryan *et al.* (1997)	– antenatal care

7.2.5. Contingent valuation studies in health care

In recent years there has been rapid growth in the number of contingent valuation studies published in the health care literature. In Box 7.9 we give some examples of these studies and the diversity of clinical areas that have been studied, ranging from arthritis to depression, and *in vitro* fertilization. It should be noted, however, that most of the published health care contingent valuation studies are experimental in nature, attempting to explore measurement feasibility issues rather than being full programme evaluations using CBA. This cautious embrace of contingent valuation is partly due to some of the inherent difficulties in measuring willingness-to-pay and partly to some ongoing conceptual debates concerning what questions should be asked of whom in health care contingent valuation studies. To review and summarize some of these issues, the next section considers some of the theoretical and practical considerations that face the analyst seeking to design a contingent valuation study to value the benefits of a health care programme.

7.3 WHAT MIGHT WE MEAN BY WILLINGNESS-TO-PAY?

The application of techniques for measuring willingness-to-Pay (WTP) is an area of growth and innovation in health care economic evaluation. But it is important to keep in mind that WTP is a measurement technique, and it is how and why this technique is applied which determines its usefulness for cost–benefit analysis. Reviews of WTP studies in health care have revealed wide variation in what questions are being asked, of whom, and how (O'Brien and Gafni 1996). There is disagreement therefore concerning how WTP should be measured and how such measures can be incorporated into cost–benefit analysis.

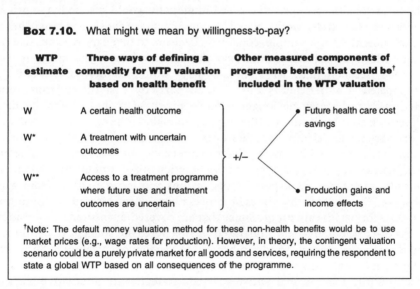

Box 7.10. What might we mean by willingness-to-pay?

WTP estimate	Three ways of defining a commodity for WTP valuation based on health benefit	Other measured components of programme benefit that could be[†] included in the WTP valuation
W	A certain health outcome	• Future health care cost savings
W*	A treatment with uncertain outcomes	+/-
W**	Access to a treatment programme where future use and treatment outcomes are uncertain	• Production gains and income effects

[†]Note: The default money valuation method for these non-health benefits would be to use market prices (e.g., wage rates for production). However, in theory, the contingent valuation scenario could be a purely private market for all goods and services, requiring the respondent to state a global WTP based on all consequences of the programme.

In this section we explore different ways in which the concept of WTP can be defined and measured for inclusion in a health care cost–benefit analysis. A simple framework is presented in Box 7.10 which distinguishes between improvements in health per se and other sources of benefit, all of which could, in theory, be valued by WTP. For the health component we also consider the nature of the commodity defined in a WTP study with particular emphasis on the role of uncertainty. We describe and illustrate this framework in the following sections.

7.3.1. Global versus restricted WTP

There are three broad categories of benefits that can arise from a health care programme: (1) intangible benefits which are the value of improved health *per se* to the individual consumer of a programme; (2) future health care costs avoided; (3) increased productive output due to improved health status. One 'restricted' perspective on willingness-to-pay is that it would be used only to value those components of benefit for which no money values existed from other market sources. In this approach, WTP estimates are restricted to quantifying the money value of changes in health *per se*, with future health care cost savings and production gains being valued using market prices.

An alternative 'global' perspective on this measurement task is to argue that the purpose of the contingent valuation study is to learn about how the individual consumer would value a specific health care programme in a world where private markets and price signals for all goods and services were operational. However, in this free market scenario for contingent valuation, consistency also calls for us to ask the respondent to consider in their valuation the future health care costs that they individually would sustain in the private market world and also work-related income effects as a consequence of ill health or treatment. As an example, consider a decision to buy a more expensive but more effective cold medication over the counter from a pharmacy. A consumer's decision (and willingness-to-pay) would be driven not only by anticipated health benefits but also, in part, by cost offsets from other medications she may no longer need to purchase if she bought the more expensive cold medications. She might also include the costs associated with work absence in deciding whether or not to buy the more expensive medications. Therefore in this simple private market consumer purchase example, my willingness-to-pay for a medication is a function not only of the health benefits but also of future out-of-pocket cost savings and income effects from work absence. By analogy this thought process can be transferred to contingent markets for health care programmes that are covered by insurance or taxation.

As discussed above and illustrated in Box 7,10, the concept of contingent markets is very powerful and can be used to assign money values to all aspects of benefit arising from a health care programme, not simply the value of health itself. While these global and restricted strategies are alternative ways to proceed, great caution needs to be exercised in how respondents are being questioned and whether there is potential for double-counting of some programme benefits. For example, when assessing an individual's willingness-to-pay for a new antihypertensive medication the respondent needs to be told explicitly whether they should be considering income effects due to work absence arising from the disease or its treatment. Double-counting would arise if the individual had considered income effects in answering the WTP questions but the analyst also valued attributable production gains using wage rate data (i.e. a human capital calculation).

7.3.2. What good or service is being valued?

Even if we focus on the restricted form of WTP based on health benefits, as shown in Box 7.10, there are at least three ways in which a good or service for valuation can be defined: (1) find the willingness-to-pay for a certain health outcome (W); (2) find the willingness-to-pay for a treatment with uncertain health outcomes (W*); (3) find the willingness-to-pay for access to a treatment programme where future use and treatment outcomes are both uncertain (W**). Consistent with the welfare economics of health care market failure as outlined by Arrow (1963), the main distinction between these three definitions of the good or service being valued is uncertainty. The difference between W and W* is the inclusion of uncertainty on the supply side with respect to outcomes for a given treatment. In moving to W** we also include uncertainty on the demand side, because individuals are being asked about their willingness-to-pay for a health care programme given they are uncertain whether they need or will demand this service in the future.

In the next sections we review these three definitions of the goods or service being valued, as illustrated in Box 7.10.

Valuing a certain health outcome (W)

Authors such as Pauly (1995) have suggested that finding the 'shadow price' for a QALY may be a useful bridge between cost–utility analysis and cost–benefit analysis. Some empirical work on the relationship between health status measures and WTP has also been undertaken (Reed–Johnson 1994). Studies that fall in this first use of WTP to value certain health outcomes would include the early work of Thompson (1986), where persons with arthritis were asked open-ended questions for the maximum they would be willing to pay to achieve a cure of their arthritis.

Valuing a treatment with uncertain outcomes (W)*

As indicated by authors such as Gafni (1991), a limitation of basing WTP estimates on certain health outcomes is that the consequences of health care programmes are inherently uncertain. Under W* therefore, the goal of measurement is to determine the maximum the respondent would be willing to pay to consume a treatment programme with outcomes that are not certainties but have specified probabilities. Although one can multiply certain health values (h) by probabilities to devise expected money values for the programme, the values collected directly on uncertain prospects (W*) will only be the same as the expected values if individuals are risk neutral with respect to income and health.

Valuing access to a treatment program (W**)

In most developed countries we observe that health care services are funded and delivered on the basis of insurance or tax contributions. This reflects an important characteristic of the health care market which is that illness and the demand for health care is uncertain. The consequence of such insurance or tax arrangements would be that persons do not bear the full cost (if any) of the service at the point of delivery. Hence it has been argued by Gafni (1991) that willingness-to-pay questions should be framed in a way that incorporates this demand side uncertainty. Specifically, in Box 7.10 we characterize W** as being the maximum an individual would be willing to pay for access to a treatment programme where both future use and treatment outcomes are uncertain. For example, this hypothetical choice might use the payment vehicle of increased insurance premiums or taxation to ensure a programme is made available. A distinction is therefore made between an ex-post perspective such as W* where the individual undertaking the valuation knows that they are a consumer of the treatment and that the only uncertainty is on the probability of outcomes, versus an *ex ante* perspective such as W** where the individuals valuation needs to incorporate the probability of sustaining the illness and needing the service in question.

Box 7.11. Willingness to pay for *in vitro* fertilization

This study illustrates two different approaches to forming contingent valuation questions. The *ex post* or user-based approach is how much you will pay at the point of consumption. The *ex ante* or insurance-based approach is how much you will pay for insurance coverage.

Ex-post perspective (user-based)
- assume you are infertile and want children
- IVF has 10 per cent chance of being successful if purchased
- mean WTP of $17 730 (if 10% chance of success)
- $28 054 (if 25% chance of success)
- $43 576 (if 50% chance of success)

Ex-ante perspective (insurance-based)
- assume you have 10 per cent chance of being infertile
- IVF has 10 per cent chance of success
- you can buy one-time insurance premium for IVF coverage
- mean WTP of $865

Implied WTP per statistical baby
- $177 730 (user-based)
- $1.8m (insurance-based)

Source: Neumann and Johannesson (1994)

In Box 7.11 we illustrate the difference between the *ex post* and *ex ante* perspective using an example of *in vitro* fertilization from Neumann and Johannesson (1994). This was a population-based survey where the authors explored willingness-to-pay for IVF services using both an *ex post* scenario (assuming infertility. what would you pay out-of-pocket) and an *ex ante* scenario (where the individuals are asked to assume they have a 10 per cent chance of being infertile and they can buy insurance coverage for IVF). What is notable from Box 7.11 is that the implied value per statistical baby is much higher for the *ex ante* or insurance-based approach ($1.8m) than the *ex post* or user-based approach ($0.17m). This is because in the insurance-based setting persons are now also incorporating their risk aversion into the valuation of access to the programme.

As a further illustration of how such *ex ante* insurance-based questions can be asked in practice, Box 7.12, taken from a study by O'Brien *et al.* (1997), shows how respondents who were enrollees in a health maintenance organization in the US were asked whether they were willing to upgrade their insurance coverage to include a new supportive drug used in cancer chemotherapy known as GCSF. The benefit of this drug is that it reduces the risk of neutropenic fever following chemotherapy; in the example in Box 7.12 the reduction in risk is from 20 per cent to 10 per cent over the six cycles of chemotherapy. A bidding algorithm was used (see below) to find the maximum additional monthly premium persons would pay to have the new drug covered.

Box 7.12. Example of ex ante insurance-based WTP

Option A: Your HMO plan covers chemotherapy	Option B: Your HMO plan covers chemotherapy and GCSF
• Assume that your chance of getting cancer over the next 5 years is 1 in 100 • You continue to pay your current monthly insurance premium for health care	• Assume that your chance of getting cancer over the next 5 years is 1 in 100 • You pay a monthly supplement to cover GCSF in addition to your insurance premium for health care

If you get cancer:	**If you get cancer:**
• You get chemotherapy but not GCSF • Over 6 cycles of chemotherapy your chance of neutropenic fever is:	• You get chemotherapy with GCSF • Over 6 cycles of chemotherapy your chance of neutropenic fever is:
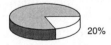 20%	10%
• You cannot buy GCSF or get it covered by another plan	• You cannot buy GCSF or get it covered by another plan

If GCSF was not currently covered by your HMO plan (Option A), would you consider paying an increased premium for coverage of GSCF (Option B)?

Source: O'Brien *et al.* (1997)

7.3.3. Connecting the Ws

The Ws in Box 7.10 are clearly connected, and the nature of the relationship depends, *inter alia*, upon the risk preferences of the respondents. For example, one could measure money values for certain health outcomes (W) and multiply these by their probabilities of arising to calculate the expected money value of a treatment programme. However, this expected value would only correspond with the measured *ex ante* value $W^{\star}$ to the extent that individuals were risk neutral (with respect to income and health) in their preferences. As was described in Chapter 6, we generally observed that individuals are risk averse and therefore the *ex ante* value would be less than the expected value. This risk preference relationship is also true for $W^{\star}$ in relation to $W^{\star\star}$, and this has been analyzed recently by Johannesson (1996).

We have already discussed the relationship between the restricted concept of WTP (W, $W^{\star}$, or $W^{\star\star}$ in this framework), with its primary focus on the value of health benefits, and the more global concept of WTP where a respondent is required to value all health and non-health benefits in money terms. It is this concept of global or overall WTP that was labelled as W' back in Figure 2.2. In practice it is unlikely that many studies will attempt to measure W', but in theory it could be done.

7.3.4. Other sources of utility for money valuation

As we discussed earlier, the work of Donaldson and Shackley (1997) has emphasized the role of non-health benefits (eg. information) for inclusion in WTP. Depending upon the programme there may be significant non-health sources of (dis)utility to capture.

Another important source of private health care market failure, identified by Arrow (1963), is due to spillovers or externalities. The concept of externality in the consumption of health care is best explained using the example of an infectious disease where one person might be willing to pay for another person to receive treatment so as to reduce the risks of disease transmission to himself or others. More generally, there might also be humanitarian spillovers in that one person derives utility from the knowledge that others can gain access to needed health care services. The implications of externalities for willingness-to-pay studies is that the sampling frame for inquiry must extend to all persons whose utility is impacted by the introduction of the programme. For example, in assessing WTP for an (elective) new vaccination programme for an infectious disease one would need to draw survey samples from all persons who would benefit from the programme, including the direct benefit to those who vaccinate and the indirect benefit of those not vaccinating but now at lower risk.

7.3.5 A simple example

To illustrate how WTP data might be used in a CBA, consider the decision context of an HMO trying to decide whether to place a new drug on its formulary. Let us suppose a WTP survey similar to that described in O'Brien *et al.* (1997) – the GCSF study described in boxes 7.12 and 7.13 – has been undertaken on a sample of HMO enrolees. The WTP scenario was the maximum additional insurance that respondents would pay to have the drug covered over a 5-year period. The first task would be to forecast the total WTP (for the HMO population) from the sample using multiple regression analysis based upon known characteristics of the sample and population. Suppose the (discounted) total WTP over the 5 years is $10m. The cost of the programme is a function, in part, of how many persons will receive the treatment, over the same time period, and this must also be forecast. Suppose the estimated cost is $7m with an estimated $2m in cost savings from health care resources not consumed by persons who receive the treatment for a net cost (discounted) of $5m. For simplicity, assume that there are no productivity losses or that gains and losses cancel out. Using these data the programme has a positive net benefit of $5m (that is, $10m – $7m + $2m). How this information can be used to inform resource allocation depends upon a number of things but particularly whether one is allocating resources within a fixed or non-fixed budget setting.

In a non-fixed budget scenario, the HMO might decide to add the new programme and actually raise insurance premiums thus increasing its budget. In a competitive market, if these marginal adjustments to coverage, which could be up or down, do not reflect consumers' values then consumers (or their employers) may elect to switch to other plans. The second scenario for WTP-based CBA is with a fixed budget. In this circumstance, knowledge that the new programme has a positive net benefit is of partial value for resource allocation and prioritising services. To implement the new program without expanding the budget, efficiency criteria would argue for a rank-ordering of existing programmes by the size of their net benefit to facilitate comparison with the new programme. Efficiency would require us to replace programmes with small net benefit by programmes with larger net benefits. The practical difficulty with this scenario is that it is hungry for data and works by comparison of net benefit; having data on the new programme is a necessary but not sufficient condition for making resource allocation decisions.

7.4. PRAGMATIC MEASUREMENT ISSUES

7.1.4. Issues of bias and precision

The goal of the contingent valuation measurement task is to obtain precise and unbiased estimates of willingness-to-pay. To pose such a question in a way that is both believable and clear to a respondent is not a trivial undertaking and is at least as complex (probably more so) as the utility measurement tasks described in Chapter 6. There are two types of general question format: open-ended and closed-ended. Open-ended questions pose a difficult cognitive task for most respondents because we are typically not used to thinking about the *maximum* we would pay for something. Experience with this approach suggests that although it may produce unbiased estimates of WTP because the respondent is not prompted, it is very imprecise with widely varying responses and many non-responses or protest responses (Johannesson 1996). Also see Donaldson *et al.* (1997*c*) on evaluation of open ended question formats.

Closed-ended question formats have been used in health care contingent valuation studies in two general formats: bidding games to find within-person maximum value and so-called 'take-it-or-leave-it' between-person surveys. Bidding games use a predetermined search algorithm to bid the respondent up or down, conditional upon how they respond to a prompted monetary value. Much like an auction, if you say yes to $50 we will ask you a higher amount; no, and we will ask you a lower amount. For example, see the study by O'Brien and Viramontes (1994). While the bidding game improves upon open-ended questions for the precision of the estimated maximum WTP, it may do so at the expense of introducing a bias in the form of starting point bias. This bias is a form of framing effect where the respondents' answers are influenced by the first numbers presented in the bidding game. Although a number of non-health and health care studies have found evidence of starting point bias (Stalhammer, 1997), this result is not conclusive because others have used bidding games and found no evidence of starting point bias, even though it was explicitly tested for (O'Brien and Visamontes 1994; O'Brien *et al.* 1997).

To illustrate this concept, we show in Box 7.13 the bidding game used in the same GCSF study mentioned in Box 7.12 from O'Brien *et al.* (1997). Respondents received one of two bid algorithms and analysis showed that the hypothesis of no starting point bias could not be rejected.

The second type of closed-ended question format is an approach used widely in environmental economic evaluation where surveys of large numbers of persons are typically undertaken to elicit values for some environmental programme or problem. (A controversial environmental example where contingent valuation methods have been used is the valuation of natural resources destroyed by the Exxon Valdez oil spill in Price William Sound.) The essence of this approach is that each respondent is only asked one question ('take-it-or-leave-it'); for example, would you be willing to pay an extra $50 per month on your taxes for this programme – yes/no? The money amount each person is asked is randomly selected from a range. So, for example, the next person might be asked if they are willing to pay $100, and so on. The data are then analyzed using econometric techniques such as probit analysis to identify a bid curve – that is, the quantitative relationship between the proportion of persons accepting/rejecting the bid at different levels of the bid. By mathematically integrating for the area under this bid curve one can determine the mean willingness-to-pay, or, alternatively, identify the median willingness to pay. For a discussion of this approach in health care see Johannesson (1996).

Box 7.13. Bidding algorithms used in the GCSF WTP study

Bid level	Insurance-based bid scale, $	Bid algorithm #1	Bid algorithm #2
1	1		
2	5		
3	10		
4	15		
5	25		
6	50		
7	100		

Notes : Y= willing to pay this bid; N=not willing to pay this bid.
Persons accepting bid-level 7 were then asked an open-ended question for the maximum they were willing to pay.

Source: O'Brien *et al.* (1997)

The 'take-it-or-leave-it' categorical approach has been used in health care contingent valuation studies by Johannesson (1994) with some success. The difficulties with this approach are in identifying the relevant range from which to sample bids and also in the large sample size one needs for precise estimation. A variant of this approach which increases precision is to ask another (random) bid question of each respondent, but the direction being conditional on the answer to the first question. In the future is is likely that interviews will be computer-based so that random bid selection (first or subsequent) is easy to achieve. However, there is still some residual risk of bias because the analyst must choose the *range* from which bids are sampled.

7.4.2 Validation of WTP by tests of scope

Is it possible to validate the findings of a WTP study? The 'gold standard' against which we would like to compare predicted WTP from CV surveys is what consumers would *actually* pay. Unfortunately, for most of the health programme benefits studied by CV methods, actual market may not exist so *criterion validity* cannot easily be established. However, there are some useful tests of *construct validity* that can be examined in WTP studies. The logic of construct validation in this setting is to determine whether the data are consistent with theoretical constructs that should be present if the WTP responses are measuring the value we intend.

There are two simple popositions ('constructs') from economic theory that can be tested. First, most goods have what is known as a positive income elasticity meaning that, other things being equal, higher respondent incomes should be associated with higher WTP. Second, the more of a positively-valued good that is supplied by a hypothetical programme, the greater should be a persons' WTP, although the marginal utility of additional units of benefit is likely to decline.

This second principle was strongly endorsed by recent guidelines for WTP studies for environmental damage assessment (National Oceanic and Atmospheric Administration (NOAA) 1993). The NOAA panel termed these validation techniques "scope tests" because the proposition is that WTP should vary with the scope of the benefit (or damage) arising from the hypothetical programme. Scope tests are an important part of WTP validation and have been recommended by European guidelines on health care WTP studies where, for example, the magnitude of a treatment effect or other health benefit can be varied in the survey (Johannesson *et al.* 1996). For examples of scope tests in health care WTP studies see Kartman *et al.* (1996), Stalhammer and Johannesson (1996), and O'Brien *et al.* (1997).

7.4.3. Payments and health care settings

One of the key difficulties with contingent valuation studies is making the scenario realistic for the respondent. Even if we adopt an *ex ante* insurance-based perspective, most consumers will not be familiar with purchasing access to individual health care programmes. It is likely that these forms of payment scenarios will work better in some health care systems such as the United States where consumers are used to paying more directly for health care than in other health care systems such as the UK which has a system of social provision based on taxation contributions. In the environmental economic evaluation literature it has been customary to characterize the decision problem as whether to vote in favour of or against a proposal to have a programme implemented which would have an associated tax contribution. In this kind of format the respondent has their mind focused on the idea of a referendum rather than an actual purchasing decision. In some settings this may be more realistic for the respondent than to consider insurance contributions.

7.5. CONCLUSIONS

As we have indicated in this chapter, CBA is, at least in theory, the most powerful of the techniques for economic evaluation because it can directly address questions of allocative efficiency which the other techniques cannot. But this advantage comes only after the analyst has overcome a number of difficulties associated with assigning a monetary value to programme benefits. Much of this chapter has focused on this thorny issue and we have described how experience with contingent valuation techniques has given rise to new enthusiasm for implementing WTP in health care programme evaluation. Whether the promise held out by these approaches is fulfilled remains to be seen. We noted that although a number of feasibility and pilot studies have appeared in the literature, there are very few complete CBA studies that use WTP as the basis for valuing all outcomes.

The further development of CBA in health care will be helped by careful use of language and definitions. Numerous published studies are termed cost–benefit analysis yet only offer a partial evaluation, comparing direct costs with and without the programme. A consistent use of the label for this technique will help focus the minds of analysts and consumers of CBA studies on the precise issues of theory and empiricism that continue to challenge this approach.

7.6. EXERCISE: DESIGNING A CONTINGENT VALUATION SURVEY FOR A NEW TREATMENT FOR OVARIAN CANCER

Scenario

The government is trying to decide whether they should reimburse a new therapy for ovarian cancer. Design a willingness-to-pay survey for a cost–benefit analysis of this new treatment for ovarian cancer. Assume that among women who receive this therapy there is a 5 per cent rate of complete cure from the cancer, but the majority will sustain some side-effects from the treatment. Data suggest there are productivity gains with more women in the treated group being able to return to work. There are also cost offsets with treated women receiving fewer health care services in the future.

Specific questions:

1. Which components of benefit arising from this treatment programme would you value using WTP? Consider the pros and cons of using a 'global' WTP estimate for valuing all programme benefits versus a 'restricted' WTP for health benefits and market prices for other components of benefit.

2. How would you define the commodity that the respondent is being asked to pay for? Consider the alternative formulations of W, W*, and W** discussed in this chapter. What kind of payment vehicle is 'believable' for each of these formulations?
3. The draft study proposal is to interview a sample of women with ovarian cancer. Would you include other subjects in the survey, and why?

Solutions/Ideas

1. Using the 'global approach' discussed in this chapter we would frame a willingness-to-pay scenario for the individual for the contingent market for the new therapy, where future attributable costs and employment effects were a personal responsibility and to be met out-of-pocket. If one used this approach and made it explicit that the respondent should consider these attributes in their valuation then it would not be appropriate to use market prices to value future health care cost savings or wage rates to value productivity effects. To do so would be double counting because the individual has been asked to consider these in a private market scenario where they are the responsibility of the individual. In practice this global approach may be a difficult cognitive task for the respondent. An easier route may be to use market prices for the future costs and productivity effects but use the willingness-to-pay approach only for the benefit of the health effects i.e. the 'restricted' approach to WTP. If this approach is adopted however, it is still important to state explicitly to the respondent that they should not consider income effects associated with work absence or future costs associated with the disease in their valuation.

2. The key difference between the three Ws is the incorporation of uncertainty into the valuation tasks. Perhaps the simplest task would be to estimate money values for the (certain) health states arising in the evaluation. More generally, however, it would be more desirable to include uncertainty with respect to outcomes such that individuals were being asked to value the treatment with probabilities of therapeutic benefit but also probabilities of harm. One of the difficulties here is the extent to which the multiple attributes of outcome and associated probabilities can be presented to respondents in a manner which will be comprehensible. The payment vehicle one might adopt for this type of money valuation could be additional out-of-pocket expense at the point of consumption (e.g. a variable co-payment on a medication). A difficulty with this payment vehicle format is that it may not be believable to respondents if the therapy is a major medical procedure that would normally be covered by a health care system at zero cost to the patient. The consequence of such a question framing might be a number of protest responses from respondents.

Formulating the valuation question to estimate W** is more complex yet. Now the respondents need to be presented with information both on the uncertain outcomes of therapy but also on probability of needing this therapy themselves in some future time period. How one frames a payment vehicle to address W** is also complex and will be conditional upon the system of health care financing that the respondent is familiar with. For example, in a predominantly private insurance system it may be most meaningful to ask the respondent to consider additional insurance premiums that they would be willing to pay to gain coverage and access to the treatment programme. In a predominantly tax-financed health care system it may be necessary to frame the question in terms of additional tax contributions (either national or local) that would facilitate the availability of the new treatment programme.

3. While it may be of interest to interview women with ovarian cancer in the estimation of W or W*, the total societal willingness-to-pay will necessitate a broader sampling. For example, to estimate W** one would need to also interview women who do not currently have ovarian cancer but are at risk of this disease. These individuals may be willing to preserve the option of having this programme available should they need it in the future. More generally, there is also the issue of externality or spillover benefits to other members of the population who are not at current or future risk of ovarian cancer (i.e. men). Men may be willing to pledge additional insurance or tax dollars to cover the ovarian cancer treatment programme either through a self-interested motivation (i.e. wives and daughters at risk) or through a general humanitarian or altruistic motivation where they are expressing a statement of value for women more generally.

REFERENCES

Appel, L.J., Steinberg, E.P., Powe, N.R., Anderson, G.F., Dwyer, S.A., and Faden, R.R. (1990). Risk reduction from low osmolality contrast media. What do patients think it is worth? *Medical Care*, **28**, 324–34,

Arrow, K. (1963). Uncertainty and the welfare economics of medical care. *American Economic Review*, **53**, 941–73.

Berwick, D.M. and Weinstein, M.C. (1985). What do patients value? Willingness-to-pay for ultrasound in normal pregnancy. *Medical Care*, **23**, 881–93.

Birch, S., Donaldson, C. (1987). Applications of cost benefit analysis to health care departures from welfare economic theory. *J. Health Economics*, **6**, 211–25.

Diener, A., O'Brien, B., Gafni, A. (1997). *Contingent valuation studies in the health care literature: A review and classification.* [Manuscript].

Donaldson, C. (1990). Willingness to pay for publicly-provided goods: a possible measure of benefit? *J. Health Economics*, **6**, 103–18.

Donaldson, C., Mapp, T., Farrar, S., Walker, A., Macphee, S. (1997). Assessing community values in health care: is the 'willingness to pay' method feasible? *Health Care Analysis*, **5**, 7–29.

Donaldson, C., Shackley, P., Abdalla, M., Miedzybrodzka, Z. (1995). Willingness to pay for antenatal carrier screening for cystic fibrosis. *Health Economics*, **4**, 439–52.

Donaldson, C., Shackley, P. (1997). Does 'process utility' exist? A case study of willingness to pay for laparoscopic cholecystectomy. *Social Science and Medicine*, **44**, 699–707.

Donaldson, C., Thomas, R., Torgerson, D. J. (1997). Validity of open-ended and payment scale approaches to eliciting willingness to pay. *Applied Economics*, 29, 79–84.

Drummond, M.F., Stoddart, G.L. (1995). Economic evaluation of health-producing technologies across different sectors: Can valid methods be developed? *Health Policy*, 33, 219–31.

Fisher, A., Chestnut, L.G., and Violette, D.M. (1989) The value of reducing risks of death: A note on new evidence. *J. Policy and Management*, 8, 88–100.

Gafni, A. (1991). Using willingness-to-pay as a measure of benefits: What is the relevant question to ask in the context of public decision-making? *Medical Care*, 29, 1246–52.

Hicks, J.R. (1939). The foundation of welfare economics. *Economic Journal*, 49, 696–712.

Hicks, J.R. (1941). The four consumer surpluses. *The Review of Economic Studies*, 11, 31–41.

Johanesson, P.O. (1995). *Evaluating health risks*. Cambridge University Press. Cambridge.

Johannesson, M. (1996). *Ex ante* versus expected willingness-to-pay. *Soc. Sci. Med.* 42, 305–11.

— (1996). *Theory and methods of economic evaluation of health care*. Kluwer, Dordrecht.

— and, Jönsson B. (1991). Economic evaluation in health care: Is there a role for cost–benefit analysis? *Health Policy*, 17, 1–23.

—, — (1991). Willingness to pay for antihypertensive therapy results of a Swedish pilot study. *J. Health Economics*, 10, 461–74.

—, —, Karlsson, G. (1996). Outcome measurement in economic evaluation. *Health Economics*, 5, 279–96.

Jones-Lee, M.W. (1976). *The value of a life: An economic analysis*. University of Chicago Press, Chicago.

Jones-Lee, M.W., Hammerton, M. and Phillips, P.R. (1985). The value of safety: Results of a national sample survey. *Economic Journal*, 95, 49–72.

Kaldor, N. (1939). Welfare propositions of economic and interpersonal comparisons of utility. *Economic Journal*, 49 549–52.

Kartman, B., Andersson, F., Johannesson, M. (1996). Willingness to pay for reductions in angina pectoris attacks. *Medical Decision Making*, 16, 246–53.

Klarman, H.E., Francis, J.O.S., and Rosenthal, G. (1968). Cost-effectiveness analysis applied to the treatment of chronic renal disease. *Medical Care*, 6, 48–54.

Koplan, J.P. *et al.* (1979). Pertussis vaccine – an analysis of benefits, risk and costs. *New Eng. J. Med.*, 301, 906–11.

Labelle, R. and Hurley, J. (1992). Implications of basing health care resource allocations on cost–utility analysis in the presence of externalities. *J. Health Economics*, 11, 259–77.

Marin, A., and Psacharopoulos, G. (1982). The reward for risk in the labour market: Evidence from the United Kingdom and a reconciliation with other studies. *J. of Political Economy*, 90(4), 827–53.

Mishan, E.J. (1971). Evaluation of life and limb: A theoretical approach. *J. Political Economy*, 79, 687–706.

Mooney, G. (1977). *The valuation of human life*. MacMillan, London.

— (1992). *The economics of health and medicine*. Wheatsheaf.

Mitchell, R.C. and Carson, R.T. (1989) *Using surveys to value public goods: the contingent valuation method*. Resources for the Future, Washington D.C.

Mushkin, S. *et al.* (1978). Cost of disease and illness in the United States in the year 2000. *Pub. Health Rep.*, 93, 493.

National Oceanic and Atmospheric Administration (1993). Natural resource damage assessments under the oil pollution act of 1990. Notice of proposed rules. *Federal register*, **58**, R4612.

Neumann, P. and Johannesson, M. (1994). The willingness-to-pay for *in vitro* fertilization: A pilot study using contingent valuation. *Medical Care*, **32**, 686–99.

O'Brien, B., and Viramontes, J. L. (1994) Willingness-to-pay: A valid and reliable measure of health state preference? *Medical Decision Making*, **14**, 289-97.

— and Gafni, A. (1996). When do the 'dollars' make sense? Toward a conceptual framework for contingent valuation studies in health care. *Medical Decision Making*, **16**, 288–99.

O'Brien, B.J., Novosel, S., Torrance, G., and Streiner, D. (1995). Assessing the economic value of a new antidepressant: A willingness-to-pay approach. *Pharma-coEconomics*, **8**(1), 34–45.

—, Goeree, R., Gafni, A., Torrance, G.W., *et al.* (1997). Assessing the value of a new pharmaceutical: a feasibility study of contingent valuation in managed care. *Medical Care* (in press).

Olsen, J. A., Donaldson, C. (1997*a*). Helicopters, Hearts and Hips: Using willingness to pay to set principles for public sector health care programmes. *Social Science and Medicine* (in press).

Pauly, M.V. (1995). Valuing health care benefits in money terms. In *Valuing health care* (ed. F.A. Sloan). Cambridge University Press, Cambridge.

Phelps, C.E., and Mushlin, A. (1991). On the (near) equivalence of cost-effectiveness and cost–benefit analyses. *Int. J. Technology Assessment in Health Care*, **7**, 12–21.

Reed-Johnson, F., Fries, E.E., and Banzhaf, H.S. (1994). *Valuing morbidity: An integration of the willingness-to-pay and health status literatures*. Working Paper No. T-G401, Triangle Economic Research, North Carolina.

Ryan, M., Ratcliffe, J., Tucker, J. (1997). Using willingness to pay to value alternative models of antenatal care. *Social Science and Medicine*, **44**, 371–80.

Sackett, D.L., Haynes, R.B., and Tugwell, P. *Clinical epidemiology: a basic science for clinical medicine*. Little, Brown & Co, Boston.

Schoenbaum, S.C., Hyde, J.N., Bartoshesky, L., and Crampton, K. (1967). Benefit–cost analysis of rubella vaccination policy. *N. Eng. J. Med.*, **294**(6), 306–10.

Stalhammar, N.O. (1996). An empirical note on willingness-to-pay and starting-point bias. *Medical Decision Making*, **16**, 242–7.

Stalhammer, N. O., Johannesson, M. (1996). Valuation of health changes with the contingent valuation method: a test of scope and question order effects. *Health Economics*, **5**, 531–41.

Sugden, R., Williams, A.H. (1979). *The principles of practical cost–benefit analysis*. Oxford University Press, Oxford.

Thompson, M.S. (1986). Willingness-to-pay and accepts risks to cure chronic disease. *Am. J. Public Health*, **76**, 392–6.

Viscusi, K. P. (1992). *Fatal trade-offs*. Oxford University Press, Oxford.

Weinstein, M.C., Fineberg, H.V., *et al.* (1980). *Clinical decision analysis,* W.B. Saunders Company, Philadelphia.

Weisbrod, B.A. (1964). Collective consumption services of individual consumption goods. *Quarterly J. Economics*, **78**, 471–7.

Williams, A. (1974). The cost–benefit approach. *British Medical Bulletin*, **30**(3), 252–6.

Zarnke, K.B., Levine, M.A.H., and O'Brien, B.J. (1997). Cost–benefit analysis in the health care literature: Don't judge a study by its label. *J. Clinical Epidemiology* (in press).

8

Collection and analysis of data

8.1. INTRODUCTION

In this chapter we review some general principles concerning the collection and analysis of data for economic evaluation of health care programmes. The intent of the chapter is to examine issues that are common to all the techniques of economic evaluation; discussion of specific issues, such as the collection and analysis of utility or willingness-to-pay data, can be found in earlier chapters. The emphasis here is to illustrate different *analytic strategies* that face a researcher embarking upon a new study. From previous chapters we have indicated what information needs to be collected, in theory, for economic evaluation. This chapter addresses two pragmatic empirical questions: (1) How do I collect relevant data? (2) How do I analyse the data when I have them?

The chapter proceeds by distinguishing between primary data collection studies such as 'piggyback' economic evaluations alongside randomized trials and integrative decision analytic models. We examine the advantages and disadvantages of measurement versus modelling and hybrid strategies where modelling is a necessary adjunct to primary measurement. We discuss why, when studies involve primary data collection, it is necessary to identify analysis plans for a research protocol and we review how the final analysis undertaken is conditional upon the costs and effects observed in the trial or clinical study. Finally, we review a number of statistical issues arising in the analysis of economic evaluation studies, including the estimation and presentation of precision around cost-effectiveness ratios using confidence intervals.

8.1.1. Effectiveness data: bias, precision, and relevance

It is important to stress at the outset that an economic evaluation of a health care programme is only as good as the effectiveness data it is built upon. Evidence on the effectiveness of the programme compared to some alternative is the necessary foundation of an economic evaluation. There are various ways in which data on effectiveness for use in economic evaluation might be collected and these can be judged according to three criteria: bias, precision, and relevance.

A hierarchy of study designs has been proposed in the clinical epidemiology literature (Sackett *et al*, 1985) for designs that yield results with differing degrees of bias. The most well-controlled study with the lowest threat of bias is the randomized controlled trial (RCT), followed by cohort studies, case–control studies and case series. Although economic evaluation can use data from any of these designs, the potential for inferential bias on effectiveness is much greater as we move away from randomized designs. The need to base economic evaluation on sound effectiveness data is illustrated by the example of heart transplantation in Box 8.1.

Box 8.1.   Cost-effectiveness of heart transplantation: effectiveness compared to what?

In a UK government-funded economic evaluation of heart transplantation, Buxton *et al.* (1984) faced the difficulty that no comparative evidence on the effectiveness of transplantation had been published. As is often the case with new surgical techniques where a case series has been developed, there was a belief that the surgery saved lives and therefore a widely-held view that it would be unethical to randomize patients to not receive transplantation. In the absence of any comparative outcomes data on the counter-factual (i.e. what would happen to a person who did not undergo heart transplantation), it was not possible to undertake a formal cost-effectiveness comparison. Rather, the study noted that data from the case series of transplant recipients indicated that, through time, there was a marked downward trend in the costs of the procedure, a marked increase in the survival of recipients, and (for survivors) an increase in health-related quality of life following the procedure.

Although randomized trials generally provide the most unbiased evidence on outcomes, they may lack precision for some clinical endpoints that are relevant to the economic evaluation. For example, if one were comparing two therapies in an economic evaluation where the main clinical (and economic) differences were associated with an adverse effect that occurred very rarely, then randomized studies may offer very imprecise information because they have been designed to show a difference in an efficacy rather than safety endpoint. In such a circumstance it may be more useful to build the economic evaluation using evidence from case–control or cohort studies where very small risk differences can be detected.

Even if a randomized controlled trial can deliver unbiased and precise data on outcomes to the health economist, the data may lack relevance to the question at hand. The RCT design generally calls for careful selection and monitoring of patients under a strict research protocol; attempts are made to 'control' the environment and treatments so that one can increase the ratio of statistical signal-to-noise. In the language of programme evaluation (Cook and Campbell, 1979) this means that the RCT has a high degree of *internal validity*. That is, we can make cause–effect inferences with a high degree of confidence.

In contrast, data from an RCT may have a low degree of *external validity* (i.e. generalizability to the real-world setting and use of the treatment) for many of the same reasons mentioned above, and this limits its usefulness for economic evaluation. This tension between internal and external validity is a theme that runs throughout the literature discussing measurement versus modelling in economic evaluation. Using the language introduced earlier, one can frame this dilemma as a trade-off between bias and relevance; by tightly controlling studies and comparisons we reduce bias but at the price of relevance to the real-world. In contrast, an uncontrolled study using observational data may produce evidence relevant to real practice but will introduce bias for making causal inferences. This trade-off is summarized in Box 8.2 which is taken from a report proposing that both sources of data add complementary information to an evaluation and that the way forward is in determining appropriate methods for the synthesis of data (US General Accounting Office 1992).

Box 8.2. Complementary strengths and weaknesses of two study designs for assessing effectiveness

Study design	Primary strength	Primary weakness
Randomized studies	Controlled comparison internal validity	Potential lack of generalizability; external validity at risk
Data base analyses	Coverage of medical practice (full payment population, full range of treatment implementations); external validity	Uncontrolled comparison; internal validity at risk

Source: US General Accounting Office (1992).

8.1.2.Working with best available data

In this chapter, with its emphasis on practical issues relating to data, it is important to state up-front that our philosophical position is that; (1) an economic evaluation is only as good as the data it is based upon, but (2) economic analysts must do the best they can with *the available data*. This second statement is not intended to relegate the option of additional primary data gathering, but it does reflect some of the constraints under which the economist typically operates. Consider, for example the technology of implantable cardiac defibrillators. Concerned about the rising use of this costly technology the UK government commissioned an economic evaluation of the devices. A cost-effectiveness study using decision analystic modelling was completed and published (O'Brien *et al.* 1992). But the major limitation of this study was the lack of reliable data on effectiveness of the device, because no randomized studies had (then) been undertaken. Policy makers need to make the best decisions they can today, recognizing that data are not (nor ever will be) perfect. Furthermore, the dynamic evolution of many health care technologies is such that we may spend additional years gathering primary data only to find that the contemporary policy question has changed. In the case of defibrillators it is only very recently that randomized studies have been undertaken (Moss *et al.* 1997).

8.2. ECONOMIC EVALUATION AND CLINICAL TRIALS

For health care interventions such as new pharmaceuticals, many countries have formal requirements for provision of safety and efficacy data prior to product licensing. The accepted standard for the collection of such data is the randomized controlled trial. In this context, it makes sense to consider how the data requirements of economic evaluation might be built in to such a programme of research. Can economic evaluation questions be simply 'piggybacked' onto existing clinical trials or do we need to adjust trial data using modelling techniques for increased external validity? As an alternative option should we recognize that, in some circumstances, the economic evaluation cannot be 'piggybacked' and a specific trial needs to be designed for economic evaluation? If so, what are the characteristics of such pragmatic trials intended to quantify effectiveness (rather than efficacy) and cost?

The advantages of having economic evaluation data collected prospectively as part of the trial are: (1) having patient-specific data on both costs and outcomes is attractive for analysis and internal validity; (2) given the (typically) large fixed costs incurred in collecting clinical data, the marginal cost of collecting economic data may be modest. However, there are numerous issues and problems that researchers face when conducting economic evaluation as part of a trial. We have already touched on one philosophical issue concerning the timing of data availability. Particularly for pharmaceuticals, it may not be possible to collect the kind of 'real world' data before the drug is in the marketplace. In the next section we highlight (using mainly pharmaceutical examples where most trial-based evaluation has been done) five different issues and then return again to these in the section on modelling. These issues are:

- choice of comparison therapy
- gold standard measurement of outcomes

- intermediate versus final outcomes
- inadequate patient follow-up or sample size
- protocol-driven costs and outcomes

8.2.1. Choice of comparison therapy

A threat to the external validity of any cost-effectiveness study exists when the comparison therapy is not the most relevant for the policy question being addressed. In many countries, placebo comparison plays an important role in regulatory approval of new medicines. For economic appraisal the relevance of a placebo-controlled study depends upon whether the new drug is intended as *adjunctive* therapy or as a *substitute* for an existing therapy that is the current standard of care. For example, in assessing the cost-effectiveness of the new antiemetic drug, ondansetron, Buxton and O'Brien (1992) made comparison (using published trials) against a widely-used and effective existing therapy, metoclopramide (Rusthoven *et al.* 1992). Trials comparing against placebo, as a proxy for no therapy (Cubeddu *et al*, 1990, Beck *et al*, 1993) were not a relevant comparison for the economic question because they do not reveal the incremental impact of the new therapy on population health.

In some circumstances, placebo comparison data may be useful for economic studies, this is typically the case where the new drug will not be a substitute for another but will be a new *adjunctive* therapy. An example would be the placebo-controlled trials of misoprostol as prophylaxis against gastrointestinal complications for persons taking anti-inflammatory drugs; a number of economic studies were undertaken using these trial data (Drummond *et al*, 1992).

In circumstances where the relevant comparison is an existing therapy and head-to-head comparative trials have been done, the active comparison used in the trial(s) may not be the most relevant for the economic analysis. For example, in Canada, the approval of the first low molecular weight heparin (enoxaparin) for prophylaxis against deep-vein thrombosis (DVT) following orthopaedic surgery, was based on trial comparisons against standard heparin. Although the cost-effectiveness of enoxaparin versus standard heparin was studied (Anderson *et al.* 1993) this may not have been the most relevant economic comparison because survey evidence suggested that low-dose warfarin was the most widely-used drug for this indication in North America (Paiment *et al.* 1987). However, a revised economic analysis based on decision analysis but comparing enoxaparin and warfarin (O'Brien *et al.* 1994) had a weaker inferential base for efficacy because no head-to-head trials of these drugs had been published. This illustrates the trade-off between internal and external validity.

8.2.2. Gold standard measurement of outcomes

Randomized trials often employ measurements for outcomes that are more detailed, invasive, or frequent than is customary in usual care. For example, in comparing alternative acid suppressant drugs, the outcome of duodenal ulcer recurrence is usually determined in clinical trials by endoscopy of all patients at fixed follow-up times (Walt *et al.* 1984); but outside of a trial, the management of such patients would be based largely upon symptoms. For an economic analysis to be externally valid, it must reflect the fact that some persons without symptoms will have ulcer recurrence (although silent) and some persons with symptoms may not have ulcer recurrence. This might require the analyst to attempt some adjustment of trial-based ulcer recurrence rates based on the proportion that are symptomatic and would be observed in clinical practice (O'Brien *et al.* 1995). (This issue was discussed in Chapter 5.)

Another example is the diagnosis of deep-vein thrombosis in clinical trials of low molecular weight heparin. The gold standard measurement in such studies is venography – an invasive, relatively expensive, often painful test involving injection of contrast media. But in routine clinical practice if venography is not universally and routinely used as the first-line test for DVT, how useful is this knowledge of the 'truth' for economic evaluation? In a study of enoxaparin (O'Brien *et al.* 1994), the true rates of DVT (by venography) were used from the trial as the prior probabilities of disease for treatment and control, in a decision analytic model which incorporated the conditional likelihood and costs of these DVT being detected by a routine diagnostic algorithm based on clinical signs and symptoms and ultrasound. Such a model includes the costs and outcomes of errors in diagnosis that will happen in routine practice but were not part of the trial because the physician will not generally use costly and invasive tests as first line therapy. Such 'adjustments' to efficacy data are necessary to make data externally valid for economic inferences but they also require some ex-trial data input, for example, on the sensitivity and specificity of clinical diagnosis and ultrasound.

8.2.3. Intermediate versus final health outcomes

In clinical trials of diseases where event rates are small, such as reduction of cardiovascular risk factors, it has become customary to report intermediate biomedical markers as outcomes because sample sizes to test for differences in final outcomes, such as cardiovascular or all-cause mortality, are often prohibitive. Trials of cholesterol-lowering drugs are a good example where the outcome is the measured change in total blood cholesterol or some subfraction (O'Brien 1991). For economic analysis to inform resource allocation we are interested in what impact such changes will have on *final* health outcomes such as mortality and morbidity. This often results in attempts to use existing epidemiologic data (e.g. cohort studies such as the

Framingham study) to construct models that can predict changes in final outcomes (e.g. deaths and myocardial infarctions) from changes in risk factors (see, for example, Edelson *et al.* 1990 on hypertension or Schulman *et al.* 1990 on blood cholesterol).

8.2.4. Inadequate patient follow-up or sample size

A feature of many clinical trials is that patient follow-up and data collection often terminate abruptly when the patient experiences one of the clinical outcome 'events' of interest. From the perspective of the economic analyst this can be frustrating because much of the cost associated with the new therapy may be incurred in the treatment of such events. Many examples can be found in cardiovascular therapy where events such as stroke or myocardial infarction are recorded but with no indication of the health care resources used to manage the cases. An advantage of the prospective economic trial is that the resource consequences of such events can be captured.

Another important design issue is determining an appropriate sample size for testing economic hypothesis. There are a number of methodological issues to be considered. For example, what size of difference in cost or cost-effectiveness is important to detect (O'Brien *et al.* 1994*b*); are we only interested in a one-tailed hypothesis that an incremental cost-effectiveness ratio is below some predetermined threshold (e.g. \$50 000 per life-year)? The heterogeneity of data on resource use is such that, to show a difference between groups at the same level of type I error, one might need a larger sample for the economic question than the clinical question. This raises some interesting ethical and design questions (O'Brien *et al.* 1994*c*). A future research agenda is to explore whether decision makers require the same level of precision for economic data (i.e. $p < 0.05$) as they do for clinical data. Framed in this way, the problem is one of determining decision-makers' preferences regarding acceptable risks for inferential errors on economic data. An interesting allied question is to explore whether the decision makers risk preference is symmetric with respect to the two types of decision error that could arise.

8.2.5. Protocol-driven costs and outcomes

A problem with basing cost estimates on data gathered as part of a clinical trial is the extent to which one is capturing resource use associated with the trial *per se* (i.e. costs of doing research) rather than the costs of providing the therapy. These so-called protocol-driven costs can arise in a number of different ways. For example, to preserve blinding in their comparison of oral gold (Auranofin) versus placebo, Thompson *et al.* (1989) required regular blood tests for patients randomized to placebo; in the analysis they excluded these costs from the placebo control group. However, excluding these protocol-driven costs may not be the only factor requiring adjustment because there may also be some form of ascertainment bias effect in that patients in both groups were seeing a physician more regularly for tests than in routine practice and therapy may have been modified based on observations that would not occur outside the trial. The point to stress is that at the outset of any clinical trial where an economic question is being addressed it is important to establish the extent to which patient management and resource use reflects regular practice.

As experience with economic evaluation alongside clinical trials increases, there will be more subtle protocol biases to consider. For example, the requirement in many trials that the physician be blind to the treatment assigned to a patient may have a bearing upon the way that patient is managed in the trial. In routine practice, *knowing* that the patient is receiving a given treatment may make the physician less cautious in terms of frequency of observation or test-ordering; this therefore poses a threat to the external validity of the cost data collected within the trial (Freemantle and Drummond 1997).

Another central feature of clinical trials is the emphasis of conforming to the rules mandated by the protocol, the principle of compliance by physicians and patients. Great efforts are typically made in the conduct of a clinical trial to ensure that patients consume their prescribed medications and that physicians prescribe such drugs according to protocol. Outside of the trial, when the drug is used in routine practice, there are no such guarantees. To the extent that patients do not comply with the prescribed therapy, there may be a dilution of the treatment effect originally observed in the trial. For example, the Lipid Research Clinics Coronary Primary Prevention Trial (Lipid Research Clinics Programme 1984) demonstrated a clear association between compliance with the study drug (cholestyramine for cholesterol lowering) and outcomes. This leads one to speculate by how much any observed treatment effect will be diluted when the drug is being prescribed outside the strictures of a trial, when compliance may drop even further.

8.2.6. Pragmatic trials for economic evaluation

Rather than attempting to 'piggyback' economic evaluation questions onto an existing clinical trial designed to address safety and efficacy questions, there is growing interest in designing specific trials to collect economic data (i.e. Why piggyback if you can go the whole hog?). Using the distinction of explanatory (i.e. can the intervention work?) versus pragmatic (i.e. does the intervention work?) trials, introduced by Schwartz and Lellouch (1967), the focus of an economic trial would be pragmatic. The intention is to offer some compromise between the goals of internal and external validity; the pragmatic trial retains the concept of subjects being randomly allocated to treatments to minimize bias, but offers fewer restrictions in how patients are recruited and followed after randomization, thus increasing external validity or generalizability.

The aim of pragmatic trials is to evaluate the effectiveness or cost-effectiveness of an intervention under the real world conditions that would prevail once the intervention was in routine use (Schwartz and Lellouch 1967). The main design features of such studies are that:

(1) patients typical of the normal caseload are enrolled;
(2) the therapy of interest is compared with current care;
(3) the settings and physicians involved are fairly representative of the totality;
(4) physicians and patients are not blind to the therapy (in order to take into account all advantages or disadvantages of therapy);
(5) all enrolled patients are followed under routine conditions,
(6) a wide range of endpoints is measured (efficacy, feasibility, tolerance, quality of life, resource use, etc.).

As an example of a pragmatic trial that examined economic endpoints, Oster *et al.* (1995) compared two strategies for lowering elevated cholesterol in a pragmatic trial based in a health maintenance organization in California. They assessed cost, clinical outcome (in post-treatment total serum cholesterol), and patient satisfaction with the HMOs current regimen (stepped care with niacin followed by other agents) compared with first-line therapy with lovastatin. Every attempt was made to make the trial reflect the real world practice and delivery of care; physicians determined the frequency of follow-up visits and the dose of the drug. Furthermore, patients incurred some expenses for their medications as they would in regular practice. (Another good example of a pragmatic trial is the FIRST study; see Schulman *et al.* 1996.)

Despite interest in the design of pragmatic trials to address economic questions, such research designs may be infeasible for some health programme evaluations (e.g. our heart transplantation example in Box 8.1). Another reality and constraint that confronts the economic analyst is that decision makers often want data today rather than tomorrow. Such considerations, and others to be discussed below, have led to the view held by some health economists that modelling in economic evaluation is 'an unavoidable fact of life' (Buxton *et al.* 1997). Whether decision analytic modelling is viewed as a substitute for a pragmatic randomized trial or a complementary exercise to adjust or adapt explanatory trial data to a real world setting, it continues to play a central role in economic evaluation of health care programmes.

8.2.7. Data collection issues

When collecting resource use data as part of a clinical trial, we have already discussed the need to identify and minimize resource consequences that are due to the research protocol and do not characterize the delivery of care in the normal setting. But how does one actually collect the resource quantities associated with therapy as part of the evaluation? The first point is that, to the extent possible, it makes sense to build upon the research infrastructure that will be already in place for collecting the clinical data. For example, many clinical trials of hospital-based acute therapies would collect data using a case report form designed for completion by a study nurse. To facilitate collection of resource quantities associated with therapy, one can add pages to this case report form and extend the responsibility of data collection by the study nurse to include key items of resources. Studies will obviously vary in the amount of detail and precision needed in the collection of resource quantities. At a minimum, for a hospital-based study, it would be desirable to know the total length of stay in hospital, the length of stay in high cost areas such as intensive care, and major diagnostic or therapeutic procedures such as CT scans or surgery. As we discussed in Chapter 3, depending upon the intervention being evaluated, the precision of costing may need to be much greater. For example, if one is comparing two alternative treatments in the intensive care unit a lot more detailed information on resources consumed in ICU would obviously be appropriate.

In addition to the resource quantities associated with the initiation of therapy, it is also necessary to capture downstream resource consequences of the treatment or the disease. Typically these downstream costs could be an exacerbation of the problem warranting readmission to hospital or a mild complication resulting in consultation with a family physician or attendance at an emergency room. Capturing these data is more problematic for a number of reasons. First, if a person is rehospitalized at a hospital that is not part of the clinical trial then knowledge of this rehospitalization and access to information on resource consumption from that hospital may be limited. To facilitate information retrieval it may be necessary to ensure that patients have given approval for such data gathering as part of the informed consent documentation. The monitoring of such events can be achieved either by patient recall or, depending upon local circumstances, it may be possible to use computerized databases of physician reimbursement claims or hospital discharges.

In many trials, ambulatory physician visits are often recorded using patient recall. For example, has the patient seen a family doctor in the past three months for a reason associated with their hypertension or its treatment? As with any survey technique, the reliability of patient recall comes into question when one is studying population groups where recall may be a problem (e.g. the elderly). Also, the method of follow-up contact could be by mail survey or telephone follow-up, and depending upon the patient group being studied there are advantages and disadvantages of both methods. Readers who are interested in more detailed discussion of principles of data collection for economic data as part of trials and design of case report forms should consult Mauskopf *et al.* (1996).

8.3. MODELLING STUDIES: APPROACHES AND ISSUES

As a set of applied quantitative techniques, economic evaluation necessarily draws upon disciplines other than economics for analytic tools. In this section we review the ways in which economic evaluation can use various modelling techniques which have been developed in disciplines such as epidemiology, statistics, operations research, and decision science. The purpose is to illustrate in what circumstances modelling techniques can be useful, either as the primary mode of enquiry or as an adjunct to adjust or project trial-based data.

8.3.1. Decision analysis models

The techniques of decision analysis are in common usage by practitioners of health care economic evaluation. A seminal contribution by Weinstein and Fineberg (1980) showed how principles of decision analysis could be applied in health care under the rubric of clinical decision analysis. The main focus of this research initiative was as a quantitative clinical epidemiology tool for physicians (and patients) who wished to quantify expected risks, benefits, utilities and sometimes costs associated with alternative treatment options for *individual* patients. This general set of methods was later adopted for structuring and analysing *collective* decisions in health care, such as programme evaluation and economic appraisal.

Decision analysis was introduced briefly in Chapter 5; for a detailed introduction to clinical decision analysis the reader should consult Weinstein and Fineberg (1980) or Sox (1987). In summary, using decision analysis for economic evaluation proceeds by careful structuring of the problem using a decision tree – a graphic schema where we begin with the decision (e.g. treatment A or treatment B) and trace out all probable pathways and consequences (e.g. health outcomes and costs) that can arise over time. An example of a decision tree can be found in Box 8.3 for treatment of duodenal ulcer. Advantages of depicting the analytic problem using a decision tree are essentially twofold: first, the analyst can quickly identify what data components are required (e.g. probabilities, costs, utilities) to complete the analysis; second, laying out the problem in this way helps to separate issues of fact from value, e.g. the probability of ulcer recurrence is a factual issue to be informed by epidemiologic data whereas the value to patients of avoiding ulcer recurrence is necessarily subjective requiring input of preference data.

The duodenal ulcer example in Box 8.3 is typical of a number of decision analytic models for economic evaluation in the literature. The model draws data from multiple sources – mainly clinical trials for probabilities such as ulcer recurrence, administrative data for costs of treatment and recurrence, and expert physician opinion concerning treatment algorithms and management conditional upon recurrence. The analyst proceeds by calculating the

Box 8.3. Decision analytic models: the example of duodenal ulcer (DU) management

Techniques of decision analysis were used by O'Brien *et al.* (1995) in their study of costs and outcomes associated with alternative treatments for duodenal ulcer. Results indicated that strategy C treatments, attempting to eradicate the bacterium *Helicobactor pylori*, either by omaprazole plus amoxillin (O+A) or triple therapy (TT), are dominant over other strategies having lower expected cost and fewer expected ulcer recurrences in a one-year period.

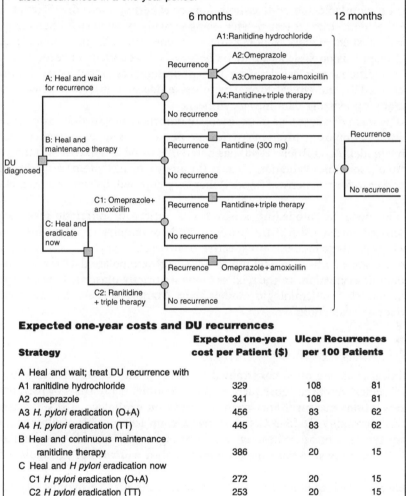

Expected one-year costs and DU recurrences

Strategy	Expected one-year cost per Patient ($)	Ulcer Recurrences per 100 Patients	
A Heal and wait; treat DU recurrence with			
A1 ranitidine hydrochloride	329	108	81
A2 omeprazole	341	108	81
A3 *H. pylori* eradication (O+A)	456	83	62
A4 *H. pylori* eradication (TT)	445	83	62
B Heal and continuous maintenance			
ranitidine therapy	386	20	15
C Heal and *H pylori* eradication now			
C1 *H pylori* eradication (O+A)	272	20	15
C2 *H pylori* eradication (TT)	253	20	15

sum of costs, weighted by their probability of occurrence, for each treatment strategy to determine the expected (or average) cost per patient. (This is known as 'averaging out the tree'.) In this example, the same process was done for the measure of outcome – expected ulcer recurrences per 100 patients. Expected costs and outcomes can then be compared between treatment strategies using the various approaches described earlier in this book.

The main advantages of such models is that they offer the analyst a flexible and timely framework for analysis. Data items that are missing or incomplete can be complemented with assumptions or expert opinion; the effect of such 'weaker data' can be tested later using sensitivity analysis. Therefore, the spirit of such models is doing the best one can with the available data. Although it is possible and may be necessary to complement secondary data with additional primary data (e.g. patient preferences for outcomes) for use in such models, the typical format is to use a decision analytic framework for integrating existing data into a synthesis.

The main disadvantage of decision analytic modelling is that various pieces of information from different studies and populations are put together into the same model. As O'Brien (1996) has noted this is the 'Frankenstein's monster' form of economic evaluation because the analyst brings (often) disparate parts together to form a monster (model) that they hope will behave in a predictable way!

The need for modelling arises for a variety of different reasons. As discussed earlier, even if the primary mode of enquiry is not an integrative decision analytic model, a prospective trial-based 'piggyback' study may still require some form of modelling to adjust or extrapolate data for use in the economic evaluation. In the next sections we briefly illustrate how extrapolation models, epidemiologic models, and Markov models can be used in economic evaluation:

8.3.2. Extrapolation models

Clinical trials are often constrained in terms of the length of follow-up for clinical and resource consequences. For example, many trials of therapeutic interventions measure short-term mortality: in cardiology, ISIS-3 recorded 30 day mortality (ISIS-3 Collaborative Group 1992), trials of ulcer medications typically measure healing rates over eight and 12 weeks (Graham *et al.* 1988). In many situations the economic analyst will wish to extrapolate data beyond the period observed in the clinical trial. This is because more general measures, such as life-years saved, are more relevant to economic evaluation than short-term measures such as percentage mortality at 30 days. Even when the clinical trial incorporates reasonably long follow-up (i.e. one year), there may still be a need to extrapolate. For example, in the economic evaluation based on the GUSTO study discussed in Chapter 3, survival was estimated in the primary analysis by assuming that the hazard of death after one year did not depend on the thrombolytic agent received. The authors constructed a statistical model based on the experience of 4379 patients in the Duke cardiovascular disease database with myocardial infarction between 1971 and 1992 who survived at least one year. This survival model was then used to extend the one-year survival data from the trial by an additional 14 years (Mark *et al.* 1995).

A second area of data extrapolation is in the area of quality-of-life measurement. A trial may have undertaken detailed measures of disease-specific quality of life and functional status but may not have measured broader concepts such as utility. It may be possible, however, to extrapolate disease-specific information into utility scales to try to estimate utility scores for patients where no primary utility measurement had been undertaken.

8.3.3. Epidemiologic models

In some disease areas where the final outcomes may take many years to develop, it is common for clinical trials to assess efficacy in terms of an intermediate endpoint. There are many examples in cardiovascular medicine, including raised blood cholesterol and raised blood pressure, where intervention studies quantify changes in risk factors such as blood pressure or cholesterol rather than final outcomes such as coronary mortality or death. The reasons for this are self-evident; the sample sizes required to show differences in mortality are often much larger than to show changes in intermediate biologic endpoints. This still poses a problem for the economic analyst who wishes to link the intermediate biologic endpoint to final health outcomes such as mortality reduction and life expectancy.

The use of epidemiologic modelling is appropriate in such a circumstance to link intermediate with final outcomes. For example, in their study of cholestyramine for treatment of hypercholesterolaemia, Oster and Epstein (1987) linked the reductions in total serum cholesterol (obtained from the Lipid Clinics Trial) to final outcomes by using the logistic equations from the Framingham Heart Study, which predicted CHD risk from pre- and post-treatment cholesterol levels. Similar epidemiologic modelling can be found in other therapeutic areas, such as osteoporosis, where analysts seek to determine the relationship between reduced bone mineral density and fractures.

8.3.4 Markov models

Some diseases and treatments are characterized by recurrence of disease states or treatment algorithms. The difficulty here is that the analyst is trying to portray, in a rather static way, the dynamic process of the continuous risk of disease recurrence. For example, in Box 8.3 we illustrated the duodenal ulcer treatment decision and showed how the analysts indicated to evaluate recurrence or no recurrence of ulcer at six-months and 12-months following

Box 8.4. Example of a Markov process for cadaveric kidney transplant

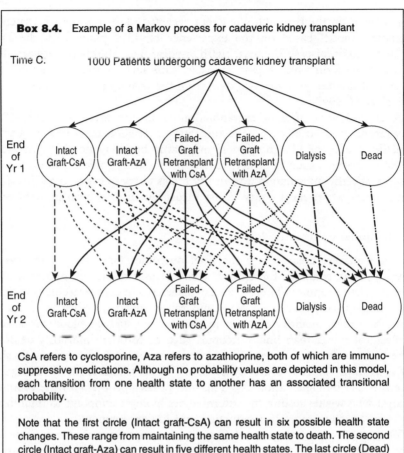

Time C. 1000 Patients undergoing cadaveric kidney transplant

CsA refers to cyclosporine, Aza refers to azathioprine, both of which are immuno-suppressive medications. Although no probability values are depicted in this model, each transition from one health state to another has an associated transitional probability.

Note that the first circle (Intact graft-CsA) can result in six possible health state changes. These range from maintaining the same health state to death. The second circle (Intact graft-Aza) can result in five different health states. The last circle (Dead) leads to only one health state (still Dead). All health states but Dead are termed 'non-absorbing' states; when no more transitions are possible, we have reached an 'absorbing' state.

Source: Example taken from Luce and Elixhauser (1990)

treatment. Clearly, patients undergoing such therapies will be at continuous risk of recurrence throughout the one-year period and will not necessarily recur at strict time-points of 6 and/or 12 months. These time-points are chosen for pragmatic reasons of simplifying the model. However, an alternative in this circumstance would have been to use what is known as a Markov model. Applied to this example, to implement a Markov model we would first need to determine the length of the Markov cycle, that is, how often the hypothetical cohort of persons being treated would be evaluated. For example, we may wish to examine presence or absence of recurrence monthly for the one-year period. The Markov model therefore proceeds by determining transition probabilities between different health states or circumstances for each cycle of the model. In principle, for the example in Box 8.3, we could draw out a large decision tree that characterized branches at each monthly point where recurrence or no recurrence were being evaluated.

There are a number of issues concerning the use of Markov models. For a detailed treatment of Markov models in medical decision-making, readers are referred to Sonnenberg and Beck (1993). The logic of a Markov model is illustrated in Box 8.4, using the example of cadaveric kidney transplantation.

In summary, Markov models require strict assumptions concerning zero memory, that is, the transition probabilities depend only upon the health state patients are in and not on how long they had been in that health state or how they got there. Whether this Markov assumption is met in practice for any given problem is often difficult to determine. Furthermore, if one considers again the ulcer problem in Box 8.3, the clinical trials for recurrence reported information at six months and 12 months. To translate these data into monthly hazard rates for transition probabilities in a Markov model, we would need to determine whether the hazard rate for recurrence was linear over the six-month period or non-linear.

8.4 ANALYSIS PLANS FOR ECONOMIC EVALUATION

A consequence of the growth in economic evaluation being conducted alongside clinical trials is that the economic analyst is asked to specify hypotheses to be tested and an analysis plan as part of the study protocol. Such requirements raise two sets of issues which we will address. First, there are conceptual issues concerning how the economic study questions should be formulated. Second, there are practical questions concerning appropriate statistical methods for analysing economic data and presenting results. In this section we address the conceptual logic of analysis plans; in the next section we examine some of the statistical issues.

As pointed out in a recent contribution by Donaldson *et al.* (1996), at the outset of a clinical trial the analyst does not know whether the experimental therapy is the same, better, or worse than the control therapy. The experiment is designed to test hypotheses concerning efficacy and safety; if we knew the answer to these questions we would not be doing the experiment. Building the economic appraisal into the trial we are adding a new outcome of cost (and maybe quality of life) for comparing the experimental and control therapies. Since differential costs are often 'driven' by differences in clinical outcomes (e.g. differential incidence of downstream events such as strokes or heart attacks) we also have uncertainty about which therapy, overall, will be more or less costly.

This state of uncertainty going into a typical clinical and economic therapy trial can be summarized as in Fig. 8.1. Compared to the control therapy the incremental costs of the experimental therapy would be more, the same, or less; similarly incremental effectiveness could be more, the same, or less (assume a single measure of outcome for simplicity). Given that the data can result in one of the nine cells in the matrix in Fig. 8.1, how should the analyst formulate a logical plan for analysis?

The first point to note is that it would not be logical to state that the plan was to conduct incremental cost-effectiveness analysis (or CUA, or CBA) because such analysis would only be appropriate in circumstances where observed costs and effects indicated non-dominance. To clarify this point, suppose the new therapy turned out to be both less costly and more effective than the control (cell #1 in Fig. 8.1); this strongly dominant solution would not require additional analysis with incremental ratios because there is compelling evidence to adopt the new programme.

The dilemma for pre-specifying the analysis protocol is that the final form of analysis is *conditional* upon the observed data for costs and effects. Hence the first hypotheses concern differences in costs and differences in effectiveness. Conditional upon these observed data it may be necessary to formulate costs and effects in an incremental form. The formal hypothesis for such an incremental ratio will depend upon how the analyst seeks to interpret such data. For example, one approach would be to hypothesize that the incremental CE ratio is less than some pre-specified threshold (e.g. $50 000 per QALY).

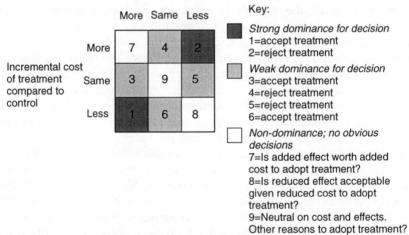

Fig. 8.1. Nine possible outcomes arising in the comparison of treatment control in terms of incremental cost and incremental effectiveness.

8.5 STATISTICAL ANALYSIS AND ECONOMIC EVALUATION

The move toward economic evaluation being alongside clinical trials led to a greater focus on issues of statistical analysis and in this section we examine some of the statistical issues that arise in the conduct of economic evaluation. While many of the basic principles of statistical inference used in the analysis of efficacy data may be applicable, there are some special issues that arise in the analysis of economic data. Framing our discussion in a general class of problem – the analysis of uncertainty – we examine a spectrum of study approaches and data types from deterministic non-sampled data to stochastic sampled data. We give an overview of sensitivity analysis and its limitations and then outline some basic principles and approaches to statistical analysis of sampled economic data that might be collected prospectively as part of a trial.

Conventional principles of statistical inference and hypothesis testing are useful when the analyst has sampled data; for example, some item of resource use, such as number of physician visits, has been measured as a random variable and can be characterized by moments of its distribution such as mean and variance. But with a decision analytic model the same item of data may not have been sampled; for example, it may have been determined by recourse to an expert panel. In this latter circumstance the analysis can be said to be deterministic rather than stochastic, and sensitivity analysis (explained below) is relevant for exploring uncertainty. Study types, based on data collected, can be divided into three groups:

1. *Deterministic cost-effectiveness analysis*: where cost and effect variables are analysed as point estimates. Sampling variation may not be available because of the source of the data (e.g. secondary data) or the variable may not have been sampled (e.g. choice of discount rate, expert opinion). Deterministic CEA models arise frequently in the early assessment of a new medical technology, where only limited data are available but some analysis is required for policy setting. For example, in their analysis of the implantable defibrillator, Kupperman *et al.* (1990) constructed a cost-effectiveness model where effect data were taken from reports of patient series in the literature as point estimates of survival probabilities and cost data were derived from a Medicare claims database and expert opinion. Given these data it was not possible to present cost and effect differences with 95% confidence intervals, but rather a deterministic point estimate of cost-effectiveness was subject to detailed sensitivity analysis, using plausible ranges for variables, to explore the impact of uncertainty.

2. *Partially stochastic cost-effectiveness analysis*: where effectiveness has been estimated from clinical trial(s) and can be expressed as a mean effect size with an associated variance, but analysis of costs is deterministic because data are non-sampled. This combination is common in decision analytic models of economic appraisal. Some studies with such data report confidence intervals for cost-effectiveness where only variation in effects has been analysed. For example, a study in ulcer maintenance therapy (Lancaster-Smith *et al.* 1992) presented 95% confidence intervals around expected one-year therapy costs including relapse management. But no

primary data had been collected to determine variation between patients in costs of managing relapse; the source of variation for the confidence interval was only that surrounding the estimated incidence of relapse on treatment and control.

3. *Wholly stochastic cost-effectiveness analysis*: where both costs and effects are determined from data sampled from the same patients in a study. If cost and effect data are sampled and variances are available then formal statistical tests can be performed on observed differences in costs (treatment–control) or effects. What is less clear is how such statistical testing might be applied to the ratio of the two estimated differences. A further issue is how to deal with economic variables, such as a discount rate, which are non-sampled but may be uncertain.

8.5.1. Beyond sensitivity analysis

Before considering the adoption of stochastic methods for economic evaluation it is necessary to review the limitations of sensitivity analysis, which was discussed in Chapter 5. This method is widely recommended for assessing problems of data uncertainty in economic appraisals of health care programmes (Commonwealth of Australia 1990; Luce and Elixhauser 1990; Ontario Ministry of Health 1991) and allied evaluative techniques such as clinical decision analysis (Weinstein and Fineberg 1980). The purpose is to examine the robustness of an estimated result over a range of alternative values for uncertain parameters. Weinstein and Stason (1977) describe the method in the following way:

'the most uncertain features and assumptions . . . are varied one at a time over a wide range of possible values. If the basic conclusions do not change when a particular feature or assumption is varied, confidence in the conclusions is increased.'

There are three major limitations with sensitivity analysis:

(1) the analyst has discretion as to which variables and what alternative values are included in the sensitivity analysis, creating the potential for selection bias (conscious or otherwise);
(2) Interpretation of a sensitivity analysis is essentially arbitrary because there are no guidelines or standards as to what degree of variation in results is acceptable evidence that the analysis is 'robust';
(3) Variation of uncertain parameters *one at a time* carries a risk that interactions between parameters may not be captured.

In the clinical decision analysis literature the limitations of traditional sensitivity analysis have led to the development of probabilistic sensitivity analysis by Monte Carlo simulation methods (Doubilet *et al.* 1985). The main application of this approach in clinical decision models has been by the statistical method of parametric bootstrapping where one assumes some distributional form (e.g. normal, Poisson, binomial) for an estimated (but non-sampled) variable; repeated samples are then drawn from these distributions to determine an empirical distribution for some construct of the variables, such as a cost-effectiveness ratio.

8.5.2. Costs and effects as point estimates

The deterministic analysis of cost-effectiveness is a comparison of point estimates. If we consider a treatment which is both more costly and more effective than control, then using the figure format introduced by O'Brien *et al.* (1994) and further developed by Gold *et al.* (1996), we can represent incremental cost-effectiveness as in Fig. 8.2. The X-axis represents the difference in effects between the experimental and control therapy (ΔE) and the Y-axis the difference in cost between experimental and control (ΔC). The slope of the line extending from the origin (the control) through our study estimate, point (e), represents the incremental cost-effectiveness of the treatment relative to control. Clearly, the steeper the slope of the line $\Delta C/\Delta E$, the greater is the additional cost at which additional units of effectiveness are gained by treatment relative to control, and the less attractive treatment becomes. In the absence of any data on sampling variation for costs or effects (point e), some form of sensitivity analysis would be useful to determine plausible ranges that may contain the true cost-effectiveness ratio.

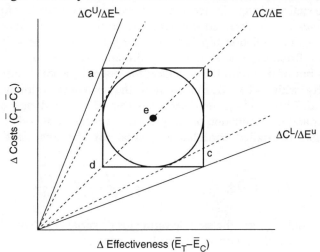

Fig. 8.2. Confidence regions for cost-effectiveness data.

8.5.3. Sampled effects and costs

In the analysis of sampled effect data with associated sampling variation, the null hypothesis is usually that there is no difference in outcome between experimental and control therapy, and this is tested against either a one-tailed alternative (usually that the experimental treatment is more effective) or a two-tailed alternative (that the experimental treatment is more or less effective than the control). For a continuous clinical variable such as blood pressure we assume, by convention, that the ratio of the difference in sample means (T – C) to the pooled standard error of the difference follows some known probability distribution such as Z or t. Critical values of this test statistic are determined by the analyst's judgement about the acceptable risk of making a type 1 (false–positive) error about a difference existing, this level conventionally being set to 5 per cent. A probability level equal or less than 5 per cent is typically referred to as 'statistical significance'. The choice of α at 5 per cent is itself a value judgement but a universal standard appears to have emerged. (Statisticians are the only profession who are allowed to be wrong 5 per cent of the time!)

A problem with hypothesis-testing as a form of stochastic analysis is that an overemphasis tends to be placed on the statistical significance of results (the size of the p value) in isolation from the magnitude of the effect size. Statistical guidelines in a number of medical journals have generally recommended that, in preference to reporting only p values, analyses should report the observed effect size with an associated confidence interval (Gardner and Altman 1989). The advantage of the confidence interval is twofold. First, it permits hypothesis testing as described above because if a 95% confidence interval for a difference includes zero then the treatment groups are not significantly different at the 5 per cent level. Second, in addition to statistical significance, the confidence interval yields information on the *magnitude* of the observed difference (quantitative significance or clinical importance). The relationship between these two parameters is important because, as Braitman (1991) notes, a difference can be highly statistically significant but of no clinical importance; for example, a small difference (say, 0.25 mm/Hg) with $p < 0.0001$. Furthermore, the concept of a minimum clinically important difference (δ) to be detected is central to the design of a clinical experiment and determination of sample size (Burnand *et al.* 1990).

A familiar two-tailed confidence interval for the treatment–effect size would be:

$$(\overline{E}_T - \overline{E}_C) \pm t_{(n_T + n_C - 2, \ 1 - \frac{\alpha}{2})} \sqrt{\frac{s^2_{ET}}{n_T} + \frac{s^2_{EC}}{n_C}}$$

where s^2_{ET} and s^2_{EC} are the sample estimates of variances. Now, lets assume that resource use was measured to enable patient-specific costs to be estimated from the same trial. Assuming patient i consumes j resources ($j = 1...\mathcal{J}$) in quantity Q_j at unit price P_j, then the costs for individual i can be expressed as:

$$C_i = \sum_{j=1}^{j} P_j Q_j$$

Note that we have made the simplifying assumption that resource prices are known with certainty and are not random variables. Summing over i patients ($i = 1...n_T$) in the treatment group mean cost per patient can be expressed as:

$$\overline{C}_T = \frac{1}{n_T} \sum_{i=1}^{n_T} C_i$$

with estimated variance:

$$s^2_{ET} = \frac{1}{n_T \ (n_T - 1)} \sum_{i=1}^{n_T} (C_i - \overline{C}_T)^2$$

Therefore, the difference between the mean cost associated with treatment and control can be expressed as a confidence interval:

$$(\overline{C}_T - \overline{C}_C) \pm t_{(n_T + n_C - 2, \, 1 - \frac{\alpha}{2})} \sqrt{\frac{s^2_{CT}}{n_T} \, \frac{s^2_{CC}}{n_C}}$$

The combination of these simple 95% confidence intervals for cost and effect differences can be portrayed as two-dimensional confidence regions for cost-effectiveness as in Fig. 8.2. The most simple and conservative definition of the confidence region is the box bounded by *abcd*. Rays from the region passing through points a and c define a slice of pie based on the upper (superscripted U) and lower (L) limits of each confidence interval. However, this combined interval is conservative because the joint probability of being at a point such as a would be less than 0.05. More precisely we can characterize a two-dimensional probability density function the circle in Fig. 8.2 – which jointly defines our confidence region for costs and effects. (Note that the slice of pie defined by the circle is smaller than that defined by the box.)

As pointed out by Gold *et al.* (1996) the precise shape of the ellipsoid confidence region will depend upon covariation between costs and effects. Seldom would we anticipate that costs and effects would be statistically independent resulting in the circle as drawn in Fig. 8.2. As shown in O'Brien *et al.* (1994) and illustrated in Gold *et al.* (1996), the result of *positive* covariation between costs and effects is a narrower slice of pie with an ellipsoid stretched from south-west to north-east; negative covariation serves to widen the confidence region with the ellipsoid stretched from north-west to south-east. This influence of covariation on the shape of the 95% confidence ellipsoid is illustrated in Fig. 8.3.

8.5.4 Confidence intervals for CE: comparing methods

The main statistical difficulty in determining the joint confidence interval for cost-effectiveness is that incremental cost-effectiveness is a ratio of two random variables ($\Delta C / \Delta E$) and so the variance of this estimate is not evaluable. There are two ways forward: (1) use of parametric methods to

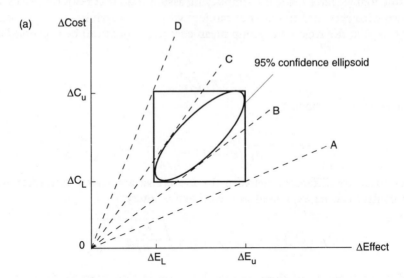

95% confidence interval on CE ratio = (slope 0B, slope 0C)

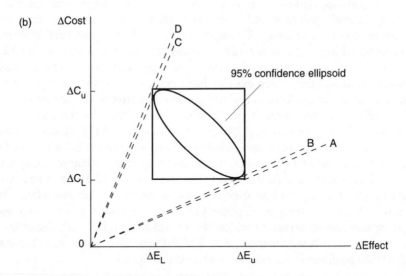

Fig. 8.3. Influence of positive and negative covariation between cost and effect differences on the shape of the confidence ellipsoid. (*Source*: Gold *et al.* 1996)

approximate the variance such as Taylor's method (O'Brien *et al.* 1994) or Fieller's method (Willan and O'Brien 1996); (2) non-parametric bootstrap methods (Chaudhary and Stearns 1996).

A detailed exposition of the various methods is beyond the scope of this chapter. However, a useful study that defines and compares these methods is available (Chaudhary and Stearns, 1996). A key conclusion from this study is that, when choosing between the various methods, the analyst needs to examine the extent to which the data are consistent with the assumptions behind the models. For example, the Taylor series method is based on the assumption that the distribution of the $(\Delta C/\Delta E)$ ratio is normal. Chaudary and Stearns (1996) also show that bootstrapping methods that rely upon assumptions of normality may also yield biased intervals. The most promising methods from their comparative analyses seemed to be Fieller's method (see also Willan and O'Brien, 1996) and a bias-corrected bootstrapping method, both yielding similar intervals. A form of the bootstrap method is outlined in Box 8.5.

Box 8.5. Non-parametric bootstrap methods

1. Draw a sample of observations from observations of the treatment group by simple random sampling with replacement. Compute $\overline{C_T^*}$ and $\overline{E_T^*}$, the bootstrap replicates of $\overline{C_T}$ and $\overline{E_T}$.
2. Draw a sample of observations from sample observations of the control group by simple random sampling with replacement. Compute $\overline{C_C^*}$ and $\overline{E_C^*}$, the bootstrap replicates of $\overline{C_C}$ and $\overline{E_C}$
3. Compute the bootstrap replicate $\hat{R}_b^*$:

$$\hat{R}_b^* = \frac{\overline{C_T^*} - \overline{C_C^*}}{\overline{E_T^*} - \overline{E_C^*}}$$

4. Repeat steps 1–3 a large number of times (say *B*) and obtain the independent bootstrap replications $\hat{R}_1^*, \hat{R}_2^*, \ldots \hat{R}_B^*$, The bootstrap estimate of and its variance (~) are simply the mean and variance of *B* bootstrap replications:

$$\tilde{R} = \frac{1}{B} \sum_{b=1}^{B} \hat{R}_b^*$$

$$\tilde{v}(\tilde{R}) = \frac{1}{B-1} \sum_{b=1}^{B} (\hat{R}_b^* - \tilde{R})^2$$

Using this result, we can construct a symmetric but crude confidence interval under assumption that is distributed normally:

$$95\% \text{ CI} = \hat{R} \pm z_\alpha \sqrt{\{\tilde{v}(\hat{R})\}}$$

8.6. RESEARCH AGENDA

The growth in economic evaluation alongside clinical trials has generated some exciting new collaborations between economists and statisticians to resolve some of the new analytic challenges. In this concluding section we highlight three statistical issues on the research agenda: sample size calculation, covariation between resource prices and quantities, and censoring of cost data.

8.6.1. Sample size

Being part of a prospective study such as a clinical trial requires the economic analyst to consider (and justify!) what sample size is required to conduct the economic analysis. At the current time there is no simple or single solution to this problem. As argued by O'Brien *et al.* (1994), if one conceives of the cost-effectiveness hypothesis as being a comparison against an acceptable CE threshold (i.e. upper bound) then one might construct a hypothesis test using one of the variance estimations previously described. But these authors argue more in favour of focusing the statistical analysis and power calculations on the *precision* of the estimate rather than a single test of a hypothesis.

There are three pragmatic considerations for sample size. First, cost data are often, but not always, more noisy (variable) than effect data and so detecting differences at the same level of inferential error will be difficult. One implication is that the analyst (and decision-maker) accepts lower levels of precision for these data and does not stick with the conventional $p < 0.05$. If one did insist on the same type I error rate as for efficacy, then one possibility is that the clinical study would have to extend beyond the point at which the clinical question can be answered, so as to collect adequate data for the economic question (at the same level of precision). If, for ethical reasons, this latter course of action is not acceptable, it may be that the analyst has to live with lower precision on cost data. Finding out what risk thresholds decision makers have for cost data is therefore an item for the research agenda. The practical issue is that, as with clinical data, it is useful to conduct some form of pilot study so that variability in costs between subjects with the disease has been estimated.

The second issue is how to determine what size of difference would be economically important or policy-relevant. (For a discussion of this issue see O'Brien and Drummond, 1995.) The third pragmatic issue on sample size for cost comparisons is that analysts should try to determine which resource quantity is the major driver of therapy costs. For example, in practice it may be more meaningful to base sample size and power on a predicted difference in total hospital days rather than some dollar amount.

8.6.2. Covariation between resource prices and quantities

In our earlier exposition of confidence intervals for (mean) cost we conveniently assumed that resource prices were known quantities rather than random variables. If the latter scenario were true, and our experiment was a sample of the population of prices, then the expression for the variance in cost would need to be based on the product of two random variables ($P \times Q$) where sampling variation and covariation would be additive, using, for example, Taylor approximation methods.

In most instances, variation in resource prices (e.g. doctors fees, nurses salaries) will not be truly random but will vary by factors such as jurisdiction. That is, the fee for a procedure may vary between the Canadian provinces of Ontario and Quebec, but is fixed within each province. Hence, one might wish to examine the economic consequences for different provinces using different vectors of price weights. This is what might be called an analysis of applicability, from one jurisdiction to another, rather than sensitivity analysis, because the source of uncertainty is driven mainly by jurisdiction.

A second aspect of covariation between prices and quantities, particularly in multi-centre studies which span multiple jurisdictions, is that cost hypotheses should be tested on total costs rather than components. For example, in producing a given therapy country A may use less doctor time and more nurse time than country B because *relative prices* between these factor inputs differ between the countries. Analyses of overall therapy costs (rather than line items) incorporate such covariation between prices and quantities and substitutions made in the production process.

8.6.3. Censored cost data

As noted by Fenn *et al.* (1996), one of the issues that can arise in collecting resource use alongside clinical trials is that patient follow-up on resources may be terminated early or censored. The authors show how the use of conventional statistical analysis based on means will be biased in the presence of censoring. They advocate and illustrate how non-parametric life table methods (e.g. Kaplan-Meier and Cox models) can be used to estimate cumulative cost distributions in the presence of censoring.

8.7. CONCLUSIONS

An important conclusion from the first half of this chapter is that measurement and modelling are complementary activities and not substitutes. While randomized controlled trials minimize threats to internal validity and bias by strict protocol adherence, they may do so at the risk of reducing the external validity or generalizability of data. We explained how economic evaluation, to produce unbiased but policy relevant data, will often need to adjust or complement trial-based data with other information. Models exist for a variety of reasons, but mainly to forecast and/or predict events where little or no data exist.

As alternative modes of inquiry we explained how economic evaluation can be 'piggybacked' onto the design of a typical safety and efficacy trial with subsequent modelling adjustments as needed, or the analyst can mount a specific pragmatic (naturalistic) trial where randomization is used but protocols for subsequent patient management are more relaxed than is conventional.

Interest in the statistical issues arising from economic evaluations alongside trials is growing rapidly. As studies move toward greater use of sampled data then analysis plans need to be based more on stochastic rather than deterministic methods. We showed a number of promising methods for the joint analysis of costs and effects and the conceptual logic behind the cost-effectiveness confidence region in two-dimensional space. Researchers are currently very active comparing the alternative methods for assessing precision around incremental costs and effects ranging from parametric methods such as the Taylor series and Fieller's theorem to more pragmatic and computer-intensive methods such as bootstrapping.

8.8 EXERCISE: ECONOMIC EVALUATION ALONGSIDE CLINICAL TRIALS – A CASE STUDY IN OSTEOPOROSIS

Scenario

You have been asked to conduct an economic evaluation of a new drug for treatment of osteoporotic fractures. A large randomized trial is planned and you have the opportunity to build economic and quality-of-life endpoints into this trial.

The drug has a positive effect on rebuilding of bones and is therefore thought to accelerate the healing of fractures. A multi-centre clinical trial in hip fracture is to be conducted in the USA and four European countries. The preliminary design of the trial is as follows:

- the trial will be randomized, double blind, and the new drug will be added from the day of the fracture to standard methods used to treat hip fractures, and compared to placebo. Drug treatment will be for three months;
- the tentative main clinical endpoints are:
  - bone building index
  - ability to stand
  - ability to walk 50 metres
  - time to hospital discharge;

- sample size calculations, based on the power to detect a clinically important difference in the clinical endpoints, suggest that there will have to be 200 patients in each group;
- patients will be assessed at baseline, one, three, and six months (end of the trial);
- because of the potentially toxic nature of the drug, additional monitoring (laboratory tests) will be performed at monthly intervals. In order to preserve blinding, tests will also be performed on the placebo patients.

Tasks

1. Comment critically on the suitability of this trial for the assessment of economic and quality-of-life endpoints (give points for and against). If necessary, propose changes to the trial design.
2. Specify the categories of data on resource use you would like to see collected as part of the trial.
3. Discuss whether you would want to collect quality-of-life data in this trial, and if so, would you use a generic or specific quality-of-life scale?
4. Specify any other data that you feel needs to be gathered in the five countries to supplement the data being collected as part of the trial.
5. Although the economic data would be collected alongside the clinical trial, do you think that there is any role for modelling in this case? If so, what kind of model would you recommend?

Solutions

1. As we have discussed in this chapter, one of the goals in designing a pragmatic economic trial is to generate evidence on costs and outcomes that are mostly likely to arise in routine practice. There are a number of limitations for this current trial for achieving this goal.

   First, this is a placebo-controlled trial which raises the question of the relevance of this comparison. Even though the placebo is adjunctive, are there any other pharmacological or non-pharmacological treatments that would be implemented in the different countries for treatment of hip fractures?

   Second, this is a double-blind trial and therefore necessitates additional tests and visits for the placebo group that would not otherwise arise but are there to preserve the blinding. Might it be feasible and desirable to have this as an unblinded trial so that both patients and physicians could be studied in a less artificial environment where they know they were either on or not on the new therapy?

   Third, is the trial long enough? Drug treatment will be for three months and follow-up will continue to six months. It is not clear whether this length of follow-up will be adequate to capture downstream consequences of therapy, such as recurrence of fracture or adverse consequences of medication. One possibility might be to end the complete follow-up at six months but continue a more streamlined follow-up for economic endpoints to one year.

Fourth, is it desirable to have this trial conducted in multiple countries? To the extent that practice patterns will vary between the USA and Europe (and even within Europe) it may not be possible to meaningfully pool the economic data. Is it possible to consolidate the trial in one continent or, ideally, in one country to reduce the heterogeneity in the economic data?

2. In addition to hospitalization data that will be collected as part of the main case report form for the trial, and depending upon the viewpoint of the economic analysis, it may be desirable to capture the following resource consequences:

   • family physician visits
   • homemaker / home help costs
   • drugs
   • nursing home costs
   • community nursing costs
   • re-hospitalization

3. A general issue in the collection of quality-of-life data in this trial is whether the period of follow-up (six months) is going to be sufficiently long to be able to ascertain clinically important changes in these hip fracture patients. In choosing among general versus disease-specific measures it might be desirable to have both a disease-specific measure which is sensitive to small but clinically important differences but also a more general measure (such as a utility measure) that will afford the study some more general comparability with other disease and treatment areas. A practical concern, however, is whether the measures chosen have been validated and are available in different countries where the study will be conducted. A further concern may be to attempt some measurement of quality-of-life in care-givers for persons with this condition. Before deciding upon any quality-of-life measures to include in the trial it is useful to review what pilot data are available that will give a perspective on whether the measures can detect the kind of changes one can expect to see in the trial.

4. In addition to the resource information being collected as part of the trial, there are at least three categories of information that will be required from each of the participating countries.

   (a) Price data to attach to resources measured. These are obvious things such as hospital prices, drug prices, and physician costs in addition to factors such as labour market wage-rates if the valuation of productive time is to be measured;

(b) Practice patterns for the management of hip fracture in each of the countries would be useful information to collect. The concern here is that the trial may be an abstraction from routine practice and also that we are seeking to combine information from five different countries where practice patterns may vary. In assessing whether the data are combinable or transferable between countries, some knowledge of variation in practice patterns for the condition will be useful;

(c) Information on reimbursement mechanisms in each of the countries would also be useful in further exploring why variation in management of patients may exist between countries. For example, are physicians paid a fee per item of service to conduct additional tests or procedures or are they reimbursed by salary? Are hospitals reimbursed on the basis of case mix groups such that there is an incentive to reduce length of stay, and so on.

5. There might be a general need for modeling to address two types of questions:

(a) modelling may be necessary to extrapolate some of the intermediate clinical endpoints to final outcomes. For example, at six months we may have knowledge regarding the extent to which bone has been rebuilt, but to what extent does this manifest itself in reduced risk of fracture recurrence in the following year? Hence there may be a need for epidemiologic models that extrapolate bone density and mass to fracture risk;

(b) modelling may also be necessary to attempt to generalize the findings from this multi country study to individual countries studied and countries not studied. The general issue here would be to ascertain whether the cost-effectiveness of the therapy was conditional upon the treatment patterns and reimbursement practices in any given country.

REFERENCES

Anderson, D., O'Brien, B., Levine, M., *et al.* (1993). Efficacy and cost-effectiveness of low molecular weight heparin versus standard heparin in the prevention of deep vein thrombosis following total hip replacement arthroplasty. *Annals of Internal Medicine*, **119**, 1105–12.

Beck, T. M., Ciociola, A. A., Jones, S. E., *et al.* (1993). Efficacy of oral ondansetron in the prevention of emesis in outpatients receiving cyclophosphamide-based chemotherapy. *Annals of Internal Medicine*, **118**, 407–13.

Braitman, L. E. (1991). Confidence intervals assess both clinical significance and statistical significance. *Annals of Internal Medicine*, **114**, 515.

Burnand, B., Kernan, W. N., *et al.* (1990). Indexes and boundaries for quantitative significance in statistical decisions. *J. Clin. Epid.* **43**, 1273.

Buxton, M. J., Acheson, R., Caine, N., Gibson, S., and O'Brien, B. J. (1985). *Costs and benefits of the heart transplant programmes at Harefield and Papworth hospitals.* DHSS Research Report No. 12, HMSO, London.

— and O'Brien, B. J. (1992). Economic evaluation of ondansetron: preliminary analysis using trial data prior to price setting *Brit. J. Cancer*, **66**, (Suppl XIX), 564–7.

— Drummond, M. F., van Hout, B. A., *et al.* (1997). Modelling in economic evaluation: an unavoidable fact of life. *Health Economics* (in press).

Chaudhary, M. A., and Stearns, S. C. (1996). Estimating confidence intervals for cost-effectiveness ratios: An example from a randomized trial. *Statistics in Medicine*, **14**, 1447–58.

Commonwealth of Australia (1990). Guidelines for the pharmaceutical industry on preparation of submissions to the Pharmaceutical Benefits Advisory Committee: including submissions involving economic analyses. Woden (ACT) Department of Health, Housing and Community Services.

Cook, T. D., and Campbell, D. T. (1979). *Quasi-experimentation: design and analysis issues for field settings.* Houghton, Mifflin, Boston.

Cubeddu, L. X., Hoffmann, I. S., Fuenmayor, N. T., and Finn, A. L. (1990). Efficacy of ondansetron (GR 38032F) and the role of serotonin in cisplatin-induced nausea and vomiting. *N. Eng. J. Med.*, **322**, 810–16.

Donaldson, C., Hurdley, V., and McIntosh, E. (1996). Using economic evaluation alongside clinical trials: why we cannot choose the evaluation technique in advance. *Health Economics*, **5**, 267–9.

Doubilet, P., Begg, C. B., *et al.* (1985). Probabilistic sensitivity analysis using Monte Carlo simulation: a practical approach. *Medical Decision-Making*, **5**, 157.

Drummond, M. F., Bloom, B. S., Carrin, G., *et al.* (1992). Issues in the cross-national assessment of health technology. *Int. J. Technology Assessment in Health Care*, **8**, 671–82.

Edelson, J. T., Weinstein, M. C., Tosteson, A. N. A., *et al.* (1990). Long-term cost-effectiveness of various initial monotherapies for mild to moderate hypertension. *J.A.M.A.*, **263**, 407–13.

Fenn, P., McGuire, A., Backhouse, M., and Jones, D. (1996). Modelling programme costs in economic evaluation. *J. Health Economics*, **15**, 115–25.

Freemantle, N., Drummond, M. F. (1997). Should clinical trials with concurrent economic analyses be blinded? *J.A.M.A.*, **277**(1), 63-64.

Gardner, M. J., and Altman, D. G. (1989). *Statistics with confidence – confidence intervals and statistical guidelines.* British Medical Association, London.

Gold, M. R., Siegel, J. E., Russell, L. B., and Weinstein, M. C. (1996). *Cost-effectiveness in health and medicine.* Oxford University Press, Oxford.

Graham, D. Y., Agrawal, N. M., and Roth, S. H. (1988). Prevention of NSAID-induced gastric ulcer with the synthetic prostaglandin misoprostol: a multi-centre, double-blind, placebo-controlled trial. *Lancet*, **2**, 1277–80.

ISIS-3 (Third International Study of Infarct Survival) Collaborative Group. (1992). ISIS-3: a randomized comparison of streptokinase vs tissue plasminogen activator vs anistreplase and of aspirin plus heparin vs aspirin alone among 41 299 cases of suspected acute myocardial infarction. *Lancet*, **339**, 753–71.

Kupperman, M., Luce, B., McGovern, B., *et al.* (1990). An analysis of the cost-effectiveness of the implantable defibrillator. *Circulation*, **81**, 91.

Lancaster, Smith, M., Gough, K., Wells, N., and Miocevich, M. (1992). An economic analysis of ranitidine versus cimetidine in the prevention of duodenal ulcer recurrence. *Brit. J. Medical Economics*, **2**, 25.

Lipid Research Clinics Programme (1984). The Lipid Research Clinics coronary primary prevention trial results: I Reductions in the incidence of coronary heart disease. *J.A.M.A.*, **251**, 351–64.

Luce, B. R., and Elixhauser, A. (1990). *Standards for socio-economic evaluations of health care products and services*. Springer-Verlag, Berlin.

Mauskopf, J., Schulman, K., Bell, L., and Glick, H. (1996). A strategy for collecting pharmacoeconomic data during phase II/III clinical trials. *PharmacoEconomics*, **9**, 264–77.

Mark, D. B., Hlatky, M. A., Califf, R. M., *et al.* (1995). Cost-effectiveness of thrombolytic therapy with tissue plasminogen activator as compared with streptokinase for acute myocardial infarction. *N. Eng. J. Med.*, **332**, 1418–24.

Moss, A. J., Hall, W. J., Cannon, D. S. *et al.* (1996). MAIDIT Trial. *New Eng. J. Med.*, **335**, 1933–40.

O'Brien, B. J. (1991). *Cholesterol and coronary heart disease: Consensus or controversy?* Office of Health Economics, London.

—, (1996). Economic evaluation of pharmaceuticals: Frankenstein's monster or vampire of trials? *Medical Care* **34**: DS99–DS108 (Supplement)

—, Buxton, M.J., Rushby, J. Cost-effectiveness of the implantable cardiometer defibrillator: an analysis of the existing evidence *British Heart J.*, **681**, 241–45.

—, Buxton, M. J., Khawaja, H. T. (1990). An economic evaluation of transdermal glyceryl trinitrate in the prevention of intravenous infusion failure. *J. Clin. Epid.*, **43**, 757–63.

—, Anderson, D., and Goeree, R. (1994a). Cost-effectiveness of enoxaparin versus warfarin prophylaxis against deep vein thrombosis after total hip replacement *Can. Med. Assoc. J.*, **150**, 1083–172.

—, and Drummond, M. F. (1994b). Statistical versus quantitative importance in the socio-economic evaluation of medicines. *PharmacoEconomics*, **5**, 389–98.

—, —, Labelle, R. J., and Willan, A. (1994c). In search of power and significance: Issues in the decision and analysis of stochastic cost-effectiveness studies in health care. *Medical Care*, **32**, 150–63.

—, Goeree, R., Hunt, R., and Mohamed, H. (1996). Cost-effectiveness of *Helicobacter pylori* eradication in the long-term management of duodenal ulcer. *Archives of Internal Medicine*, **155**, 1958–64.

Ontario Ministry of Health (1991). *Guidelines for preparation of economic analysis to be included in submission to Drug Programs Branch for listing in the Ontario Drug Benefit Formulary Comparative Drug Index*. Ministry of Health, Toronto.

Oster, G., and Epstein, A. M. (1987). Cost-effectiveness of anti-hyperlipemic therapy in the prevention of coronary heart disease. The case of cholestyramine. *J.A.M.A.*, **258**, 2381.

—, Borok, G. M., Menzin, J., *et al.* (1996). Cholesterol-reduction intervention study (CRIS). *Archives of Internal Medicine*, **156**, 731–9.

Paiment, G. D., Wessinger, S. J., and Harris, W. H. (1987). Survey of prophylaxis against venous thromboembolism in adults undergoing hip surgery. *Clinical Orthopedics*, **223**, 188–93.

Rusthoven, J., O'Brien, B. J., and Rocchi, A. (1992). Ondansetron versus metoclopramide in the prevention of chemotherapy-induced emesis and nausea: a meta-analysis. *Int. J. Oncol.*, **1**, 443–50.

Sackett, D. L., Haynes, R. B., and Tugwell, P. (1985). *Clinical epidemiology: A basic science for clinical medicine*. Little, Brown and Co, Boston.

Schulman, K. A., Kinosian, B. P., Jacobson, T. A. *et al.* (1990). Reducing high blood cholesterol level with drugs: cost-effectiveness of pharmacologic management *J.A.M.A.*, **264**, 3025–33.

—, Glick, H., Buxton, M. *et al.* (1996). Results of the economic evaluation of the FIRST study: a multinational prospective evaltuation *Int. J. Technol. Assess. Health Care*, **12**: 4.

Schwartz, D., and Lellouch, J. (1967). Explanatory and pragmatic attitudes in therapeutic trials. *J. Chronic Disease*, **20**, 637–48.

Sonnenberg, F. A., and Beck, J. R. (1993). Markov models in medical decision-making: a practical guide. *Medical Decision Making*, **13**, 322–38.

Sox, H. C., Blatt, M. A., Higgins, M. C., and Marton, K. I. (1988). *Medical Decision Making*. Butterworth-Heinemann, Boston.

Thompson, M. S., Read, J. L., Hutchings, H. C., and Harris, E. D. (1989). The cost-effectiveness of auranofin: results of a randomized clinical trial. *J. Rheumatology*, **15**, 35–42.

United States General Accounting Office (1992). *Cross design synthesis: A new strategy for medical effectiveness research*. GAO/DEMD-92-18, Washington, D.C.

Walt, R. P., Hunt, R. H., Misiewicz, J. J., *et al.* (1984). Comparison of ranitidine and cimetidine maintenance treatment of duodenal ulcer. *Scand. J. Gastroenterology*, **19**, 1045–7.

Weinstein, M. C., and Stason, W. B. (1977). Foundations of cost-effectiveness analysis for health and medical practices. *N. Eng. J. Med.*, **296**, 716.

Weinstein, M. C., and Fineberg, H. V. (1980). *Clinical decision analysis*. W.B. Saunders, Philadelphia.

Willan, A., and O'Brien, B. J. (1996). Confidence intervals for cost-effectiveness ratios: An application of Fieller's theorem. *Health Economics*, **5**, 297–305.

9

Presentation and use of economic evaluation results

9.1. INTRODUCTION

The implicit or explicit objective of economic evaluation is to improve decisions about the allocation of health care resources. Therefore, in this penultimate chapter we discuss issues relating to the presentation and use of economic evaluation results.

In Chapter 3 we pointed out that, in order to assess the usefulness of economic evaluation results, readers (users) of studies needed to answer the following questions:

(1) are the methods employed in the study appropriate and are the results valid?
(2) if the results are valid, would they apply to my setting?

The problems and prospects for using economic evaluation in health care decision-making have been widely debated in recent years, following the attempts to use it in priority setting in the State of Oregon's plan to revise its Medicaid programme (Eddy, 1991) and the inclusion of a formal requirement for economic analysis in the process for reimbursement of pharmaceuticals in Australia (Commonwealth of Australia, 1995) and the province of Ontario (Ontario Ministry of Health 1994).

It is not the purpose here to provide a detailed policy commentary on these developments, since the formal position *vis-à-vis* economic evaluation is likely to change over time. Rather, the intention is to draw out the methodological lessons from the use of economic evaluation in decision making, particularly as these relate to the conduct and reporting of studies.

The next two sections of the chapter deal with aspects of *validity*. First, the various proposed reporting frameworks for economic evaluation are reviewed, with an emphasis on the methods for ensuring transparency in the reporting of results. Then the practice of comparing economic evaluation results in cost-effectiveness rankings or 'league tables' is discussed and the major pitfalls identified.

The following two sections of the chapter deal with aspects of *applicability* of economic evaluation. First, the issue of transferring results from one setting to another is discussed, along with some examples. Then the problems and prospects for using economic evaluation are explored, based on the experience gained so far. The chapter ends with a reminder about the limitations of economic evaluation in health care decision-making.

9.2. REPORTING FORMATS
FOR ECONOMIC EVALUATION

9.2.1. Why insist on a common reporting format?

Several of the published guidelines for economic evaluation include a suggested reporting format. There are a number of reasons why a common reporting format for economic evaluations would be desirable. First, it may increase the transparency of studies; that is, it would be easier to assess precisely what the analyst had done and, hence, whether the methods were appropriate. Secondly, it might facilitate comparisons between studies; that is, if all analysts reported their results in a similar fashion, the user could be more confident that differences (say) in cost-effectiveness ratios reflect the characteristics of the interventions or programmes being evaluated, rather than differences in study methodology. Thirdly, it might improve the general quality of evaluations undertaken, since the requirements of the reporting format would lead analysts to address important methodological considerations.

Some of the arguments for a common reporting format are not clear-cut. For example, as we shall discuss later in Section 9.3, comparisons between studies, especially in 'league tables', can be problematical. Also, it might be argued that, far from stimulating methodological improvements, a common reporting format might stifle them if analysts interpreted this a maximum, rather than a minimum, standard that had to be achieved.

The transparency argument is probably the strongest one in favour of a common reporting framework and this was one objectives of the Public Health Services Panel on Cost-effectiveness in Health and Medicine (Gold *et al.* 1996) and the prime motivation for the recommendations of the *British Medical Journal* Working Party on Economic Evaluation (1996). The Public Health Services Panel recommended that reports of economic evaluations should always include the Panel's chosen 'reference case'. The *BMJ* Working Party acknowledged that there are still many methodological debates in economic evaluation and that it may therefore be difficult to develop standards in all areas. However, it would be possible to standardize the reporting, thereby increasing the transparency of studies. Therefore, it specified reporting guidelines that would be used by peer-reviewers of articles submitted to the *BMJ*.

9.2.2. The 10-point checklist as a reporting framework

The 10-point checklist introduced in Chapter 3 is primarily intended as a structure for the critical appraisal of published papers. However, the same questions can serve as a guide to analysts seeking to improve the quality of their study report. If the report is written in a way that would enable the reader to answer all the checklist questions, the analyst would be a long way towards satisfying the basic requirements of transparency.

9.2.3. Similarities and dissimilarities of existing reporting formats

The proposals of the *BMJ* Working Party on Economic Evaluation and the checklist in Chapter 3 represent but two of a growing number of suggested reporting formats for economic evaluation. There are a number of different motivations for the various proposals. Some, like the reporting formats suggested by the Commonwealth of Australia (1995), the Ontario Ministry of Health (1994), and the Canadian Coordinating Office for Health Technology Assessment (1994), are linked to a formal requirement for the provision of economic data prior to the reimbursement (public subsidy) of pharmaceuticals. Others, such as that suggested by the US Public Health Service Panel on Cost-effectiveness in Health and Medicine (Gold *et al.* 1996), are more concerned with the maintenance of methodological standards in published work and the interpretation of economic evaluation results by decision makers. Yet others, such as the proposals of the Task Force on Principles of Economic Analysis of Health Care Technology (1995), also stress the importance of procedural issues, including the contractual relationship between analyst and research sponsor.

The precise content of the various proposals, especially the level of detail, reflects their different objectives (Drummond 1994). Several reviews comparing and contrasting the different suggestions have already been published (Jacobs *et al.* 1995) and others will follow as additional recommendations are made in the future. However, two general points have already emerged.

First, although there are differences among the various proposals, there are a number of recommendations common to many of the existing reporting formats. These include the provision of details on:

- the background (importance) of the question (problem);
- the viewpoint for the analysis;
- the reasons for selecting a particular form of analysis;
- the (patient) population to which the analysis applies;

- the comparators being assessed;
- the source of the medical evidence and its quality;
- the range of costs considered and their measurement (in physical and money terms);
- the measure of benefit in the economic study (e.g. life years gained, QALYs gained);
- the methods for adjusting for timing of costs and benefits;
- the methods for dealing with uncertainty;
- the incremental analysis of costs and benefits;
- the overall results of the study and its limitations.

This list should come as no surprise to readers of this and other texts on economic evaluation of health care programmes. It signifies that there is now a fair amount of agreement on the major elements of study methodology, although many of the details are still open to debate.

The second general point to emerge is that full reporting on all relevant aspects of economic evaluation methodology would require considerable space, certainly more than is typically available in mainstream medical journals. One possible solution is to produce a separate technical report that would be made available to interested parties (Gold *et al.* 1996). Another possibility is that detailed analyses of published studies could be provided by structured databases of economic evaluations, two of which already exist in the United Kingdom (NHS Centre for Reviews and Dissemination, 1996; Office of Health Economics, 1996). However, the reality is that most users of economic evaluations will be consulting the journal publication, so analysts should ensure that this version of study report is as informative as possible, using the 10-point checklist or another reporting format as a template.

9.3. INTERPRETING COST-EFFECTIVENESS 'LEAGUE TABLES'

9.3.1. Motivations behind the 'league table' approach

In recent years it has become fashionable to make comparisons between health care interventions in terms of their relative cost-effectiveness, in cost per life-year or cost per quality-adjusted life-year gained. The first published ranking or 'league table' for the United Kingdom was that derived by Williams (1983). League tables of interventions in North America have been published by Torrance and Zipursky (1984) and Schulman *et al.* (1991). An example of a league table is given in Table 9.1

There are two, quite distinct, motivations behind the league table approach. First, analysts undertaking an evaluation of a particular health treatment or programme often seek, quite appropriately, to place their findings in a broader

Table 9.1.   League table of costs and QALYs for selected
health care interventions

	Cost/QALY (£ Aug 1990)
Cholesterol testing and diet therapy only (all adults, aged 40–69)	220
Neurosurgical intervention for head injury	240
GP advice to stop smoking	270
Neurosurgical intervention for subarachnoid haemorrhage	490
Anti-hypertensive therapy to prevent stroke (ages 45–64)	940
Pacemaker implantation	1100
Hip replacement	1180
Valve replacement for aortic stenosis	1140
Cholesterol testing and treatment	1480
CABG[1] (left main vessel disease, severe angina)	2090
Kidney transplant	4710
Breast cancer screening	5780
Heart transplantation	7840
Cholesterol testing and treatment (incrementally) of all adults aged 25–39 years	14,150
Home haemodialysis	17,260
CABG[1] (1 vessel disease, moderate angina)	18,830
CAPD[2]	19,870
Hospital haemodialysis	21,970
Erythropoietin treatment for anaemia in dialysis patients (assuming a 10% reduction in mortality)	54,380
Neurosurgical intervention for malignant intracranial tumours	107,780
Erythropoietin treatment for anaemia in dialysis patients (assuming no increase in survival)	126,290

Source: Maynard (1991)

context. For example, Schulman *et al.* (1991) compared their estimates of the
cost per life-year gained from early treatment of asymptomatic people with
HIV infection with a broader range of interventions, including treatment for
elevated cholesterol, mammography, and renal analysis. Secondly, some
analysts seek to inform decisions about the allocation of health care resources
between alternative programmes. For example, Williams (1983) calculated the
cost per QALY of a range of health care interventions and divided them into
strong candidates for expansion and less strong candidates for expansion,

although in part his analysis was designed to illustrate what could be achieved by using available data and to argue for further refinements. Also, in Canada Laupacis *et al.* (1992) argued that the adoption and utilization of new health technologies could be classified into five grades of recommendation based on their incremental cost per QALY, although they acknowledged that many other issues apart from cost-effectiveness, such as ethical and political considerations, affect the implementation of a new technology.

Most of the criticisms of league tables are directed at the second of these two potential motivations. However, in reality most analysts quoting league tables have either not been clear about their motivation, or had the first, more limited, objective in mind. Nevertheless, the concerns need to be addressed.

9.3.2. Methodological considerations in the construction and use of league tables

For the information in league tables to be of any use to decision makers, we need to be confident that the methodology of the source studies (contained in the table) is sound and that it is relatively homogenous among the various studies.

Drummond *et al.* (1993) explored these issues with particular reference to the league table shown in Table 9.1. They found that there was considerable variation in methodology among the source studies generating the 21 estimates of cost per QALY in the table. They argued that in interpreting the league table a number of methodological features are particularly important. These are: (1) the discount rate; (2) the method for estimating health state preferences; (3) the range of costs and consequences considered and; (4) the choice of comparison programme. The methodological issues surrounding the choice of discount rate, the inclusion/exclusion of costs and consequences, and the estimation of health state preferences have been discussed elsewhere in this book. However, the fourth issue, the choice of comparison programme, is probably the most important in the interpretation of league tables and is discussed in Box 9.1.

9.3.3. Broader objections to the use of league tables

Notwithstanding the methodological challenges outlined above, a number of authors have argued that the second use of league tables (i.e. to allocate resources) is flawed. The objections relate to: (1) whether cost-effectiveness decision rules are really workable in practice (Birch and Gafni 1992, 1993; Johannesson and Weinstein 1993) and (2) whether the adoption of a cost-effectiveness threshold (Laupacis *et al.* 1992) is wise (see Gafni and Birch 1993; Laupacis *et al.* 1993; Naylor *et al.* 1993).

Box 9.1. Is the programme cost-effective? It all depends on what we compare it to

Suppose our interest is in programme A_2. This could be because it is a new screening programme proposed by public health specialists or a new drug suggested for reimbursement. Compared with doing nothing, A_2 costs an additional $100,000 and generates 11 extra QALYs, with an incremental cost-effectiveness ratio of $9100 per QALY. This might be the figure included in a league table for comparison with other interventions. (The cost per QALY ratio between two points is given by the slope of the line and is indicated on the graph.)

However, suppose current practice is to have programme A_1. This costs $50,000 yet generates only one QALY. If we chose to compare A_2 with A_1 we would obtain a more attractive incremental cost-effectiveness ratio of $5000 per QALY. But A_1 is a dominated programme (see Chapter 5) and should not feature in the relevant set of alternatives. Therefore the incremental analysis of A_2 over A_1 would be misleading.

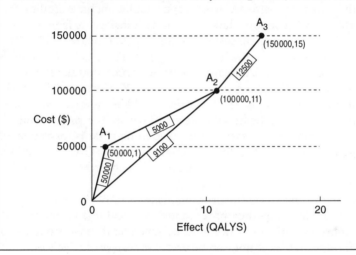

(1) Are cost-effectiveness decision rules workable in practice?

In Chapter 5 (Section 5.5) we presented a hypothetical example of how alternative treatments could be ranked in terms of their incremental cost-effectiveness ratio. We showed how decision rules could be applied, either to determine how a fixed budget could be spent or to determine which alternatives would be adopted, given different levels of willingness to pay for a unit of effectiveness (eg a lifeyear or a QALY). Essentially, this is the approach implied by the second use of league tables outlined above.

In the simple hypothetical example we did not discuss issues of *divisibility* or *returns to scale*; that is, we did not discuss whether each alternative treatment could be given in part (e.g. to fewer people), rather than in total, and, if so, whether the partial application would have the same cost-effectiveness ratio as the whole.

In objecting to the approach outlined in Section 5.5, Birch and Gafni (1993)

argue that the two simplifying assumptions, perfect divisibility of pro-grammes and constant returns to scale, are unlikely to apply in practice and that therefore the decision rules will not apply. Johannesson and Weinstein (1993) argue that the methods of dealing with indivisibility of programmes, through interger programming or dynamic programming, are well-known and that, in any case, the simple rules give good approximations. This is an empirical point which, to our knowledge, has not been explored in the context of actual health care resource allocation decisions.

(2) Is adopting a cost-effectiveness threshold wise?

Here the objections are numerous. First, the outcome measure used in most cost-effectiveness league tables (i.e. the QALY) may not capture all the relevant benefits of health care programmes (see the discussion in Chapter 2). Secondly, most cost-effectiveness league tables include studies from a range of settings and economic data may not be transferable from one setting to another. (This issue is discussed in Section 9.4 below.) Thirdly, the adoption of a threshold implies a 'shadow price' for a QALY. (This issue was raised in Section 5.5.) Whereas it might be argued that the shadow price represents society's willingness to pay for a QALY, Gafni and Birch (1993) argue that it is unlikely that the shadow price would be independent of the size of the health programme being considered. That is, the programme's true opportunity cost can only be assessed by examining what is forgone in other sectors (e.g. education). Therefore, a single cost per QALY threshold is meaningless and may be a recipe for unconstrained growth of health care expenditures.

Of course, in the real world the decision maker is unlikely to know the costs and benefits of all competing programmes in health and other sectors. Therefore, more consideration needs to be given as to how economic data, presented in league tables or not, can be useful in real-world decision-making. This is discussed further in Section 9.5 below.

9.4. TRANSFERRING ECONOMIC EVALUATION RESULTS FROM SETTING TO SETTING

In the discussion of league tables we mentioned that the studies being compared often come from a range of settings. In interpreting economic evaluation results, decision makers need to form a view on whether the results apply in their own setting. Some scientific data are clearly transferable. For example, the clinical effect of a patient taking a given medicine is likely to be similar in the USA and Canada. However, the same may not be true of the same operation performed by different surgeons. Also, in some cases the clinical endpoints may not be totally independent of the health care setting. For example, the EPIC trial of a new drug in cardiology (EPIC Investigators,

1994) used a combined endpoint of death, non-fatal myocardial infarction, unplanned surgical revascularization, unplanned repeat PTCA, unplanned insertion of an intra-aortic balloon pump for refractory ischaemia, and unplanned implantation of a coronary stent. Because of these issues, the applicability of economic evaluation results from one setting to another has been widely debated and is an issue both within countries and between countries.

With the growing international literature on economic evaluation and the rapid international spread of new health technologies, there is a need to undertake, or at least interpret, economic evaluations on the international level. For example, health care decision makers, especially in those countries having limited resources for health technology assessment, may wish to reinterpret in their own setting the results of an economic evaluation that was done elsewhere. Also, controlled clinical trials are often mounted on an international basis in order to recruit sufficient numbers of patients or to satisfy the needs of different national medical and regulatory agencies which like to see evidence of efficacy in their own patient population. Increasingly, these trials may incorporate the gathering of economic data.

However, the gathering of economic data poses different challenges and the results of studies may not be transferable from one setting to another. Indeed, one of the countries to require economic data in support of submissions for government reimbursement of pharmaceuticals has pointed out that the data need to be relevant to local circumstances (Commonwealth of Australia 1995). The suggestion is that demonstrating the cost-effectiveness of a new medicine in (say) the USA may not of itself prove that the same product would be good value for money in Australia.

There are a number of reasons to suppose why economic data may not be easily transferable. These include differences in the availability of alternative treatments, in clinical practice patterns, in relative prices, and in the incentives to health care professionals and institutions. The next section discusses in more depth the differences, between countries or locations, likely to affect cost-effectiveness.

9.4.1. Factors likely to affect cost-effectiveness

Basic demography and epidemiology of disease

Countries differ in respect of the age structure of their population and the incidence of various diseases. In some cases this will affect the cost-effectiveness of health care programmes, particularly those delivered on a population basis. For example, programmes of immunization or screening and treatment of disease are likely to be more cost-effective in populations where the incidence of the disease in question is high. Different age structures between countries are likely to lead to different levels of incidence in various countries and hence the size of the overall economic burden. The cost-effectiveness of treatment is also likely to vary by patient characteristics, including age, lifestyle, and medical history. Therefore, when discussing the cost-effectiveness of health care treatments and programmes, it is important to specify the patient population to which any statements apply.

Availability of health care resources and variations in clinical practice

Countries differ in respect of the range of treatments and health care facilities available to their populations. In the case of treatment for ulcer, the availability of surgery could vary from place to place. In some countries with national health care systems, such as Sweden and the UK, rationing takes place, with waiting lists for hospital admission. The availability of important diagnostic facilities, such as endoscopy, could also vary from one location to another. In turn, the availability of resources may affect the way medicine is practised. For example, if there are long waiting times for endoscopy, a clinician may try a therapeutic dose of a drug for a patient experiencing ulcer-type pain without waiting to confirm the diagnosis. Another difference between countries, more directly related to drug therapy, is the range of licensed products and availability of generics.

Although clinical practice is partly constrained by the available alternatives, it is known that practice varies among clinicians in the same geographical area facing essentially the same range of treatment options (McPherson *et al.* 1982). To the extent that clinical practice varies systematically between countries, this is likely to affect the relative cost-effectiveness of therapies.

Incentives to health care professionals and institutions

In some health care systems the level of remuneration of health care professionals and institutions is largely independent of the level of service delivered. For example, hospitals are given a global budget and physicians are paid by salary. In other systems physicians are paid by fee per item of service and hospitals reimbursed by the number of cases in each category treated.

It has often been suggested that physicians operating under a fee-for-service system are more likely to generate extra demand for their services, whereas those paid by salary or capitation are more likely to deter demand. This may affect the number of physician visits and diagnostic tests performed for a given patient suffering from (say) ulcer-type pain.

In the case of hospital treatment for ulcer, the method of reimbursement could affect which services are delivered on an out-patient basis and also the length of stay for in-patients. A hospital being paid a fixed amount for treating a given case has more incentives to free the bed for the next patient than a hospital being funded through a global budget.

Relative prices or costs

It is well known that absolute price levels vary between countries. However, from the point of view of cost-effectiveness assessments, the critical issue is whether the *relative* prices of health care resources differ. Most obviously, if the relative prices of the main drugs for a given condition differ between countries, then their relative cost-effectiveness will differ.

Perhaps less obvious is the fact that the relative cost-effectiveness of drugs will differ if the relative prices of *other* health care resources differs between countries. For example, a drug with greater efficacy, a better side effect profile, or more convenient route of administration, will appear better value for money in a country where the costs of investigations, hospitalizations, surgery, and physician visits are relatively higher, since consumption of these items is likely to be reduced. For example, Hull *et al.* (1981) found that the relative price of venography (a diagnostic test for deep-vein thrombosis) differed between the USA and Canada. This affected the relative cost-effectiveness of alternative diagnostic strategies for DVT in the two countries and would also affect the estimates of the value for money of drugs to prevent DVT.

It should also be remembered from Chapter 4 that the prices of health care resources do not always reflect costs, although it is often a tacit assumption of economic evaluations that they do. Therefore, in arguing that savings in other health care resources, such as surgical time, justify a more expensive but more efficacious drug, some consideration should be given to whether the prices of those resources really reflect their true opportunity costs.

9.4.2. Ways of adapting results from setting to setting

An analyst seeking to adapt economic evaluation results from one setting to another could be faced with one of three situations. First, only clinical data may have been collected in the clinical trials and there is a need to produce economic evaluations for more than one country or setting. Here the only option is to undertake a modelling study, where the clinical data are combined with cost (and possibly quality of life) data from a number of sources (e.g. routinely available statistics, free-standing cost studies, etc.).

Secondly, economic data (e.g. quantities of resource use) may have been collected alongside a clinical trial undertaken in one country, but economic evaluations are required for other settings. Here, a modelling study using only the clinical data could be undertaken, as above. Alternatively, the resource use data could be adapted in some way in order to make them relevant to another setting.

Thirdly, economic data may have been collected alongside a multi-national clinical trial and economic evaluations are required for all the countries enrolling patients in the trial. Here the analyst has a number of options for using the resource use data. Either they could be pooled, as is common for the clinical data, and priced separately for each country; or alternatively, the resource use data for patients from each country could be analysed separately and then priced for each country as above. In this case the analysts would also have the option of calculating cost-effectiveness ratios for each country using the pooled clinical results or the individual clinical results for each country.

All three situations present analytical challenges and there are currently very few examples in the published literature. However, some studies are discussed below.

Using modelling to adapt results from one setting to another

An example here is the study by Drummond *et al*. (1992) of misoprostol, a drug for prophylaxis of gastric ulcers in patients on long-term non-steroidal anti-inflammatory drug use experiencing abdominal pain. A clinical trial, undertaken in the USA (Graham *et al*. 1988), had shown that patients given misoprostol (400μg daily) for three months had a lower rate of endoscopically determined lesions than those receiving placebo (5.6 per cent versus 21.7 per cent). With the higher dose, of 800μg daily, the rate of lesions fell to 1.7 per cent.

Apart from conferring clinical benefits, a lower rate of gastric lesions is likely to generate economic benefits. Namely, if fewer patients have lesions it is likely that fewer will require diagnostic work-up for suspected ulcer and fewer will require treatment in ambulatory care or in hospital. Therefore, an economic evaluation could assess whether these potential savings in resources justify the costs of adding misoprostol.

Drummond *et al*. wanted to conduct economic evaluations in Belgium, France, the United Kingdom and the USA. However, whereas the clinical data might be considered applicable in all countries, other factors might differ. These could include the compliance with therapy, the method of diagnostic work-up, the nature and extent of ambulatory care for ulcer, the rate of hospitalization for ulcer, the level of surgical intervention, and the length of hospital stay. In addition, it was known that the prices of resources, including the acquisition cost of misoprostol, differed from place to place. Whereas the drug price was broadly similar in the three European countries studied, it was around 40 per cent higher in the USA.

In order to model the expected cost of adding three months prophylaxis, Drummond *et al*. devised a decision tree (see Box 9.2). This provided a framework for combining the clinical data from the trial with other data obtained by additional study. For example, the nature of diagnostic work-up and ambulatory care was ascertained by asking expert panels of physicians in the four countries. Hospital admission rates for ulcer were determined from epidemiological surveys, whereas surgical rates and length of hospital stay were obtained from routine hospital statistics. The method of obtaining the relevant financial data varied from country to country. In some countries data on fees and charges were available; in others free-standing costing studies were carried out.

The results (see Table 9.2) showed that indeed there was some variation between countries. It is particularly interesting to note that in the USA, where the acquisition cost of misoprostol is highest, the overall economic results are

Box 9.2. Using a decision tree to adapt data from setting to setting

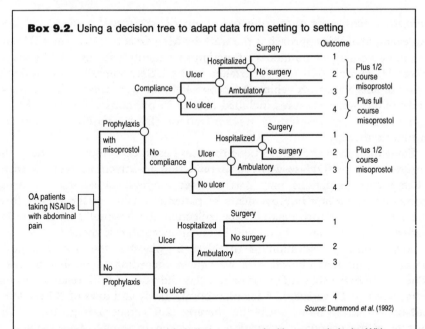

Source: Drummond *et al.* (1992)

In the decision tree above prophylaxis is compared with no prophylaxis. With no prophylaxis it was assumed that the ulcer rate approximated to that in the placebo group in the clinical trial, although an adjustment was made for the fact that around 40% of lesions discovered endoscopically will be silent (i.e. not bothersome to the patient). Thus, these will not require costs in diagnostic workup or therapy. In the treatment arm the non-compliers were also assigned the trial placebo ulcer rate. The difference in expected cost is driven by the clinical data, but the calculation in both arms requires data that was not gathered in the trial.

the most favourable. At the high dose the expected cost of adding three months prophylaxis is the lowest in the four countries and at the lower dose there is a net saving. This is because of the relatively higher cost of *other* resources in the US health care system, especially surgery. However, it should be remembered that the savings in this case represent the value of resources that could potentially be freed for other uses.

Table 9.2. Expected costs (savings) per patient for three months prophylaxis ($)*

	Belgium	France	UK	USA
High dose	32	61	55	22
Low dose	5	15	3	(40)

* Ulcers 0.3cm or larger, silent ulcer rate of 40%.

Adapting economic data collected alongside a clinical trial

An example of this approach is the work by Menzin *et al.* (1995) on rhDNase for improvement of pulmonary function in patients with cystic fibrosis. A phase III clinical trial was undertaken in the USA comparing two different doses of rhDNase with vehicle (placebo). Patients were treated for 24 weeks and the outcome measures included change in pulmonary function (FEV$_1$) and incidence of respiratory tract infections (RTI$_S$) requiring parenteral antibiotic therapy.

Since the treatment of infections requires health care resources, one of the arguments for rhDNase was that a reduction in infections reduces costs. (These cost reductions may partly offset the cost of adding the drug, notwithstanding any improvements to patients' quality of life.) Therefore, the trial included prospective data collection for hospital admissions, in-patient days, and days of oral and intravenous antibiotic therapy.

Apart from the addition of rhDNase or placebo, the trial was fairly naturalistic in that clinical care was given according to normal practice. The trial showed that rhDNase once a day did reduce RTI-related hospital admissions (0.41 versus 0.56 for placebo; p < 0.05) and days of RTI-related out-patient intravenous antibiotic therapy (2.9 versus 4.4; p < 0.05). The results of the economic evaluation undertaken in the USA are shown in Fig. 9.1. Compared with placebo, the cost of treating RTIs over 24 weeks was $1682 less among patients receiving rhDNase once daily, primarily due to reductions in the cost of hospitalization (Oster *et al.* 1995).

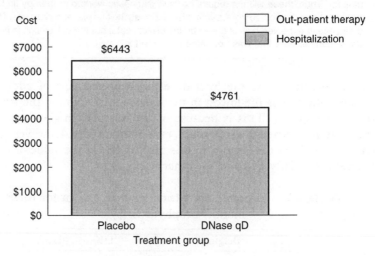

Fig. 9.1. Economic evaluation of DNase therapy in the USA. Mean total costs of care related to respiratory tract infection over 24 weeks by treatment group. (*Source*: Oster *et al.* 1995.)

In addition, there was interest in conducting the same economic evaluation in France, Germany, Italy, and the UK. One approach would be to take the reductions in resource use observed in the trial and to price these in local currency. Table 9.3 shows the results. It can be seen that the savings range from £434 ($711) in the UK to 7011FF ($1 064) in France, all being less than the corresponding figure in the USA, presumably reflecting relative price levels.

Table 9.3. Difference in mean cost of RTI-related care (placebo minus rhDNase) excluding cost of study medication, over 24 weeks in local currencies and US dollars, by country

Component of cost	Country			
	France (FF)	Germany (DM)	Italy (L)	UK (£)
		Costs in local currency		
In-patient care:				
days in hospital	4540	711	982000	300
antibiotic therapy	806	1259[1]	122000	50
Out-patient care	1665	−[1]	181000	84
TOTAL	7011	1970	1285000	434
		Costs in US $[2]		
In-patient care:				
days in hospital	693	337	660	477
antibiotic therapy	123	607[1]	82	79
Out-patient care	254	−[1]	122	134
TOTAL	1070	934	864	690

[1] A detailed breakdown of inpatient and outpatient antibiotic costs was not available.
[2] Calculated using 1990 Purchasing Power Parities. Organization for Economic Cooperation and Development (OECD): OECD Health Data File, 1992.
Source: Menzin *et al.*, (1996)

However, it could be argued that, because of variations in local practice patterns, these *trial-based* estimates for other countries might be misleading. For example, few patients may be admitted to hospital for treatment of RTI in Italy, as there is extensive use of injectable antibiotics in ambulatory care. Also, length of stay in hospital could differ from that in the USA, as the hospitals may be operating under different financial incentives, or have a greater or lesser pressure on beds. Therefore, the analysts in the four other countries were asked to consider whether a *practice-adjusted* estimate of resource use and cost should be presented alongside the trial-based estimates. The adjustments were made by:

(1) seeking expert opinion on likely treatment patterns for RTI;
(2) analysing a series of patient case notes (charts) to estimate length of hospital stay and resource use for treatment of RTI.

The outcome of this exercise was that in the UK no adjustments (to the trial-based estimates) were considered necessary. However, in Germany, length of stay was considered to be, on average, 14.4 days rather than 12.3 days. In France and Italy, both the rate of hospitalization and the length of stay were adjusted. The overall effect was to reduce slightly the estimates of savings in Italy (from $908 to $607) and in France (from $1064 to $850). In Germany, there was a very small increase in the savings from treating RTI.

The problem with this approach is in justifying the adjustments made. One might argue that the savings observed in the trial, whilst not very generalizable, are relatively free of bias. This is an example of the conflict between internal and external validity mentioned in Chapter 8. In this case the main saving grace was that, in the main, the adjustments made were conservative (i.e. reduced the estimates of the savings from rhDNase). If the results had gone the other way there might have been more criticism of the adjustments made. Therefore, analysts wishing to make adjustments to trial-based data might be advised to state these up-front in the analysis plan for the study, prior to seeing the data. Any adjustments should also be based on empirical data rather than guesswork.

Analysing economic data from multinational trials

One response to the problem over the lack of transferability of cost-effectiveness data would be to undertake clinical trials with economic data collection in all relevant countries and settings. In part, this is achieved by undertaking multinational trials, except that often relatively small numbers of patients are included from some countries. Indeed, one of the motivations on the clinical side for undertaking multinational trials is to enroll sufficient numbers of patients within a relatively short period of time. Since the intention is usually to pool the clinical data, it is likely that the trial will be underpowered for analysing differences between treatment groups in any single country or centre. Although ultimately an empirical question, it is likely that a multinational trial will also be underpowered for the analysis of resource data at the individual country level.

Currently there are few examples of multinational economic clinical trials in the published literature and there has been little discussion of how the data from these studies should be analysed. One option would be to approach the problem in the same way as it is handled in the analysis of clinical data. Namely, statistical tests could be performed to check for the existence of an interaction between treatment effect and country (or centre).

Normally, these tests turn out to be negative, although they themselves may be short of statistical power. However, a negative test on the resource data may be sufficient grounds to pool them. Economist analyses could then be undertaken by using the overall data set and by applying prices for each individual country.

If the tests for an interaction between the effect on resources and country (or centre) turn out to be positive, the analyst would then have to explore two options. First, country-specific resource data could be used to calculate the cost-effectiveness ratios using the overall clinical data set. The main argument for this approach is that there would be sufficient statistical power, at least for the clinical part of the cost-effectiveness ratio. Alternatively, country-specific resource use data could be used to calculate cost-effectiveness ratios with country-specific clinical data. The main argument for this approach would be that impacts on resource use in a given country are likely to be driven, at least in part, by the clinical differences between the therapies. Therefore, country-specific data should form both the numerator and denominator of the ratio.

As can be seen from the discussion above, many issues in the analysis of economic data collected alongside multinational clinical trials remain unresolved. Therefore, it is impossible to give firm guidance at present. However, given the large number of studies currently underway, progress in this methodological area is likely in the near future.

9.4.3. Exercise: undertaking an economic evaluation of non-steroidal anti-inflammatory drugs (NSAIDs) in three countries

The objectives of this exercise are:

(1) to illustrate how decision trees can be useful in modelling the cost-effectiveness of therapies and in transferring results from one setting to another;
(2) to illustrate how differences between clinical trials and clinical practice, and between countries, can affect cost-effectiveness estimates.

Problem

One of the critical differences between NSAIDs is their gastric side-effects. These can affect both the level of tolerability of the drug and its economic impact. (For example, gastric side effects may have resource consequences if treatment is required.) Whereas there may be little to choose between NSAIDs in terms of their relative efficacy, exploration of the impact of gastric side effects could be important. In particular, it may mean that a choice of therapy based on acquisition cost alone could be inappropriate.

Data

Data are presented in Table 9.4 on the acquisition costs and rates of gastric ulcers for three NSAIDs in three countries. The acquisition costs are expressed in US dollars for six months therapy and vary by country. This could be for historical reasons (e.g. the time at which the various products were launched) and the level of income in the countries concerned. Two rates of gastric ulcers are presented – the rate determined endoscopically in clinical trials and the rate adjusted to exclude silent ulcers. (The latter rate reflects the

Table 9.4.   Acquisition costs and rates of gastric ulcers with three NSAIDs

	Acquisition costs ($)			Rate of gastric ulcers over 6 months (%)	
	Country 1	Country 2	Country 3	Endoscopically -determined	Adjusted to exclude silent ulcers
Mobifren	225	75	121	23.9	14.3
Osteotec	294	100	134	17.8	10.7
Voldene	300	136	126	10.2	6.1

fact that around 40 per cent of the lesions discovered by endoscope may not result in treatment since they are asymptomatic.)

Table 9.5 gives data on the treatment of gastric ulcers in the three countries. This contains data on treatment practices and unit costs. Country 3 is obviously one with a less well developed economy, where price levels are lower. Finally, Fig. 9.2 provides a decision tree that can be used to combine the data on probabilities and costs to calculate the expected cost of six months' therapy.

Table 9.5.   Data on treatment for gastric ulcers in three countries

	Country 1	Country 2	Country 3
Probabilities			
Patients with ulcers treated in hospital	0.086	0.053	0.050
Patients hospitalized for ulcers requiring surgery	0.12	0.43	0.20
Unit costs ($)			
Ambulatory care for ulcer	901	540	87
Medical hospital care for ulcer	3450	1548	133
Surgical hospital care for ulcer	15700	2533	555

Tasks

The decision tree shown in Fig. 9.2 can be used to calculate the expected cost $(C^\star)$ of six months of therapy.

1. Calculate the expected cost of six months of therapy for each of the three NSAIDs in each of the three countries.
2. Explain why the relative cost of therapy varies by country.
3. Imagine that you are an economist working for the company that produces Voldene, the NSAID with the lowest rate of gastric side effects. In a country where this therapy does not give the lowest expected cost, what other economic analyses would you consider?

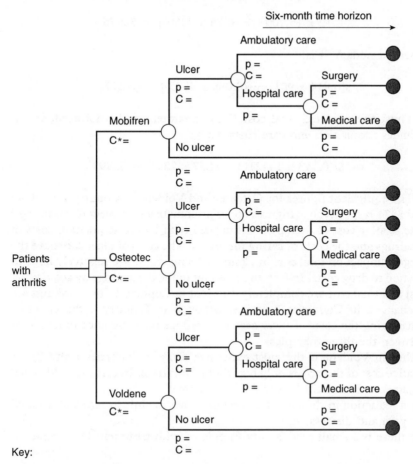

Six-month time horizon

Key:

C* Expected total cost for six months' therapy, including complications ($)
C The cost of each event ($)
p Probability

Fig. 9.2. Decision tree for assessing the cost-effectiveness of NSAIDS. *Patients developing an ulcer are assumed to incur half of the six-month cost of therapy.

Solutions

1. To calculate the expected cost of six months therapy, the decision tree model is completed using the data in Tables 9.4 and 9.5. This is done for Country 1 below. Note that the rate of ulcers adjusted to exclude silent ulcers is used since it is more likely to reflect what would happen in regular practice.

    The probabilities at each node sum to one and the expected cost calculations are made by rolling back the tree from *right to left*. For example, the expected cost at node X is:

$$\$[0.12 \times 15,700) + (0.78 \times 3450)] = \$4575$$

Then, at node Y it is:

$$\$[0.914 \times 901) + (0.086 \times 4575)] = \$1217$$

Thus, the expected total cost C for treatment with Mobifren, which includes acquisition and care costs, is:

$$\$[(0.143 \times 1442) + (0.857 \times 225)] = \$399$$

The equivalent figures for Osteotec and Voldene in Country 1 are $242 and $374 respectively. (Figures are approximate and subject to rounding.)

2. The relative cost of therapy is influenced both by the acquisition costs of the drugs and the costs of caring for ulcers. The costs of ulcer care have the biggest impact on total cost in Country 1 since these are relatively large in relation to drug costs. In fact, the rankings of the three drugs by acquisition cost and total cost are completely different in Country 1. The rankings are unchanged in Countries 2 and 3, although in Country 2 the effect of considering the costs of ulcer care is to reduce the difference in total cost between the three therapies.

3. Although Voldene is the most expensive drug in Countries 1 and 2, the relative cost of therapy is only highest in Country 2. In this case additional arguments that might be considered are that:
   (a) a reduction in the rate of ulceration is worthwhile in terms of avoided pain and distress;
   (b) there is a small case fatality associated with treatment for ulcers.

9.5. PROBLEMS AND POTENTIAL FOR USING ECONOMIC EVALUATION IN DECISION-MAKING

Although this book is primarily about the methods of economic evaluation, it is important to address the potential for using study results. If the problems of using economic evaluation are not understood, it may not be worthwhile investing resources in undertaking the studies in the first place. Much of the potential for using economic evaluation and the related problems are situation-specific, but it is possible to make a few general observations.

9.5.1. In what situations could economic evaluation be used?

Haan and Rutten (1987) provide a taxonomy of decision making situations where economic evaluation could be used to encourage a rational diffusion and use of health technology (see Box 9.3). They divide these into situations where regulation (of the health care system) is by directive and those where regulation is by incentive. The extent to which these apply is likely to vary by health care systems. For example, in some socialized health care systems where central control over the finance and planning of the system is possible, it may be feasible to regulate by directive, e.g. deciding on the number and location of specialist facilities like heart transplant centres. Clearly, economic evaluation can inform such decisions (see Buxton *et al.* 1985).

Box 9.3. Taxonomy of decision making situations where economic evaluation could be used to influence the diffusion and use of health technology (After Haan and Rutten (1987)

Regulation by directive (central/ regional government)	**Regulation by incentive**
Pre-market controls for drugs and devices	Reforming payment schemes for health care institutions (e.g. hospitals)
(Conditional) exclusion from public reimbursement	Budgetary reform within institutions
Planning of specialist facilities or specific technologies	Changing payment systems for health care providers
	Cost-sharing arrangements
	Encouraging competition in the health care system
	Medical audit and utilization review systems

   There are many health care decision making situations where economic evaluation could potentially be used. The range of possibilities depends on the health care system operating in a given country. National, socialized, health care systems have a greater potential for using regulation by directive. Liberal, market-based health care systems are more likely to rely on regulation by incentive in order to encourage a rational diffusion and use of health technologies.

However, the worldwide trend is currently towards managed competition in health care. In this case, regulation by incentive is likely to be a much more fruitful way of encouraging a rational diffusion and use of health technology.

9.5.2. Where has economic evaluation actually been used?

Drummond (1994) discusses a number of examples where economic evaluation has been used to inform some of the decisions outlined in Haan and Ruttens taxonomy. In general, the actual use of economic evaluation is still quite limited in relation to the potential. Coyle (1993) suggests a number of reasons why this would be the case. These include lack of dissemination of findings, lack of recognition (by decision-makers) of their importance, lack of understanding of study results, and a lack of mechanisms to use them in decision-making.

The two most widely publicised uses of economic evaluation to date are in the Oregon Medicaid Plan (Eddy, 1991) and in decisions about the reimbursement of pharmaceuticals in Australia (Commonwealth of Australia 1995) and Ontario (Ontario Ministry of Health 1994). Both instances illustrate that the application of economic evaluation is not just a technical issue. In Oregon, a cost-per-QALY league table was constructed in order to inform the public debate about which treatments to include in the states Medicaid package. Although there were undoubtedly imperfections in the economic analyses carried out, the main problem was that the league table became a focus of political debate. Therefore, the arguments focused not on the role of economic evaluation, but on whether it was right to ration and, if so, the best way of rationing.

In Australia the provision of data on the cost-effectiveness of pharmaceuticals has been mandatory since 1993. Pharmaceutical companies applying for public subsidy of their product, through inclusion on the governments Pharmaceutical Benefits Schedule, must make a submission comparing the costs and consequences of their drug with a relevant alternative (comparator). A similar procedure is followed in the province of Ontario in Canada. Mitchell and Glasziou (1996) have reported on the first two years of operation of the scheme in Australia. It has proved workable although there have been disagreements about the choice of comparator, the valuation of productivity changes and the level of feedback that should be given to applicant companies. The ultimate test of economic evaluation will be whether it improves the quality of decision making about the pricing and reimbursement of medicines in Australia.

9.5.3. In what ways could economic evaluation be used?

We tend to think of economic evaluation as a basis for undertaking studies and this is what the book has been mainly concerned with. However, from the discussion in Section 9.5.2 above, it is clear that the formal use of economic evaluation in health care decision making is still quite limited.

Clearly, it is not possible to undertake a formal economic evaluation for every conceivable decision. Sometimes the time horizon for making the decision is very short and this would preclude a study. (However, Schoenbaum et al. (1976) did undertake a study within three weeks in order to help the US government decide whether or not to launch an immunization campaign for swine influenza.)

On other occasions a formal study may be inappropriate because the cost of the study may be large in relation to the importance of the decision. There is no point in spending $100 000 on a study to decide how to spend $50 000, although this has probably been done somewhere! Therefore, it is worthwhile recognizing two other possible ways of using economic evaluation. First, it could be used as *a way of assessing proposals* for the use of resources. Box 9.4 contains a checklist of questions similar to the methodological checklist outlined in Chapter 3. However, the questions have been reformulated as a management checklist to be used by someone considering a proposal being made (e.g. by a clinician wishing to expand a service). Probably, this is the way that many decision makers use economic evaluation, since it is unlikely that a published study exists, or could be commissioned, to inform a given decision directly. To date there has been little study of how decision makers actually use economic evaluation. The special journal issues edited by Drummond *et al.* (1994) and Grabowski and Sloan (1997) are a useful starting point for anyone wishing to pursue this further. Secondly, decision makers may use economic evaluation more generally as a *systematic way of thinking*, or as a way of structuring problems. Understandably there is little published data dealing with this potential way of using economic evaluation, since the processes for arriving at particular decisions are rarely documented.

9.5.4. What should be our overall philosophy for the use of economic evaluation?

In Chapter 2 we discussed three hypothetical analysts, each having a slightly different perspective on the role of economic evaluation. Two perspectives in particular, those of Analysts A and C, merit more discussion here.

Analyst A was the one who thought that economic evaluation ought to be firmly grounded in the theory of welfare economics. The role of the evaluation is therefore to give decision makers a 'theoretically correct' answer to their question, at least according to the criterion of economic efficiency. On the other hand, Analyst C saw the role of economic evaluation as identifying, measuring, and where possible, valuing a wide range of costs and consequences. However, the valuations of costs and consequences would not necessarily be consistent with welfare economics theory, as they could come from decision-makers acting on behalf of individual members of society, rather than the individuals themselves.

These two perspectives on the role of economic evaluation have been called respectively the *Paretian* and the *decision-making* approaches (Sugden and Williams 1979). Clearly, the Paretian approach has the theoretical high ground, although even the most committed Paretians acknowledge that distributional issues as well as efficiency issues need to be dealt with. This is particularly important since the criterion for a potential Pareto improvement – that the gainers from a particular project should be able to compensate the losers – does not require the compensation to take place in practice.

Box 9.4. Questions to ask of anyone making a proposal for the use of resources

Consideration of alternatives
What is the main justification for the proposed service; what would be the consequence of doing nothing at all?

Does the proposal contain an explicit comparison of alternative treatments or programmes, or is the implicit alternative the existing service provision?
If a completely new alternative treatment or programme is proposed:
• is it adequately described?
• why was this particular option chosen?
• were other options rejected, if so why?

Assessment of cost and benefits
In evaluating the proposed service against alternatives, what range of costs is considered? Does this include:
• capital as well as operating costs?
• costs other than those resulting in money expenditure (e.g. the opportunity cost of space denied other uses)?
• costs outside the immediate department where the service will be provided?
• costs on other parties (e.g. patients, other public or private agencies)?

What is known about the effectiveness of the health treatments or programmes discussed in the proposal?
• have these been evaluated by a randomized controlled trial or similar method?
• are there plans to monitor the effectiveness of any new procedures; if so, how?
• have all relevant dimensions of outcome been considered and will any attempts be made to assign preferences or values to them?

Would costs and benefits be substantially different if the proposed service provision were of a different scale? That is:
• if the service provision could be larger, what would be added and what would be the additional costs and benefits?
• if the service provision had to be smaller, what aspects of it would be cut and what would be the reductions in costs and benefits?

Is it claimed that the proposal will be party self-funding, in that savings will be generated? If so, what specific actions need to be taken to realise such savings (e.g. closing hospital wards or other institutions) and what are the likely resource costs associated with taking these actions?

Other important issues
Does the proposal acknowledge any differences in the *timing* of costs and benefits between the alternatives assessed? If so, how is this dealt with in the proposal?

What are the main sources of uncertainty surrounding the proposal (e.g. in the effectiveness of new medical procedures, or in expected revenue costs or savings)?
• what happens to costs and benefits if the analysis is re-worked using more pessimistic assumptions?
• what could be done, perhaps at a slight increase in cost, to reduce uncertainty (e.g. by additional information gathering)?

The above checklist does not comprise a comprehensive range of questions. It is the intention that the questions themselves, and the responses they solicit, will suggest further questions pertinent to the evaluation of choices in the use of health service resources.

Sugden and Williams defend the decision making approach on the grounds that: 'there is a fairly strong argument that, at least in a fairly centralized, public, decision-making system, the objective chosen will normally correspond to that implied by the potential Pareto improvement criterion'. They also argue that, through the control of the tax system, government decision makers can convert potential Pareto improvements to actual improvements.

Departure from the strict Paretian framework would imply that estimates of individuals willingness-to-pay for health care programmes are *just another piece of relevant information* in reaching a decision about the allocation of health care resources, alongside data on effects (in physical units) and health state preference scores. Therefore, one does not have to subscribe to the Paretian value judgement in order to be interested in willingness-to-pay, although those analysts undertaking these measurements clearly believe that individuals' valuations are important in health care resource allocation decisions.

A related issue concerns whether CEA or CUA and CBA are nearly equivalent (Phelps and Mushlin 1991). The logic is that if, at the end of the day, decision makers must apply their values in reaching a decision, this suggests that presenting a cost-effectiveness ratio is almost the same as undertaking a CBA, since decision makers will make their own assessment of the societal willingness to pay for a life-year or a QALY.

It should be clear from the discussion in Chapters 2 and 7 that CEA and CBA are not necessarily equivalent. For example, CBA may include the value of aspects of health programmes that are not related to changes in health status (see Fig. 2.2). Secondly, the total societal willingness-to-pay for a given health care programme will include the value placed on it by altruistic individuals whose own health state is not directly affected.

Of course, it would in principle be possible to extend the cost-effectiveness or cost–utility analysis to include the gains in quality of life that altruistic individuals experience from observing others who receive health care. However, most CEAs and CUAs consider only the changes in health state (or preference score) for those directly affected by the programme. Usually this means the patient only, although some studies have considered the QALYs gained by caregivers (Drummond *et al.* 1991). On the other hand, the decision-maker, as society's representative, may consider that, for allocation of public resources for health care, only the value directly related to changes in health state is relevant and that, for equity reasons, a gain of a QALY should be valued the same no matter to whom it falls. (This would be close to the position adopted by Analyst B in Chapter 2.) In this case the decision maker may be happy to use CEA/CUA and to maximize the gains in health status from the allocation of health care resources. (Ideally, the consideration of these gains should extend beyond the individual patient if it can be shown that there are externalities in the consumption of health care.)

We have taken a broadly-based view in this book, because we feel that it is important for the reader to become familiar with all the forms of economic evaluation. The objective of economic evaluation is to be an *aid* to decision making, not a complete basis for making decisions. Therefore, it is important to expose the strengths and weaknesses of all the approaches rather to suggest that there is but one theoretically correct approach.

9.6. CONCLUSIONS

In this chapter we have explored a range of issues relating to the presentation and use of economic evaluation results. Some issues are relatively straightforward and would command a broad consensus. For example, it is important for the analysts to present their results in a transparent manner. Also, it is important to explore those factors likely to cause the costs or consequences of treatments to vary from one setting to another.

There is more disagreement about other issues, such as the overall philosophy for the use of economic evaluation. Some analysts (like Analyst A) believe that economic evaluations should only be performed in a manner consistent with the theoretical foundations of welfare economics. Others believe (like Analyst C) that the role of economic evaluation is to encourage systematic thinking about costs and consequences of health care treatments and programmes.

Very little is known about decision-makers' attitudes to these issues and the ways in which the results of economic studies, however performed, are used in decision-making. This is likely to be a priority for research in the future.

REFERENCES

Birch, S., and Gafni, A. (1992). Cost-effectiveness/utility analyses: do current decision rules lead us to where we want to be? *J. Health Economics*, **11**, 279–96.

—, — (1993). Changing the problem to fit the solution: Johannesson and Weinsteins (mis)application of economics to real world problems. *J. Health Economics*, **12**, 469–76.

BMJ Working Party on Economic Evaluation (1996). Guidelines for authors and peer reviewers of economic submissions to the *BMJ*. *Brit. Med. J.*, **313**, 275–83.

Buxton, M. J., Acheson, R., Caine, N., Gibson, S., and O'Brien, B. (1985). *Costs and benefits of the heart transplant programmes at Harefield and Papworth Hospitals.* DHSS Research Report No. 12, HMSO, London.

Canadian Coordinating Office for Health Technology Assessment (CCOHTA) (1994). *Guidelines for the economic evaluation of pharmaceuticals: Canada.* CCOHTA, Ottawa.

Commonwealth of Australia (1995). *Guidelines for the pharmaceutical industry on preparation of submissions to the Pharmaceutical Benefits Advisory Committee: including economic analyses.* Department of Health and Community Services, Canberra.

Coyle, D. (1993). Increasing the impact of economic evaluations on health care decision making. *Discussion Paper 108*, Centre for Health Economics, University of York, York.

Drummond, M. F. (1994). Evaluation of health technology: economic issues for health policy and policy issues for economic appraisal. *Soc. Sci. Med.*, **38**(12), 1593–600.

— (1994). Guidelines for pharmacoeconomic studies: the ways forward. *PharmacoEconomics*, **6**, 493–7.

—, Mohide, E. A., Tew, M., Streiner, D. L., Pringle, D. M., and Gilbert, J. R. (1991). Economic evaluation of a support programme for caregivers of demented elderly. *Int. J. Technology Assessment in Health Care*, 7(2), 209–19.

—, Bloom, B. S., Carrin, G., Hillman, A. L., Hutchings, H. C., Knill-Jones, R. P., *et al* (1992). Issues in the cross-national assessment of health technology. *Int. J. Technology Assessment in Health Care*, 8, 671–82.

Drummond, M. F., Torrance, G. W., and Mason, J. M. (1993). Cost-effectiveness league tables: more harm than good? *Soc. Sci. Med.*, **37**(1), 33–40.

—, Davies, L. M., and Rutten, F. F. H. (ed.) (1994). From results to action: the role of economic appraisal in developing policy for health technology. *Soc. Sci. Med.*, **38**(12), 1591–688.

Eddy, D. (1991). Oregons methods: did cost-effectiveness analysis fail? *J.A.M.A.*, **266**(15), 2135–41.

EPIC Investigators (1994). Use of monoclonal antibody directed against the platelet glycoprotein lib/111a receptor in high-risk coronary angioplasty. *N. Eng. J. Med.*, **330**, 956–61.

Gafni, A., and Birch, S. (1993). Guidelines for the adoption of new technologies: a prescription for uncontrolled growth in expenditures and how to avoid the problem. *Can. Med. Assoc. J.*, **148**(6), 913–17.

Glasziou, P. and Mitchell, A. (1996). Use of pharmacoeconomic data by regulatory authorities. In *Quality of life and pharmacoeconomics in clinical trials* (ed. B. Spilker). Lippincott-Raven Publishers, Philadelphia.

Gold, M. R., Siegel, J. E., Russell, L. B., and Weinstein, M. C. (ed.) (1996). *Cost-effectiveness in health and medicine*. Oxford University Press, New York.

Grabowski, H., and Sloan, F. (ed.) (1997). Cost-effectiveness in health care decision-making. *Soc. Sci. Med.* (In press.)

Graham, D. Y., Agrawal, N. M., and Roth, S. H. (1988). Prevention of NSAID-induced gastric ulcer with the synthetic prostaglandin misoprostol: a multi-centre, double-blind, placebo-controlled trial. *Lancet*, 2, 1277–80.

Haan, G., and Rutten, F. F. H. (1987). Economic appraisal, health service planning, and budgetary management for health technologies. In *Economic appraisal of health technology in the European Community* (ed. M. F. Drummond). Oxford University Press, Oxford.

Hull, R. D., Hirsh, J., Sackett, D. L., and Stoddart, G. L. (1981). Cost-effectiveness of clinical diagnosis, venography and non-invasive testing in patients with symptomatic deep-vein thrombosis. *N. Eng. J. Med.*, **304**, 1561–7.

Jacobs, P., Bachynsky, J., and Baladi, J.-F. (1995). A comparative review of pharmacoeconomic guidelines. *PharmacoEconomics*, **8**, 182–9.

Johannesson, M., and Weinstein, M. C. (1993). On the decision rules of cost-effectiveness analysis. *J. Health Economics*, **12**, 913–17.

Laupacis, A., Feeny, D., Detsky, A. S., and Tugwell, P. X. (1992). How attractive does a new technology have to be to warrant adoption and utilization? Tentative guidelines for using clinical and economic evaluations. *Can. Med. Assoc. J.*, **146**(4), 473–81.

—, —, —, and — (1993). Tentative guidelines for using clinical and economic evaluations revisited. *Can. Med. Assoc. J.*, **148**(6), 927–9.

McPherson, L., Wennberg, J. E., Hovind, O., *et al.* (1982). Small area variation in the use of common surgical procedures: an international comparison of New England, England and Norway. *N. Eng. J. Med.*, **307**, 1310–14.

Menzin, J., Oster, G., Davies, L., Drummond, M. F., Greiner, W., Lucioni, C., *et al.* (1996). A multinational economic evaluation of rhDNase in the treatment of cystic fibrosis. *Int. J. Technology Assessment in Health Care*, **12**(1), 52–61.

Naylor, C. D., Williams, I., Basinski, A., and Goel, V. (1993). Technology assessment and cost-effectiveness: misguided guidelines? *Can. Med. Assoc. J.*, **148**(6), 921–4.

Ontario Ministry of Health (1994). *Ontario guidelines for economic analysis of pharmaceutical products.* Ministry of Health, Toronto.

Oster, G., Huse, D. M., Lacey, M. J., Regan, M. M., and Fuchs, H. J. (1995). Effects of recombinant human DNase therapy on health care use and costs in patients with cystic fibrosis. *Annals of Pharmacotherapy*, **29**, 459–64.

Phelps, C. E., and Mushlin, A. (1991). On the (near) equivalence of cost-effectiveness and cost–benefit analyses. *Int. J. Technology Assessment in Health Care*, **7**, 12–21.

Schoenbaum, S. C., McNeil, B. J., and Kavel, J. (1976) The swine-influenza decision. *N. Eng. J. Med.*, **295**, 759–65.

Sugden, R., and Williams, A. (1979). *The principles of practical cost–benefit analysis.* Oxford University Press, Oxford.

Task Force on Principles of Economic Analysis of Health Care Technology (1995). Economic analysis of health care technology: a report on principles. *Annals of Internal Medicine*, **122**, 60–9.

10

How to take matters further

10.1. ECONOMIC EVALUATOR'S SURVIVAL GUIDE

10.1.1. Introduction

Like most other resources, the resources required to undertake economic evaluations are scarce. Therefore, it is important to ensure that these resources are used profitably. (From the individual evaluator's point of view it is also important to avoid wasting one's time when this could be better spent on other activities.)

In this short section we present a list of questions the economic evaluators should ask themselves, or another party requesting an evaluation, when embarking on a new study. The object is to minimize the following two difficulties:

(1) evaluators becoming involved in inappropriate or unprofitable evaluations;
(2) evaluators spending longer than necessary on any given evaluation.

There is no strong scientific basis for the suggested questions proposed in Section 10.1.2, although some of them mirror quite closely the checklist for critically assessing the literature presented in Chapter 3. Rather, our questions reflect years of experience in participating in economic evaluations and the mistakes we have made. We can make no guarantees of course; disease and infirmity among the evaluation team, changes in government, and world wars can disrupt the best laid plans! However, we feel that the guidance here at least gives the evaluator a fighting chance.

Here's hoping that you survive and can do better than ourselves in the future!

10.1.2. Some questions to ask yourself when beginning a study

1. Who needs this study and why?
   (a) What viewpoints are legitimate/feasible?
   (b) Is the person requesting the evaluation arguing for an unnecessarily restrictive viewpoint?

(c) Is anyone serious about the evaluation; that is, are the results likely to change any actions/policies that are being contemplated?

(d) Will it be possible for someone to act on the results of the evaluation, whatever these turn out to be; that is, are the necessary management procedures or decision-making procedures in place?

(e) In general, do people have an open mind with respect to the evaluation results?

2. *How did we arrive at these alternatives for consideration?*

(a) Is more than one alternative programme proposed, or is the implicit comparison the *status quo*?

(b) What would happen if the *status quo* were maintained?

(c) Have any important alternatives been omitted?

(d) Is this particular approach to meeting the given service objectives suggested by previous research, or does it represent someone's pet scheme?

(e) Would slightly more or slightly less of the proposed programme be preferable; what would we lose if the programme were pruned; what could be gained if extra features were added?

3. *What do we know about the effectiveness of the proposed alternatives?*

(a) Have any of the alternative programmes, especially the one(s) now being proposed for economic evaluation, been shown to do more good than harm by controlled study (especially involving random allocation of subjects to programmes or treatments)?

(b) If so, what do we know about the methodological quality of that study and how do we know the same results would be obtained in our setting?

(c) If not, are the supporters of this economic evaluation serious about undertaking a controlled study of effectiveness of the new programme compared to existing approaches? (If not, are you serious about them?)

(d) What justification can be given for going ahead with an economic evaluation without generating the effectiveness evidence?

4. *What do we know about the likely costs and funding implications of the proposed alternatives?*

(a) What would be your quick estimate (to the nearest $25 000) of the additional resources required to fund the new programme (if found to be effective)?

(b) Is this sum large in comparison to the likely costs (especially in your time input) of the evaluation? (If not, why are you involved at all?)

(c) Is there any hope that the extra resources needed to implement the new programme will be found, either through cost savings generated by the programme, resources redeployed from elsewhere, or new funding?

(d) Would any such redeployment or new funding be hard to achieve?

5. *How would we carry out such an evaluation?*

(a) What resources would be needed for the evaluation (e.g. personnel, computing)?

(b) Are these already available or would extra support be required? (If so, has any thought been given as to where support might come from; in particular, are people aware of the methods of obtaining research grants?)

(c) What kind of moral support can you expect from those requesting the evaluation, especially within your own organization?

(d) When are the results of the evaluation required? Is everybody clear on what can be achieved (with the evaluation resources at your disposal) within the given time period?

(e) Whose cooperation do you need to undertake your study? (Will they give it willingly, or only if forced to?)

(f) Do you like the other people involved well enough to spend extended periods of time with them? (You may have to!)

6. *How will the results of the evaluation be disseminated?*

(a) Are there any obstacles to the widespread dissemination of the results?

(b) Is a publication planned? If so, will you be able to meet the criteria for reporting the study?

(c) Will dissemination of the results be in time to influence the relevant decisions?

10.2. ADDITIONAL LITERATURE

A number of references have been given at the end of each chapter. In particular, the reader should consult the recent books by Gold *et al.* (1996), Johannesson (1996), and Sloan (1995), which all contain a wide range of additional references.

Further examples of economic evaluations can be located by normal literature searches. In addition, there are two economic evaluations databases that offer a rich source of information.

The *Health Economic Evaluation Database (HEED)* is a joint venture between the Office of Health Economics and the International Federation of Pharmaceutical Manufacturers' Associations. It contains structured abstracts of studies, methodological papers and reviews. Further details can be obtained from:

OHE-IFPMA Database Limited
12 Whitehall
LONDON SW1A 2DY
United Kingdom
Tel: +44 171 930 9203
Fax: +44 171 747 1419

The *NHS Economic Evaluation Database* is maintained by the NHS Centre for Reviews and Dissemination. It contains detailed structured abstracts and critical reviews of studies, plus citations for methodological papers, cost studies and reviews. Further details can be obtained from:

NHS Centre for Reviews and Dissemination
University of York
Heslington
YORK YO1 5DD
United Kingdom

Also, the database can be accessed on-line by dialling +44 1904 431732, or through the WorldWide Web: http://www.york.ac.uk/inst/crd/info.htm

REFERENCES

Gold, M. R., Siegel, J. E., Russell, L .B., and Weinstein, M. C. (ed.) (1996). *Cost-effectiveness in health and medicine*. Oxford University Press, New York.
Johannesson, M. (1996). *Theory and methods of economic evaluation of health care*. Kluwer, Dordrecht.
Sloan, F. (ed.) (1995). *Valuing health care*. Cambridge University Press, New York.

Author Index

Wilkinson, M. 145
Willan, A. 255
Williams, 268, 269–70
Williams, A. 176, 181, 182, 205, 207,
208, 287, 289

Wolfson, A. D. 149

Zarnke, K. B. 206
Zipursky, 268

Subject Index